ROBERT R. LINTON, M.D.

VISITING SURGEON AND CONSULTING SURGEON,
MASSACHUSETTS GENERAL HOSPITAL, BOSTON

Atlas of
VASCULAR SURGERY

Illustrated by Jerome T. Glickman and Gayanne DeVry

W. B. SAUNDERS COMPANY

PHILADELPHIA · LONDON · TORONTO 1973

W. B. Saunders Company: West Washington Square
Philadelphia, Pa. 19105

12 Dyott Street
London, WC1A   1DB

833 Oxford Street
Toronto 18, Ontario

Atlas of Vascular Surgery   ISBN 0-7216-5783-4

Print No.:   9   8   7   6   5   4   3   2   1

Dedicated to my loving wife,
Emma Bueermann Linton
and, in memory, to my teacher of surgery
Edward Pierson Richardson, M.D.

PREFACE

This Atlas of Vascular Surgery is an attempt to provide a detailed illustrated presentation of the technical aspects of some of the newer surgical procedures that are possible today for the treatment of the common peripheral vascular diseases. It is hoped, therefore, that it will be of chief value to the young surgeon in helping him to perform these vascular procedures without having to try methods that have been used and abandoned because of the poor results obtained with them. In addition, it may be of value to some surgeons who have entered this new field of surgery but have not had the opportunity to obtain special training in it. The well established vascular surgeon will view it with some interest but in many instances may feel that his particular method of doing a given procedure is better. No priority is claimed for the majority of the techniques described, and it is impossible to give credit to all those who have contributed to the development of this new field of surgery, both past and present, because there have been so many. For fear of leaving out names that should be included, only a very few are mentioned and no bibliography is included. As much as I wish I could, it is impossible to give credit to everyone, both in the profession and in industry, who has made it possible to perform the life- and limb-saving operative procedures that we are able to do today. For myself, my training in general surgery under Dr. E. P. Richardson and in the peripheral vascular field with Drs. Arthur W. Allen and Leland S. McKittrick, all at the Massachusetts General Hospital, has proved invaluable to me in providing a basis from which I could continue on with the newer developments in vascular surgery.

The book is divided into two main parts. Part I deals with diseases of the venous system, and Part II with those affecting the arterial system. It is also presented mainly in pictorial form to demonstrate some of the standard and time-tested methods of treating the most common of the peripheral vascular diseases. It includes those procedures that can be performed without the use of a cardiopulmonary bypass, and so excludes both cardiac surgery and those intracranial vascular procedures that should be done by the neurosurgeon. The presentation of the illustrations is somewhat unique in that they demonstrate, with few exceptions, the operative field and the techniques used for the different operative procedures from the position the operating surgeon almost invariably takes, if he is right-handed. This method of presentation, with the utilization of four basic colors to demonstrate the blood vessels and anatomical structures, was chosen for clarity.

It is fully realized that the publication of a work of this type by an individual would be impossible without help from the many surgeons who have aided in the development of this new field of vascular surgery both in the United States and abroad. It is difficult to give credit to all who deserve it, but I must express my gratitude for their assistance to the following: the members of the Vascular Clinic at the Massachusetts General Hospital that was organized as a surgical group in 1928; my assistants and the resident surgeons who have helped me to perform these procedures; the members of the department of anesthesia who have made it possible to perform safely many of the long, complex procedures; Dr. Charles E. Huggins, head of the blood bank, who has made unlimited frozen blood and platelet transfusions available; the members of the chemistry and blood laboratories who have given us reports on vital tests at any time of day or night; the nursing department, especially those nurses who take such wonderful and expert postoperative care of the patients in the recovery and intensive care units, and all the other nurses, including those of the intravenous group; and the department of radiology which cooperates so efficiently in the work-up of the patients. I am also indebted to Mr. Jerome T. Glickman for his excellent medical illustrations prepared with the assistance of Miss Gayanne DeVry; also to my secretaries, Miss Marion E. Shea, Mrs. Barbara Welwood and Mrs. Louise A. Kelly, for their untiring and excellent help in preparing the manuscript for this Atlas. I also wish to express my appreciation for the great cooperation I have received from Mr. John L. Dusseau of the W. B. Saunders Company in arranging for the illustrations to be reproduced in color.

ROBERT R. LINTON

CONTENTS

Contents

Contents

x

Contents

xiii

Contents

xiv

xv

xvii

Contents

Introduction

Great advances have been made during the past three decades in the surgical treatment of diseases of the major arteries and veins. Many of the operative procedures performed today, in fact, were inconceivable of being accomplished as short a time as 20 years ago. As a result of our increased knowledge, the improvement in technical skills and the development of new equipment with the help of industry, such as synthetic vascular prostheses and sutures, vascular surgery has mushroomed into being one of the largest, if not the largest surgical specialty. The differentiation between general and vascular surgery is difficult; all surgery is vascular in that the surgeon spends the greater part of the operative time in controlling blood vessels that must be divided and ligated to provide a clean operative field. The major portion of vascular surgery performed today involves reconstruction of the major arteries and the major veins, which demands a specialized knowledge and experience in performing these highly technical procedures. It seems justifiable, therefore, to speak of the surgeons doing them as "vascular surgeons."

The Vascular Surgeon

The first requirement for becoming a vascular surgeon should be a four- to five-year period of thorough training in general surgery that includes the cervical, the thoracic, the abdominal, the pelvic and the extremity regions. This should be followed by one or two years of apprenticeship with a competent vascular surgeon, not only to learn the techniques of the operative procedures, but also the necessary preoperative studies and postoperative care of the patient. In the arterial field one is dealing in the vast majority of patients with a chronic progressive disease, atherosclerosis, so the best possible long-term results should be the goal rather than speed in performing the operative procedure in an effort to do as many cases as possible. The vascular surgeon must learn to remain calm in all emergencies and not become tense and nervous when things do not seem to be going well. He and his patients will all live longer if he is confident that he has each step of the operation under proper control, so that when the procedure is completed he will have accomplished to the best of his ability what he had planned to do and, as a result, the patient will be relieved of his symptoms and in many cases cured. In order to meet these requirements he must adhere to the adage, "It must be done right."

History and Examination of the Patient

A careful history and physical examination of the patient are of extreme importance in the diagnosis of peripheral vascular diseases. Many patients are elderly, so it is important to determine if they are satisfactory

1

risks for major surgery. This should include an investigation of the cardiac, pulmonary and renal functions, or any other serious symptoms unrelated to what appears to be their main vascular disease. It should be remembered, however, that age alone is not necessarily a contraindication to many of these major procedures. A history of angina pectoris, emphysema, bronchitis or impaired renal function, if serious enough, can be a definite contraindication to some of the more serious surgical procedures. In order to properly evaluate many of these patients, it is advisable to admit them to the hospital several days prior to surgery so that the necessary studies and indicated consultations from other members of the profession can be obtained.

OBESITY

Most patients with vascular disease are obese and overweight, a serious impediment to obtaining the best results in reconstructive surgery for diseases of the arteries because it is technically much more difficult to isolate the blood vessels than in thin individuals. In addition, good hemostasis is more difficult to accomplish and, as a result, postoperative hematomas and infections are more liable to develop. To offset these disadvantages of obesity, it has been my custom to insist that the patients who are overweight reduce to the normal weight for their height, and I place them on a strict 1000 calorie, low cholesterol diet and an appetite-depressant drug.

Obesity is also common in patients with diseases of the veins, making operative procedures on them difficult and unduly hazardous to perform. In many cases it is the cause of poor results even for the surgical treatment of varicose veins and the postthrombotic syndrome of the lower extremity. For these reasons they also are placed on the same reducing regimen. Fortunately the treatment in the majority of patients with peripheral vascular diseases, both arterial and venous, can be classified as elective surgery, so that it is not hazardous to postpone operations on them for two or three months in order to get them to reduce to the normal weight for their age and height. In some cases the weight loss on this regimen has been as much as 40 pounds in two months. This also has the advantage that it makes the patient a much better operative risk and there are fewer postoperative complications, especially pulmonary problems. The reason for the weight reduction is explained to the patient carefully and I tell them I will not operate on them until they have lost the necessary amount of weight. This gives them an incentive to reduce, and it is seldom that a patient does not cooperate. All patients who are treated for peripheral atherosclerotic disease of the arteries are advised to stay on a low cholesterol diet indefinitely, since it is believed that a high cholesterol intake plays a part in the etiology of the disease.

USE OF TOBACCO

The majority of the patients with serious arterial disease are found to be heavy cigarette smokers, so it is necessary to make them stop smoking several weeks before going into the hospital in order to improve their pulmonary function and to prevent the postoperative pulmonary complications so common in the heavy smoker. There seems little question that tobacco does play an etiological role in peripheral atherosclerosis, so all these patients are advised they must give smoking up permanently and not go back to it after the operation.

The Examining Room

For the most satisfactory examination of a patient with peripheral vascular disease, either arterial or venous, it is important that the examining table be so placed in the examining room that the surgeon can examine the patient from both sides equally well (Plate 1). This is especially important for the evaluation of pulses in the cervical region, the abdomen, and the upper and lower extremities. At the foot of the table there should be a platform the width of the examining table that measures 18 inches high and 18 inches in depth. Another small stool is placed beside it to enable the patient to step up easily onto the higher one. This platform is valuable for many reasons, especially for examining the patients' lower extremities in the erect position. It may also be used for the injection of sclerosing solutions in varicose vein therapy, with the surgeon sitting on the stool that is shown. This position is useful also to determine if a patient has a suitable saphenous vein for an autogenous venous femoropopliteal bypass graft. In addition, the platform affords a place for the patient to rest his feet while he is having his lower legs and feet examined in the dependent position. The table can be lengthened for examination of the patient in a supine position by pulling out the sliding panel by means of the small knob underneath it, as is shown in the inset. In addition to the sphygmomanometer shown on the wall, an oscillometer should be available as shown on the small side table at the right.

Examination of the Peripheral Pulses

A standard technique should be developed for the palpation of the peripheral pulses throughout the body, since their presence or absence gives important information with reference to the condition of the arteries. The methods that have been found most satisfactory are shown in Plates 2, 3, 4 and 5.

A reliable oscillometer is necessary to obtain oscillometric readings in addition to palpation of the pulses in the extremities, especially the lower. The most important determination is the maximum oscillation, which is recorded along with the systolic blood pressure at which it comes through. These observations are an excellent check on the acuity of one's fingers in determining the pulses, since occasionally one finds an excellent oscillation at the ankle in the absence of pedal pulses. Further examination may reveal that the pedal pulses are present or that there is one in the peroneal artery at the external malleolus or in the anterior tibial artery proximal to the level of the malleoli. The reverse can also be true when one thinks he feels pulses in these arteries but is not sure; the oscillometer will tell without question that they are not there because of the very low oscillometric readings. It is also helpful in following patients after reconstructive arterial surgery because one can often detect reductions in the oscillometric readings as time goes on. If this occurs, it usually indicates that there is a slowly developing obliterative process in the reconstructive procedure or in the arteries proximal or distal to it; this can then be corrected by reoperation before it develops into complete occlusion.

Requirements for Successful Vascular Surgery

Arteriosclerotic diseases of the arteries, including the aorta, secondary to degenerative changes in them is the most common of the vascular diseases, the result of the increase in the life span of humans during the past few decades. The great advances in vascular surgery that have been made in the treatment of these diseases have been made possible through the improvement of surgical instruments and the development of synthetic grafts, especially those of knitted Dacron, and synthetic vascular sutures. The discovery of penicillin by Sir Alexander Fleming has, without question, been one of the main factors, if not the greatest, permitting surgeons to perform this new type of reconstructive vascular surgery of major arteries and veins without postoperative infections in the operative field, the lungs and the kidneys. The subsequent development of other antibiotics has also been important.

The discovery of the anticoagulant, heparin, and its ready availability have helped greatly in the performance of many of the prolonged arterial reconstructive procedures by prevention of arterial thrombosis during the operation. The warfarin group of drugs has been useful for prolonged anticoagulant therapy; for the most part it is used in the treatment of deep venous thrombosis and occasionally for postoperative anticoagulation following arterial surgery. The development of the modern blood bank, with the ready availability of blood and human albumin solutions, has played an important role in making many of the major arterial and aortic procedures possible.

Anesthesia

Improved methods of anesthesia and better trained anesthesiologists with a fuller understanding of the fluid and electrolyte requirements during the operation and in the postoperative period have also contributed greatly to the successful results obtained in this field. It is important, however, that the anesthesiologist and the surgeon cooperate in selecting the best type of anesthesia for the operation that is to be performed. The most satisfactory method for the majority of major vascular procedures performed at the Massachusetts General Hospital is induction with intravenous pentothal, with maintenance with a muscle relaxant and nitrous oxide and oxygen administered through an endotracheal tube, sometimes supplemented with ether. Cyclopropane is indicated for patients with liver disease. Halothane, because of its toxic effects in some patients, is not the best choice for prolonged operative procedures and should never be administered a second time within a four month period, nor should it be used for patients with severe liver disease. Planned hypotensive spinal anesthesia has a definite place in portasystemic venous shunt surgery to reduce blood loss and to facilitate the performance of the surgical procedure. It is important, however, to maintain the arterial pressure at the normal level for the great majority of arterial reconstructive procedures to prevent thrombosis of the arteries proximal and distal to those in the operative field; therefore, anesthetic agents should be selected that will maintain the normotensive state. Local anesthesia is seldom used except for angiography. Finally, it is important for the surgeon to have an anesthetist he knows and can trust at the head of the table so that he does not have to worry about the anesthesia and can have the peace of mind to concentrate and perform the operation to the best of his ability.

Angiography

Great advances have been made in angiography by the radiologists' use of radiopaque nontoxic iodine-containing solutions. It is possible with these techniques to pinpoint the location of the disease processes, especially in the arteries and to some extent in the veins, thereby enabling the surgeon to plan his operative procedure prior to the actual surgery. Many of these are performed best by the radiologist in his own department with modern roentgenographic equipment. The procedure includes visualization of the aortic arch and its great vessels, the carotid, subclavian and upper extremity arteries, the abdominal aorta and iliac arteries with selective angiograms when necessary, and the celiac axis, superior and inferior mesenteric and renal arteries. In addition, the specially trained roentgenologist is able to perform phlebography of the inferior vena cava, the veins of the extremities and the portal venous system. The latter is visualized by means of the venous phase of selective celiac and superior mesenteric artery angiography. It is important, however, that a vascular surgeon do the majority of femoral angiograms on patients with femoral popliteal obliterative atherosclerosis. These procedures can be accomplished in the operating room under local anesthesia. Not only does this enable the surgeon to obtain the ones that will be of the most use in helping him to decide which operative procedure will be the best for the patient, but he can also develop a reliable technique for use when he finds it necessary to perform femoral angiograms during an operation, which occurs quite frequently. Angiograms of arteries for arteriosclerotic disease frequently do not show the disease process to be as serious as the surgeon finds it; because the majority of radiologists are rarely able to come to the operating room to see the actual pathology, the surgeon is usually better able to evaluate the angiograms.

Operative Technique

Every surgeon must develop his own operative technique. The exposure of both arteries and veins requires meticulous dissection in order to clear their walls down to the adventitia. It has been found that this can be accomplished most readily by using scissors for the dissection and the cutting away of the tissues surrounding the blood vessels. These are put under tension by traction with forceps held by both the surgeon and his assistant. This frequently means picking up the adventitia of the blood vessel, or the entire vessel, to retract it while separating it from adjacent structures such as a large vein or surrounding fibrous tissues. The scissors should have slightly curved blades similar to the curved Mayo type. The tips should be rounded and not pointed. The most important characteristic is that the blades move freely and close with only the slightest finger pressure without friction so that the tips can actually indicate to the sensitive fingers of the surgeon what type of tissues they are cutting through, thus sometimes warning him, before it becomes visible, that there is a structure such as a blood vessel that should not be cut. The blades of most scissors are screwed together so tightly that much pressure is needed to close them and it is impossible to tell what one is cutting. This may result in troublesome complications, which can be avoided by the use of sharp, loose-bladed scissors. It is important that the scissor edges be exceedingly sharp. I have learned that it is best to sharpen one's own scissors, which is readily accomplished by use of an electrically driven, flat-surfaced, revolving fine hone. One must at the same time keep the blades at the right degree of tension by not screwing them together too tightly.

KNOT TYING

Another important aspect of operating technique is knot tying. It is of fundamental importance because an insecurely tied knot may result in serious hemorrhage, or even loss of life. It is to be emphasized also that the first half of any knot, whether it is a one- or a two-handed type, is the most important part of the knot. It should be a perfect overhand knot without a kink in either end of the ligature, such as the knot in Plate 6; otherwise, it will not snug down tightly on the vessel or the ligature may break. Whether it is tied as a square or a granny knot, under these conditions it will often be an ineffective hemostatic ligature. The control of very small blood vessels with ligatures, which is frequently necessary in vascular surgery, demands a special technique. Many times in tying a knot the ends of the ligature can be kept tight between the two halves of the knot. This cannot be done, however, in ligating fragile vessels such as small arteries arising from major arteries because the ligature will either slip off or tear the vessel. It is necessary, therefore, to learn the technique whereby, after making the first half of the knot and pulling it tight, the ends of the ligature are left loose for threading through each other to make the second half of the knot; they are then pulled taut to complete the knot (Plate 11 *E*). This technique can best be accomplished by either the two-handed method or the German seamstress one-handed method because, with other methods, the ends of the ligature must be kept too taut between the first and second halves of the knot. Another important rule is that as each part of the knot is pulled taut, the ends of the suture or ligature and the knot must all be kept in a straight line, as shown in Plate 11. Because of the poor cohesion of some of the newer types of vascular sutures, especially the monofilament sutures and the Dacron type coated with Teflon, it is important to put at least four or five throws into the knots, making sure that each throw is very snugly set.

The two-handed shuttle type made with the thumb and forefinger of each hand is a standard technique and should be mastered first. Another method is a one-handed type that some surgeons do not think makes a secure knot, but these are usually those men who have not mastered the technique. Many surgeons also believe that the square knot (Plate 7 *A*) is the most secure, which certainly is true if it is tied correctly; however, if not correct it can be less secure than a granny knot (Plate 7 *C*). Many times, especially in deep narrow wounds, it is difficult to tie a square knot. As a result the knot may end up as a "barrel sling" type (Plate 7 *B*), which is one of the most slippery of the slip knots. On the other hand, under these conditions a granny knot will be more secure tied by the one-handed or the two-handed method, although it may end up as two half hitches (Plate 7 *D*). These can be made secure by snugging them tight and especially by putting two extra throws in the knot. There are many occasions during an operation when in tying small blood vessels it is justifiable to use the granny knot tied by the one-handed method once the technique has been mastered. Even adding an extra throw will result in the saving of time without sacrificing security if the technique is mastered. The so-called "surgeon's" knot (Plate 7 *E*) has little if any use in vascular surgery.

There are a number of techniques for tying the one-handed knot. It has been found that the "German seamstress" knot is the one which can be performed most smoothly and effectively since both hands can be maintained in the pronated position, thereby facilitating the necessary finger motions as shown in Plate 8. Two other methods in popular use are shown in Plates 9 and 10. The technical details of each method can easily be followed from these illustrations. It should be noted that if it is necessary to tie a square knot by the one-handed method, it can be readily accomplished by combining two of the methods. It is of utmost importance that whichever methods the surgeon in training decides to use, he should learn and perfect them outside the operating room and not at the operating table. To keep in practice he can use the different techniques for tying the overhand knot when he begins the knot in his shoelaces each time he puts on his shoes or on any other occasions of knot tying. Other useful methods of hemostasis and blood vessel control are shown in Plates 12 and 13.

PROSTHESES

Aortic and arterial prostheses function best if they are porous rather than blood tight, since this will allow the fibroblasts of the host to grow through the interstices of the graft and to incorporate it as part of the body. For this reason, the knitted type is superior to the woven. In addition, knitted prostheses are much easier to implant because the edges do not unravel. The most commonly used are made of Dacron or Teflon. The only possible advantage of the latter would be that it is woven so tightly that it does not leak after implantation, so that preclotting of it is unnecessary. However, this is actually a disadvantage because the Teflon prosthesis does not become incorporated in the host tissues; furthermore, it requires only three to five minutes to preclot a knitted graft to make it blood tight. The most satisfactory protheses today are made of Dacron. To my knowledge none has disintegrated from host tissue reaction over the period of 15 years since they were first used.

SUTURES

The suture makers have been a great help in perfecting synthetic sutures. At present the braided type coated with Teflon seems to be the most satisfactory. A single strand synthetic suture would be better, but difficulties have been encountered in maintaining knot security, and at present they are not so commonly used as the other. It is recommended that the sutures that are used to implant the synthetic grafts be made of Dacron because silk is an animal protein which gradually disintegrates in the body. The anastomotic suture lines have been known to disrupt when this type of suture has been used. This is especially true for Teflon grafts which, because of their inertness and tight weave, do not become incorporated in the host tissues and are held in place only by the sutures. Silk sutures should never be used to implant them.

Many sizes of arterial sutures are now available. The most commonly used are 6-0 to 3-0 Teflon-coated Dacron; it is seldom that a smaller or larger suture is necessary. The needles are all swaged on to the suture to aid in the passage through the tissues and grafts. They also come with tapered or cutting points. The former are necessary when lightweight Dacron grafts are implanted because the cutting point ones tend to tear the fabric, causing troublesome bleeding from the needle holes. The cutting needles are necessary for the thicker grafts and also for the implantation of saphenous vein bypass grafts, or while working on thick-walled arteries.

The most common type of needle is the curved one, which has definite advantages when working in a deep surgical wound. However, for the majority of suturing of vascular anastomoses it has been found that a straight needle is far superior.

TECHNIQUE OF VASCULAR SUTURING

In preparing a blood vessel for a grafting procedure, it is important not to clear away too much of the adventitia because this represents the strongest part of the vessel wall and prevents it from dilating and becoming aneurysmal. However, any loose, stringy pieces of tissue should be removed with a fine pair of scissors because they tend to catch in the suture and to make the vessel walls wrinkle at the point of anastomosis. This is especially true when suturing autogenous venous grafts and small arteries. Wrinkling interferes with the streamlining of the blood flow and may cause occlusion from thrombosis. In addition, whenever possible the needle of the suture should pass from the intimal side through to the outside of the vein graft when making the anastomosis to prevent wrinkling from occurring. If the needle must be passed in the opposite direction from the outside to the inside of the vessel wall, it is of extreme importance to retract the adventitia with forceps very firmly behind each stitch as the suture is pulled through to prevent kinking of the vessel wall. These seem like minor details but they can make the difference between a successful anastomosis and one that fails. It is of extreme importance, therefore, to have good surgical assistance in the construction of anastomoses to prevent these errors from occurring. It has been found from experience that the use of the straight arterial needle facilitates greatly the construction of the majority of vascular anastomoses (Plate 14).

It is much easier to pass a straight needle through tough tissues without its bending than it is to use a curved needle, because the curved needle so frequently bends without going through the vessel walls. The straight needles are much easier to place accurately since the action is one chiefly of pointing with the end of the needle and the needle holder at the structures that are to be sutured. The needle holder rests on the near edge of the incision, which steadies it, and it is possible to use it as a lever. The tip of the needle is readily grasped with the needle holder as it comes through the tissues and the suture is pulled through. It can then be replaced accurately in the right position in the needle holder without its having to be picked up by the left hand, which is so necessary when a curved needle is used. As a result, a pair of fine pointed forceps can be used in the left hand to maintain tension on the vessel while the needle holder remains in the right hand. This is demonstrated in Plate 14. Another advantage of the straight needle is that it can be bent into a curve or a ski type of needle very readily and then straightened again if desired, whereas it is very difficult to make a curved needle perfectly straight.

It is helpful in anastomosing small blood vessels to use a binocular loupe that gives two and a half to three times magnification; a binocular dissecting microscope is especially necessary for anastomosing blood vessels that are 2 mm. or less in diameter.

INSTRUMENTS

The instruments that are used to perform many of the new operative procedures in vascular surgery include many of the standard ones that have been used for many years in general surgery. In addition, it is necessary to employ some of the instruments that have been developed in the last 20 years specifically for vascular surgery. There are many of these latter, so each surgeon must select from among them the ones with which he can best accomplish these highly technical operative procedures. Both the standard and the new instruments I have found most useful are shown in Plates 15 to 22. The different stapling instruments that have been devised are not shown because they cannot be used satisfactorily with atherosclerotic arteries (work on which constitutes so much of the reconstructive vascular procedures), and especially since the suture technique when done properly can give such excellent results.

It has been a wonderful experience to have been able to take part in these new horizons in surgery that have developed in the past three decades. The most dramatic results have been obtained in the saving of the lives of patients with abdominal aortic aneurysms. This has been done by excision of the aneurysm and implantation of vascular grafts of synthetic prostheses. Prior to the development of this technique, the aneurysm would commonly have ended in rupture and the death of the patient. The prevention of hemiplegia by operating for atherosclerotic disease of the carotid artery has been another great milestone. It has also been exceedingly gratifying to salvage by the means of blood vessel grafting procedures the lower limbs of patients with impending gangrene or, in many cases, with actual gangrene of the feet that before would have necessitated major amputations. It has been equally rewarding to have been able to improve the surgical treatment of diseases of the veins, including varicose veins and stasis ulcers of the lower extremities, to save the lives of patients with bleeding esophageal varices, and to help to prevent or to treat thromboembolic disease, with considerable improvement in the mortality rate from pulmonary embolism. For the present, and probably for some time in the future, the operative procedures that are described and illustrated in this book will continue to be performed as the best available forms of therapy. Without any question there is much yet to be learned, and there will be additional improvements in the various techniques described as new and better operative procedures are devised and performed. There seems little doubt, however, that through further research the etiology of some of these diseases, especially atherosclerosis, will be discovered and that therapy will become prevention rather than correction.

For the present, however, in order to treat the patients who are so afflicted it is necessary to have surgeons well trained in this new field of major blood vessel surgery with knowledge of the best procedures that can be performed and with the ability to carry them out with the meticulous attention to technical details that is so necessary for success. At this time, in order to give the best treatment possible for some of the major complicated operative procedures, it seems best that many of the operations should be performed in the larger medical centers rather than in community hospitals. The large medical centers are better staffed with more competent vascular surgeons and with other trained personnel, and have all the other ancillary services available both day and night. This includes adequate blood banks that can supply large amounts of blood on short notice, a service frequently necessary in many of the cases, especially emergency procedures. The postoperative condition of many of the patients during the first few days requires the most skillful care in the recovery and intensive care units by the anesthesiologist, the resident surgeons and specially trained nurses, in addition to the surgeon in charge, and this is more readily available in hospitals where large numbers of vascular surgery patients are treated.

Plate 1

THE EXAMINING ROOM

A. This is a drawing showing the best arrangement for the equipment in an examining room for patients with peripheral vascular disease. It is important that the examining table be placed midway between the side walls of the room, so that the surgeon is able to examine the patient from each side and the foot of the table. This greatly facilitates digital examination of the arterial pulses because it permits the surgeon to stand on the right side of the patient to examine the arterial pulses on the right side and on the left side of the patient for those on the left. The table has a sliding panel (a) which can be pulled out to increase its length so that the patient can lie down with the lower extremities extended. There is a large platform (b) at the foot of the table which is 18 inches high and deep and is the width of the table. The smaller one (c) is 8 inches high and deep and 12 inches wide, so that the patient can step up readily to the larger one and turn to sit down on the end of the table. The large platform is used as a foot rest and permits examination of the feet and lower legs in the dependent position. The patient also can stand erect on it for examination of the superficial veins of the lower extremities; it also permits a better examination of the posterior aspect of the lower limbs to prevent overlooking varicosities of the short saphenous vein and other lesions, which may occur if this routine is not carried out. This platform also enables the patient to stand or sit with the feet resting on it for injection of a sclerosing solution in the treatment of varicose veins. It is useful for the patient to stand on while the lower extremities are examined to determine if the long saphenous veins will be satisfactory for autogenous venous femoropopliteal bypass grafts. It is important to evaluate the size and quality of these vessels when the patient is first examined at the surgeon's office, because this examination is usually made in the afternoon or after the patient has been ambulatory all day, which results in maximal dilatation of the vessels. The stool (d) in the foreground is used by the examining surgeon while he performs these examinations. A sphygmomanometer (e) is on the back wall above the examining table. An oscillometer (f) is shown on the smaller table at the right. This instrument is an invaluable aid in the examination of the arterial circulation. It has been found exceedingly helpful in checking the accuracy of one's digital examination of the pulses, both preoperatively and as follow-up in the postoperative period.

B. This shows the table after the sliding panel (a) has been pulled out, thus allowing the patient to lie down with the legs extended so that they can be examined more satisfactorily for pulsations and by oscillometry.

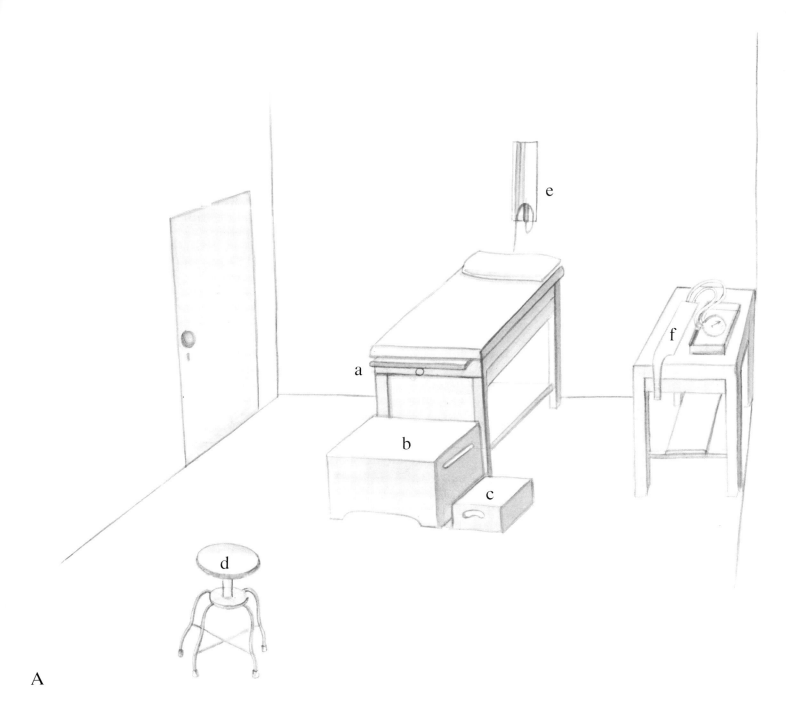

A

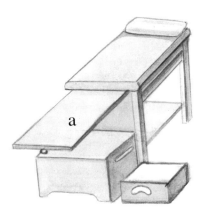

B

11

Plate 2

PALPATION OF ARTERIAL PULSES

I. Extracranial Arteries

Atherosclerotic disease of the extracranial arteries is frequently heralded by minor cerebrovascular symptoms and in some instances unfortunately by a complete hemiplegia. Some indication of whether these symptoms are due to intracranial or extracranial arterial disease can be obtained by a careful examination of the pulsation of the palpable extracranial arteries.

A. The superficial temporal artery is readily palpated by pressure with two or three fingers against the temporal bone just in front of the ear and above the zygoma. The absence of pulsation in this artery usually means occlusion of the external carotid artery or the common carotid artery. Another check on the external carotid is palpation of the external maxillary artery as it crosses the mid portion of the mandible.

B. It is not possible to palpate separately the external and internal carotid arteries because of their juxtaposition. The common carotid artery is most readily palpated in the middle part of the neck, preferably while standing behind the patient, by pressing it against the transverse processes of the cervical vertebrae. Occasionally one may feel a thrill over the bifurcation of the artery, indicating a greatly narrowed lumen at this site from atherosclerotic disease.

C. Auscultation with a stethoscope over the carotid arteries is of help in detecting an area of stenosis. If it is heard loudest in the base of the neck at the circle (1), this usually indicates narrowing of the origin of the common carotid artery or the innominate artery on the right side and on the left, the origin of the common carotid artery from the aorta.

One must be careful to examine both carotid systems, and if severe disease is present on both sides care must be taken not to apply pressure too long, thereby inducing occlusion of the common carotid artery, because syncope may develop and there is also the possibility that a small thrombus may break off to embolize one of the intracranial arteries.

II. Upper Extremity Arteries

D. The subclavian artery is palpated at the base of the neck above the clavicle by compressing the second and third portions of it against Sibson's fascia and the upper part of the first rib. Auscultation over the artery at circle (2) in *C* will help to ascertain if there is occlusive disease proximal to this level, since it is not possible to palpate the first portion of the artery.

E. The brachial artery is palpated in the mid upper arm by utilizing the fingers of both hands to press the artery against the humerus, well distal to the profunda brachia. If a pulse is palpated at this level, the palpation is continued distalward to the antecubital space where the brachial artery bifurcates into the radial and ulnar arteries. The radial and ulnar arteries are palpable only at the wrist; the former is more readily palpable since it can be compressed against the radius.

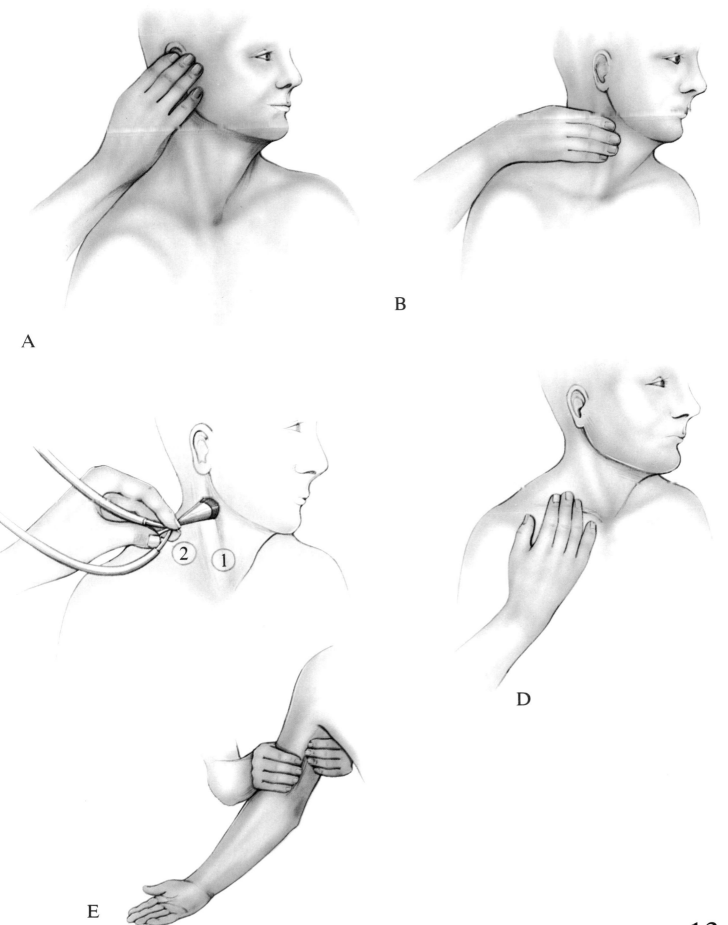

A

B

2 1

D

E

13

Plate 3

PALPATION OF ARTERIAL PULSES
(Continued)

III. THE ABDOMINAL AORTA

A. The abdominal aorta is palpable distal to the renal arteries in most patients except obese individuals. It is the largest artery in the body that can be palpated, and yet it is surprising how frequently it is not included in a routine physical examination. As a result, abdominal arteriosclerotic aneurysms are quite frequently not diagnosed until roentgenograms of the abdomen are taken during a gastrointestinal or a genitourinary work-up. This part of the aorta is subject to occlusive disease in some patients and to aneurysmal disease in others, so that palpation is important, especially to detect aneurysms. Should a large aneurysm be found, it should be removed while it is still asymptomatic. Palpation of the aorta is best performed from the right side of the patient, using both hands at the level of the umbilicus and just cephalad to it. By moving the hands into the right and left lower quadrants the common iliac arteries can be palpated. Auscultation is frequently helpful when obliterative disease is present, but less so with aneurysms.

B and C. The right external iliac and common femoral arteries are palpable in the groin region, the former above the inguinal ligament and the latter below it. Palpation of these arteries is best carried out on the side they lie in, that is, the right ones from the right side and the left ones from the left side of the patient, as in *C*. A more accurate quantitative analysis of the pulses can be obtained by utilizing the fingers of both hands. As the examiner gains experience he will learn to grade the volume of the pulsations. This can be an important observation because a pulse of less than 3 plus means that serious proximal occlusive disease is present in the aorta and/or the iliac arteries. This should be endarterectomized or replaced by a synthetic graft before attempting to correct any superficial femoral artery block that may be present.

Rectal examination can often be helpful in determining the presence of aneurysms of the hypogastric arteries, and also in evaluation of congenital arteriovenous fistulas that involve these arteries and its branches. Occasionally the distal end of a large and elongated abdominal aortic aneurysm may be palpable with the fingertip.

Palpation of the superficial femoral artery in the mid thigh is possible but difficult to evaluate quantitatively. It perhaps is most helpful in determining if a bypass femoropopliteal graft is still functioning. It should be palpated while standing at the outer side of the extremity that the artery lies in.

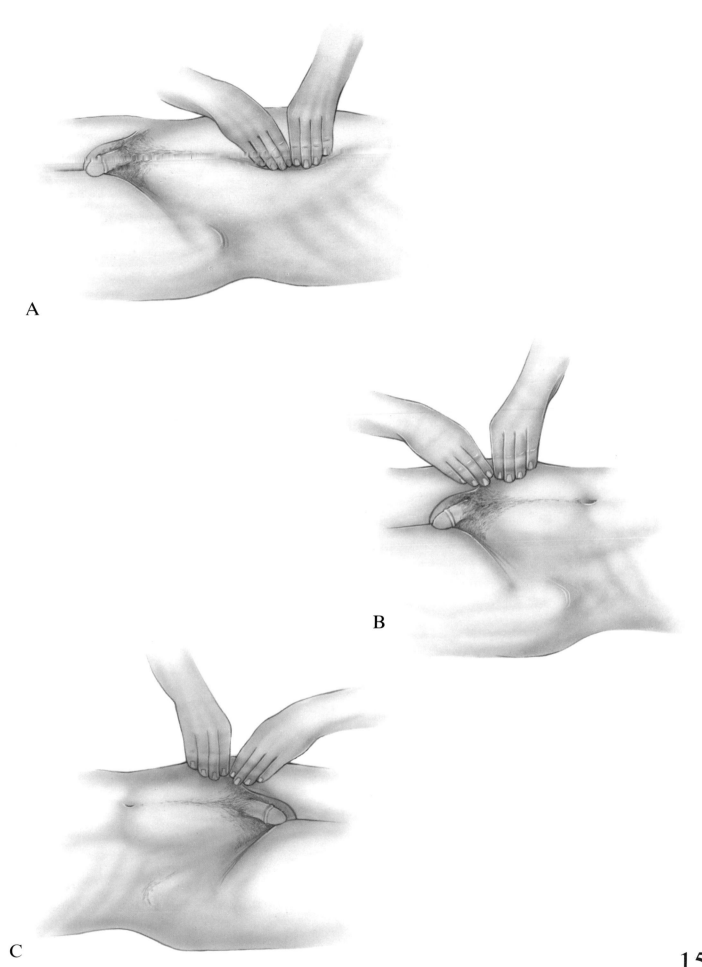

A

B

C

Plate 4

PALPATION OF ARTERIAL PULSES
(Continued)

IV. THE LOWER EXTREMITY

A and B.   *A* shows the position of the hands for examination of the right popliteal artery, and *B* shows it for the left. The popliteal artery is more difficult to palpate than most arteries because it is not possible to compress it directly against firm or bony structures. As a result, each examiner must develop his own technique. The one I have found most useful is to stand on the right side of the patient for both right and left extremities, with the knee completely extended but in a relaxed state.

C and D.   *C* shows the position of the hands for the left popliteal artery and *D* demonstrates the position of the fingers of both hands in the left popliteal space, with rotation of the extremity for demonstration purposes. The fingers of the right hand are used to palpate the pulse and those of the left hand force the popliteal artery and the tissues of the popliteal space against the right hand fingers so that the artery is compressed between them, making it possible to palpate it and grade the pulse if it is present.

Auscultation at this level is seldom of much aid except to differentiate between an arteriovenous fistula and an aneurysm. The gastrocnemius and soleus muscle mass prevents accurate palpation beyond the popliteal space except in the presence of aneurysms extending distal to this level. Palpation of the popliteal artery with the patient in the prone position with the lower leg flexed to 90 degrees has been advocated, but I have not found this as satisfactory as the procedure described.

16

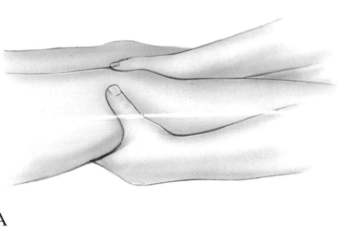

A

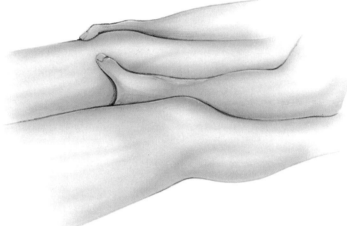

B

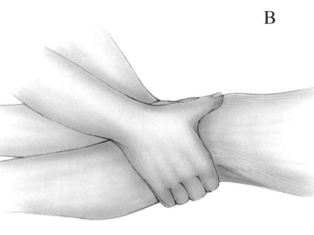

C

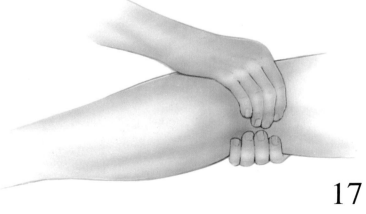

D

17

Plate 5

PALPATION OF ARTERIAL PULSES
(Continued)

IV. THE LOWER EXTREMITY *(Continued)*

A.   The posterior tibial artery is palpable only at the level of the ankle. One's ability to determine the presence or absence of a pulse in it is frequently important in estimating the state of the peripheral arterial circulation to the lower leg and foot. It may be difficult to palpate, especially in a patient with an obese or edematous ankle. In addition, its location in the concavity between the medial malleolus and the os calcis makes it more difficult to palpate than most of the peripheral arteries. It is best examined by using the tips of the second, third and fourth fingers of the right hand for the left posterior tibial artery as illustrated, and those of the left hand for the right artery. The fingers are placed midway between the internal malleolus and the prominence of the os calcis, with pressure exerted against this bone. The thumb of the examining hand is placed above the external malleolus, so actually one is grasping the ankle in the examining hand. In this way one can accurately control the pressure applied over the posterior tibial artery. This pressure will vary, depending on the volume of the pulse, and then be graded according to its volume.

B and C.   The dorsalis pedis artery lies on the dorsum of the foot. The examination is best carried out by standing below the patient's foot or on the opposite side of the patient and using the same hand as the foot that is being examined, that is, the right hand for the right foot and the left for the left. The second, third and fourth fingers of the examining hand are placed on the dorsum of the foot, using the flexor surfaces of the terminal phalanges and not just the tips of them. The thumb is placed against the plantar surface (*C*) so that one is actually grasping the foot during the examination. The fingers are moved from side to side in search of the dorsalis pedis pulse and at the same time the pressure applied is varied in order to pick up the weaker pulses. A search should also be made for the anterior branch of the peroneal artery lying just anterior to the lateral malleolus by moving the examining fingers to this area.

If no pulses are encountered, the examining hand is moved cephalad to the external malleolus, and finger pressure is made between the tibia and fibula to determine whether the anterior tibial artery is pulsating. The pulses in all these arteries are graded from 0 to normal, or 4 plus.

Despite the fact that the dorsalis pedis artery is readily palpable to the experienced examiner, it frequently is inaccurately recorded by the inexperienced. It is surprising how many nondiabetic patients are referred to me with gangrenous areas on the toes whom the referring doctor reported as having palpable dorsalis pedis pulsations, which, of course, they did not have. The absence of this artery in a normal-appearing foot should give no cause for concern, because it is congenitally absent in about 10 per cent of persons with normal circulation.

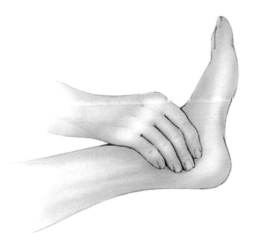

A

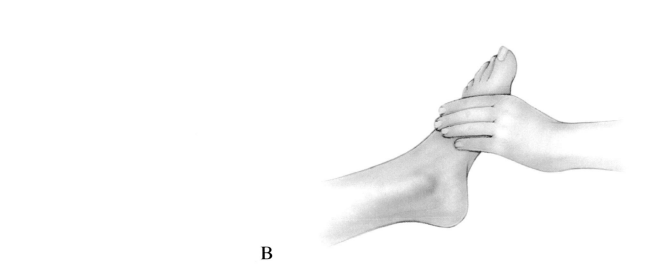

B

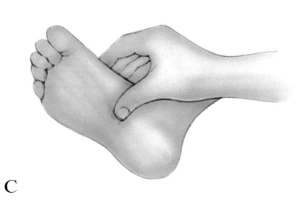

C

Plate 6

KNOT TYING

BASIC TECHNIQUE

A. The first half of a knot, whether it be a square knot or a granny knot, is the most important part of the knot. The ligature is looped around the end of the hemostat that is holding the blood vessel, as is illustrated, so that the end (b) in the right hand crosses underneath end (a) in the left hand. End (b) is then grasped with the thumb and forefinger of the left hand and shuttled through the loop to make the overhand knot. It should be a perfect overhand knot without any kink in either end of the ligature, as shown.

B. The two ends are then pulled taut, making sure that the three points — the site of the bleeding blood vessel held by the hemostat, and the thumb and forefingers of each hand holding the ends of the ligature — are all in a straight line. This gives the most secure control of the bleeding blood vessel, and after the knot is pulled tight, the hemostat can be removed and the knot completed either as a square knot or a granny knot.

C. This demonstrates the wrong way to perform the first half of the knot. Note that the ligature to be tied is simply passed behind the hemostat without being formed into a loop. The end (b) is crossed over end (a) and shuttled through beneath it to create the first half of the knot.

D and E. This shows the type of knot that results from this method, demonstrating that end (b) forms a loop around end (a). As a result, the ligature often is not pulled tight enough, or when it is pulled tightly, it breaks end (a) at the knot because of the shearing force of the loop in end (b), as shown in *E*. This method is definitely the incorrect way of starting any type of knot that is to secure a blood vessel and should never be used.

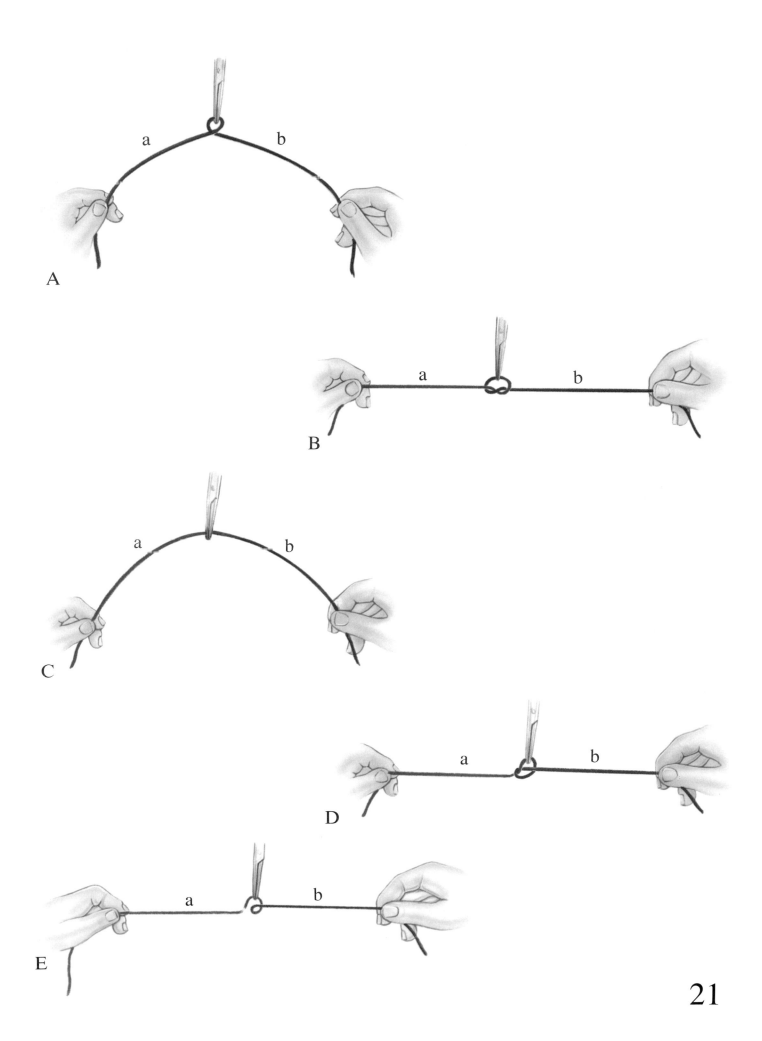

A

B

C

D

E

21

Plate 7

KNOT TYING *(Continued)*

The Square Knot, the Granny Knot and the Surgeon's Knot

A. This demonstrates the well known square knot which, if tied perfectly, is the most secure knot and one which will not untie or slip. Notice that traction is exerted on the ends of the ligature by the two hands in exactly opposite directions in a straight line with the vessel to be tied to obtain this perfect square knot.

B. This demonstrates a square knot which has been tied improperly, exerting traction at an angle instead of in a straight line, and with more tension being applied by the left hand than the right. Under these conditions the square knot then becomes one of the most slippery of slip knots, ending up as shown in the form of a "barrel sling" type of knot. This error in the tying of the square knot occurs commonly when it is tied carelessly; it may also occur even while attempting to tie it correctly when the ligature must be placed in a deep narrow part of the operative field. Under these conditions it is not as safe as a granny knot.

In order to tie the square knot perfectly it is necessary after completing the first half of the knot to reverse the direction of the hands, or to change the ends of the ligature from one hand to the other so that the knot may fall evenly. The insecure square knot occurs most frequently when this change of position of the hands or the ends of the ligature is not carried out.

C. This demonstrates the granny knot. It is shown tied in the same manner as the square knot in *B*, pulling the ends of the ligature at an angle. Both halves of the knot, however, are tied by shuttling the end of the ligature in the right hand through with the forefinger and thumb of the left hand for both the first and second halves of the knot, whereas in the correct square knot the second half is tied by reversing the direction of the shuttle of the thumb and forefinger of the left hand. The granny knot makes a safe secure knot if one or two extra throws are placed in it.

D. If the granny knot is tied as shown in this illustration, which is frequently done, especially in deep parts of a wound, it ends up as two half hitches which, if pulled tightly, produce a much more secure knot than the barrel sling type that one ends up with if the square knot is tied improperly. For this reason it is believed that the granny knot, if tied with one or two extra throws in it, is a safer knot than a carelessly tied square knot.

E. This is the so-called surgeon's knot. It has little if any use in surgery, since the first half of the knot cannot be pulled tight because of the extra throw placed in this half of the knot. There are some instances in which it is useful, however, and that is in tying a ligature around a stiff object such as a catheter or a piece of glass tubing, because the first half of the knot when pulled tightly holds more securely while the second half of the knot is being completed.

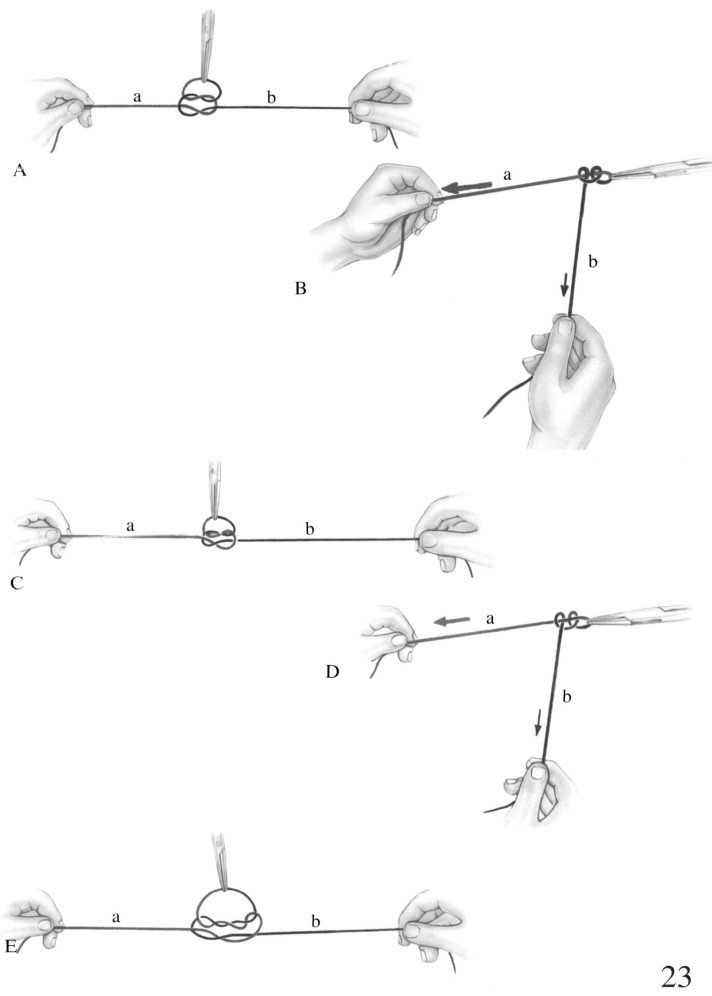

A

B

C

D

E

23

Plate 8

KNOT TYING *(Continued)*

ONE-HANDED "GERMAN SEAMSTRESS" TYPE OF KNOT

A one-handed knot is not a generally accepted method of tying for all surgeons. It is believed, however, if the methods of one-handed knot tying are mastered, these knots can be made as secure as the two-handed type. It should be pointed out that the latter, of course, should be well mastered before using the one-handed types. This plate demonstrates the most useful and expeditious method of tying a one-handed knot known as the German seamstress type. The advantages of this method of knot tying are that the hands are in the pronated position throughout the various steps of completing it; also, it is possible to tie it with very loose ends, which is important in ligating very small blood vessels or tender bleeding points in order not to pull away the first half of the knot from the bleeding point while tying the second half.

A. The ends of the ligature are held as shown, with the thumb and forefinger of each hand making a loop around the hemostat.

B. The end (b) held with the right hand is then loosely looped around the ends of the third and fourth fingers of the left hand.

C. In actually performing this part of the knot the hand remains pronated, but in order to demonstrate how it is done, the left hand has been rotated for clarity. Note that the fixed part of end (a) held in the left hand has now been grasped between the ends of the third and fourth fingers of the left hand, as demonstrated, so that it can be pulled through the loop of end (b) made around these two fingers and held in the right hand.

D. This demonstrates the end of loop (a) being released by the thumb and forefinger of the left hand so that it can be pulled through the loop that was made around the third and fourth fingers of the left hand.

E. The pull-through has been completed and the first half of the knot has been formed with end (b) still held between the tips of the third and fourth fingers.

F. This shows the completion of the one-handed knot by pulling the ends of the ligature held in each hand and the end of the hemostat holding the blood vessel all in a straight line. It is customary to repeat this maneuver two or three times, creating a granny knot; with these extra throws this makes a very secure knot. If the surgeon desires to make a square knot this can be done by using one of the other one-handed methods to complete the square knot, as in Plates 9 and 10.

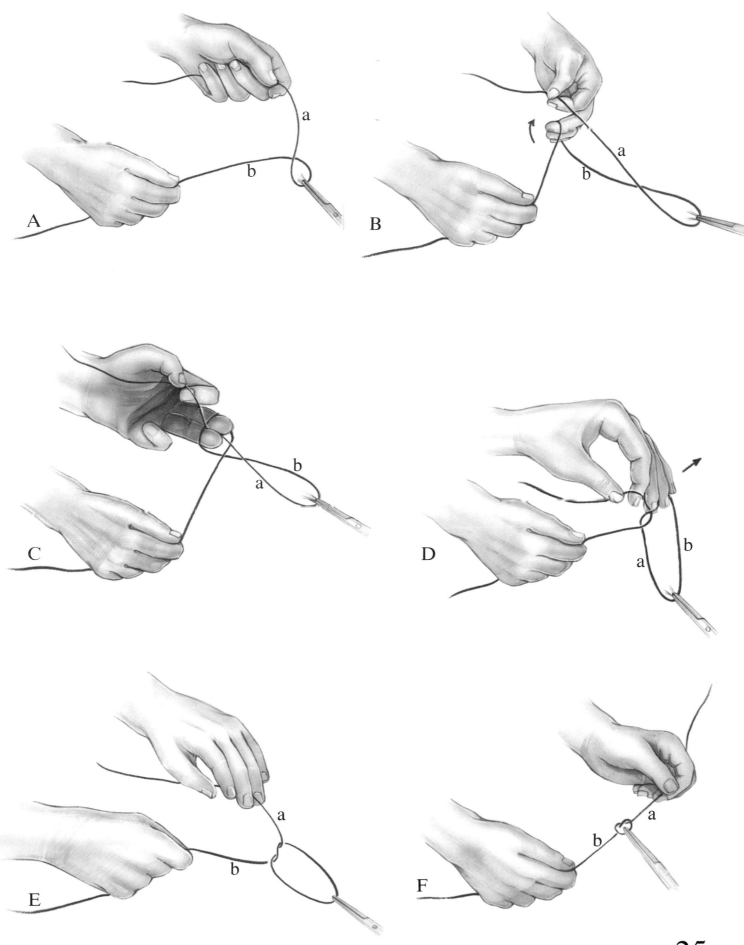

A

B

C

D

E

F

25

Plate 9

KNOT TYING *(Continued)*

ONE-HANDED KNOT TYING

This is another method of one-handed knot tying which is much more commonly used than the German seamstress type. The reason for this is difficult to understand, since this method is not so versatile as the other and requires tying with the hands in the supinated position. It is useful at times, however, and should be learned.

A. This demonstrates the method of creating the loop by passing the two ends of the ligature around the third, fourth and fifth fingers of the left hand. It has the disadvantage that there must be tension on the ends of the ligature during most of the knot tying, so it is not so useful in tying fragile bleeders.

B. After creation of the loop, the ligature end (b) is caught by threading the tip of the middle finger underneath it, then bringing it through the loop.

C. This demonstrates the advance of the finger to obtain better control of the end (b).

D. This demonstrates that the end of (b) held by the thumb and forefinger of the left hand has been released so that it can be pulled through the loop.

E. This demonstrates how it is pulled through further by flexing the middle finger to control it.

F. The end is finally pulled through and the two ends (a) and (b) are then lined up with the blood vessel held by the hemostat so that all three are in a straight line as it is pulled taut. Again, the knot can be completed as a granny knot by a similar throw or by making a square knot out of it, using the German seamstress type of one-handed knot.

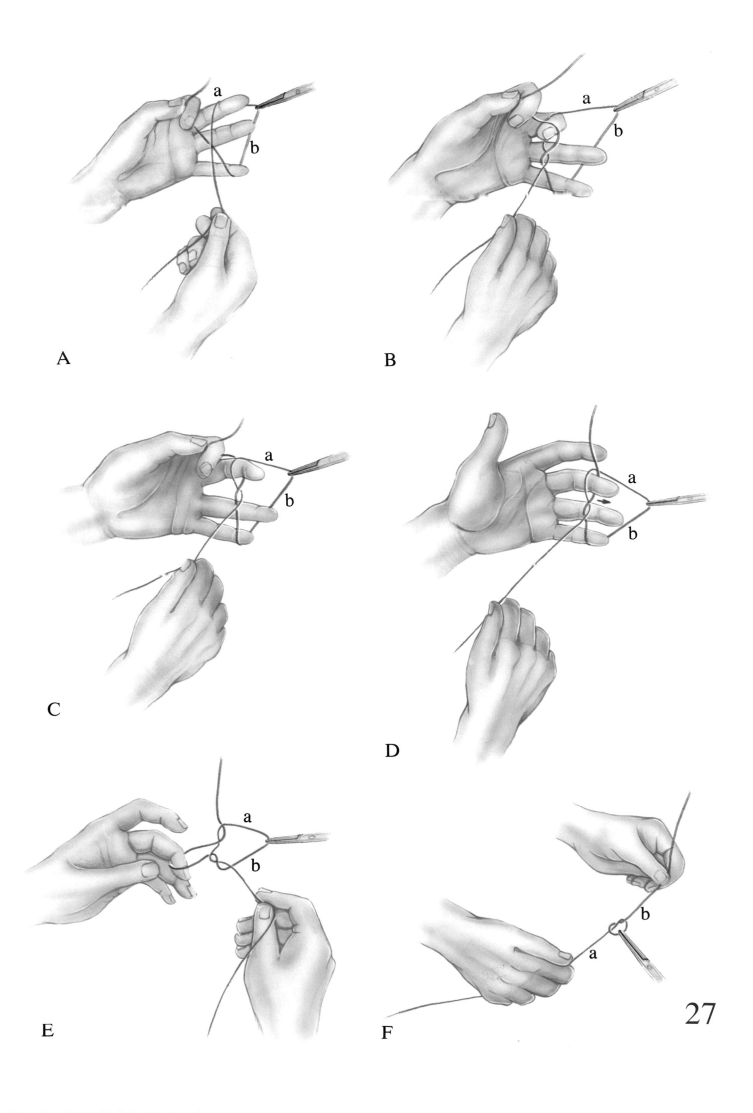

A

B

C

D

E

F

27

Plate 10

KNOT TYING *(Continued)*

ONE-HANDED CRILE KNOT

This method of knot tying is useful under certain conditions, but again it is necessary to keep the ends of the ligature taut, so it is not so useful for tying fragile blood vessels.

A.   This demonstrates one method of tying the knot by making a loop around the end of the forefinger of the left hand.

B.   End (b) is then caught across the back of the terminal phalanx of the forefinger of the left hand as shown to bring it through the loop.

C and D.   These show (b) being pulled through further to complete the overhand first portion of the knot.

E.   This demonstrates the knot being pulled taut by keeping the ligature in a straight line between the two hands and the hemostat on the blood vessel.

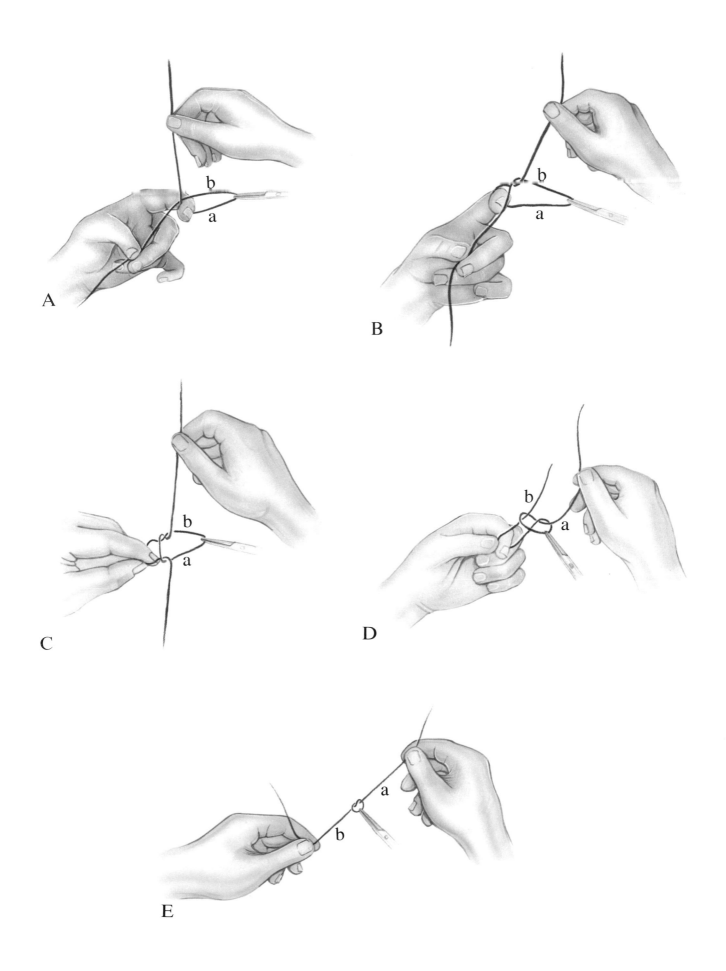

Plate 11

KNOT TYING *(Continued)*

A. This demonstrates a faulty method of ligating a blood vessel irrespective of the type of knot that is being tied. The error is that the forefinger of the right hand is pushing against a hemostat and the blood vessel to be tied, so that as the hemostat is removed the blood vessel may be partially pushed away from the knot, which makes it insecure even if it remains on the blood vessel. Furthermore, the forefinger hides the knot so that it is difficult for the surgeon to know how much force to apply to each end of the ligature, or to be certain when it has been tied securely enough to permit removal of the hemostat. Again it must be emphasized that the three points, the fingers of the two hands holding the ligatures and the blood vessel which is being tied, not only must be in a straight line, but all three should be visible to the surgeon tying the knot.

B. This demonstrates another unsatisfactory method of ligating a blood vessel. It is used most frequently by the inexperienced surgeon while tying bleeders or sutures in the depth of an incision. The mistake is that the ends of the ligatures are held across and above the incision, thus making a "V" out of the three points, the fingers of the two hands holding the ligature ends and the blood vessel being tied. As a result of this method of ligation, as soon as the hemostat is removed, the first overhand knot will almost invariably pull away from the blood vessel because it will take a straight line between the surgeon's two hands.

C. This demonstrates the correct way of ligating a vessel or placing a suture in the depths of a wound in order to keep in a straight line the three cardinal points of the ligature or suture that is being tied. In a long incision it is possible to place the fingers of both hands in the incision so that the ligature is parallel to the long axis of the incision as it is pulled taut, keeping the knot and the two ends of the ligature all in a straight line.

D. Another method of tying in a deep incision is shown in which one end of the ligature is held above the incision and the other at a deeper level beyond the blood vessel, but all three points are still kept in a straight line.

E. This demonstrates a method of ligating very fragile blood vessels, which is so frequently necessary in vascular reconstructive surgery. The illustration shows the first overhand portion of the knot tied and the hemostat removed from the bleeder. It should be noted that the ends of the ligature are then left loose and not pulled taut in completing the second half of the knot. If this precaution is taken, it is rare for the first portion of the knot to loosen while the second half is being completed. Invariably if the ends are kept taut while making the second half of the knot the ligature will slip off the vessel that is being tied.

The importance of hemostasis in vascular surgery cannot be overemphasized, so that the adherence to these simple rules of correct methods of knot tying will facilitate the carrying out of vascular surgery and save troublesome operative and postoperative complications.

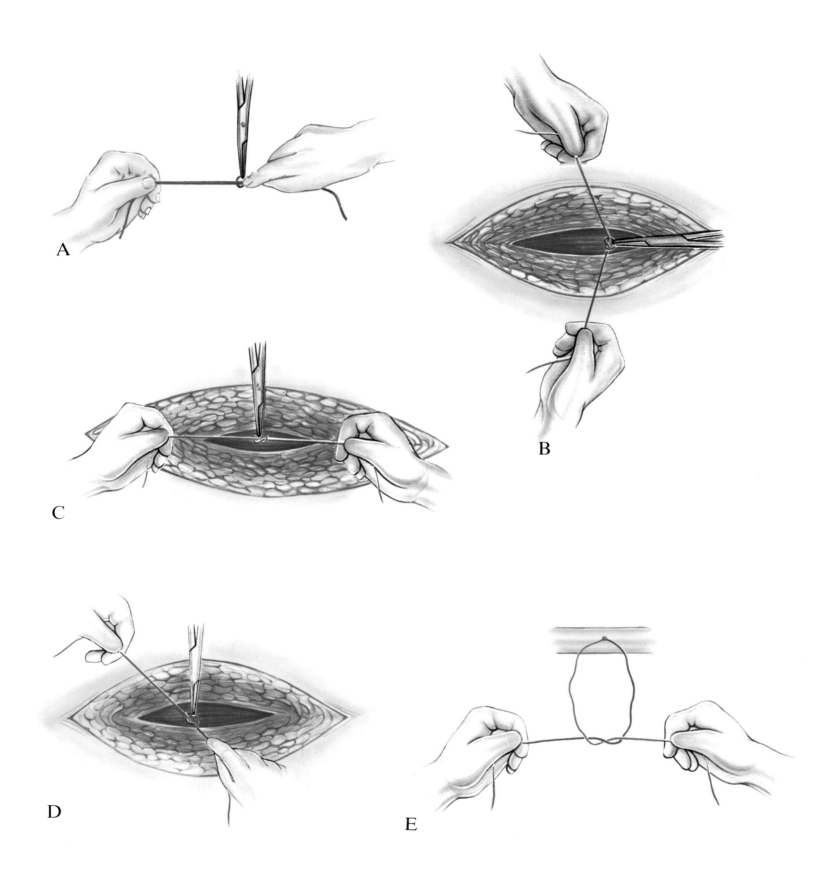

A

B

C

D

E

31

Plate 12

METHODS OF TEMPORARY CONTROL
OF MAJOR ARTERIES

A. This demonstrates a method that should never be used to occlude a major artery because so much pressure must be exerted to control the arterial blood flow that it will frequently cause a fracture of the arterial wall, with secondary thrombosis. The drawing shows a rubber catheter or tubing that has been placed around a major artery. To stop the blood flow it has to be pulled, with upward traction on the two ends, hard enough to impinge the lower wall of the artery against the upper. This requires a great deal of force because of the elasticity to the artery and, as a result, will invariably cause a fracture of the media and intima.

B. The more acceptable methods are utilization of some means of forcing the anterior and posterior walls of the artery together by pressure from both sides. It is always surprising how little force is necessary to control a large artery, even the abdominal aorta, by pressing it between the thumb and forefinger. This method is demonstrated by the utilization of a bulldog or a serrefine type of clamp. These small clamps are most useful in dealing with the peripheral arteries such as are found in the limbs. The bare metal blades are so slippery they tend to slip off an artery, and covering them with rubber tubing adds to the slipperiness. A small section of a white hollow, cloth tube shoelace slipped over and tied to the blades of the larger bulldog clamps, as is shown, will prevent them from slipping.

C and D. For larger arteries a tourniquet clamp that works on the same principle is found to be of great value. It gives excellent control, with minimal chance of damage to the arterial wall. It can be released and reapplied so easily that it is of great use in working with such structures as the abdominal and thoracic aortas. The metal end of this clamp should also be wrapped with a cloth covering to cushion it and to help prevent it from slipping. This is readily accomplished by winding several layers of umbilical tape around it smoothly, then tying the ends at the back of clamp to keep the knot out of the way.

E. Another method of controlling a small to moderate-sized artery is the passing of a large ligature around the vessel to be controlled. Both ends are passed through a tube of stiff polyvinyl. The tubing is then pushed down and the ligature pulled upward, which readily controls the blood vessel. A hemostat grasps the ligature taut at the end of the tube to maintain the blood vessel control. The disadvantage of this method is that it tends to pucker the blood vessel, making it much more traumatic than the bulldog or tourniquet clamp if the vessel is calcified.

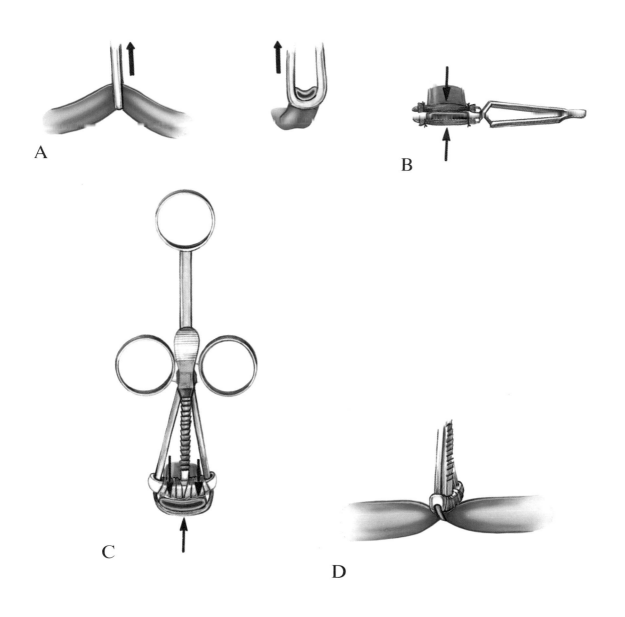

A

B

C

D

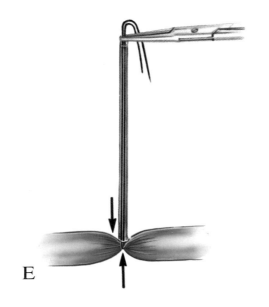

E

33

Plate 13

SPECIAL METHODS OF SECURING BLOOD VESSELS

A.   There are conditions in which ligature control of bleeding vessels is difficult to obtain. This is especially true when the end of the vessel is just barely caught in the hemostat or a previously placed ligature has slipped off and the end of the vessel has retracted out of sight. Under these conditions bleeding is readily controlled with a simple double over-and-over suture, usually fine chromic catgut on an atraumatic needle (1). This ensures that the suture will not slip off (2).

B.   This demonstrates a method of controlling an end of a completely divided large vein. There is always a large amount of venous blood that wells up, so it may be difficult to see the vessel. It is a mistake to attempt to clamp the end blindly because of damage that may be done to adjacent vital structures. It can be readily controlled, however, by inserting a finger in the wound against the vein or in its vicinity, then with suction clearing the field enough to catch the cut end of the severed vein at any place in its circumference with a hemostat (1). This instrument is then gently turned as shown in (2). This immediately controls the bleeding because the venous pressure is low, so that an adequate ligature, or transfixion ligature, or both, can be applied.

C.   This demonstrates a similar method of control of a laceration in a large vein. Again it is a simple matter to grasp the edge of the laceration after temporary control with finger pressure proximally and distally by the first assistant. Or with a fingertip on the site of bleeding, the end of a hemostat can be directed to the edge of the laceration, grasping it at a point as shown in (1) then twisting it as in (2). This immediately stops the flow of blood and permits the surgeon either to repair the vein or to ligate it doubly.

D.   This shows the most satisfactory method of repairing a lacerated vein by using an Allis clamp to obtain immediate control of it. The laceration should then be closed with mattress sutures of 5-0 or 4-0 arterial silk. These methods of using a hemostat or Allis clamps are not applicable to arteries since their walls are too fragile.

A laceration at the origin of a small arterial branch, or a branch that may have been torn off too short to ligate, is best secured by the same type of small mattress sutures of fine silk, by passing them only through the arterial adventitia and not the entire arterial wall. It is important that during the placement and the ligation the artery be kept in a flaccid state by proximal control of it.

E.   This shows the method most commonly employed to secure the end of a large artery or vein with a nonabsorbable ligature of linen or cotton. It should be placed proximal enough to leave a generous cuff beyond it to ensure that the ligature does not slip off. In addition, a transfixion ligature of the same material should be placed in the cuff distal to the primary one, still leaving an adequate cuff beyond it.

F.   This shows the securing of the end of a large artery or vein by the suture technique. It requires temporary proximal control. The end of the blood vessel is then closed with a double row of arterial sutures as shown. This method is safe because the sutures cannot slip off.

G.   This shows the safest method of securing the proximal end of the abdominal aorta, if it needs to be interrupted. It consists of multiple mattress sutures of Teflon-coated, braided Dacron placed through all layers with an adequate distal cuff. They are placed close together but should not interlock. The aortic wall must be flaccid, with adequate proximal control, as shown, while the sutures are being placed. If this technique is used, it is unnecessary to use buttressing pieces of synthetic fabric.

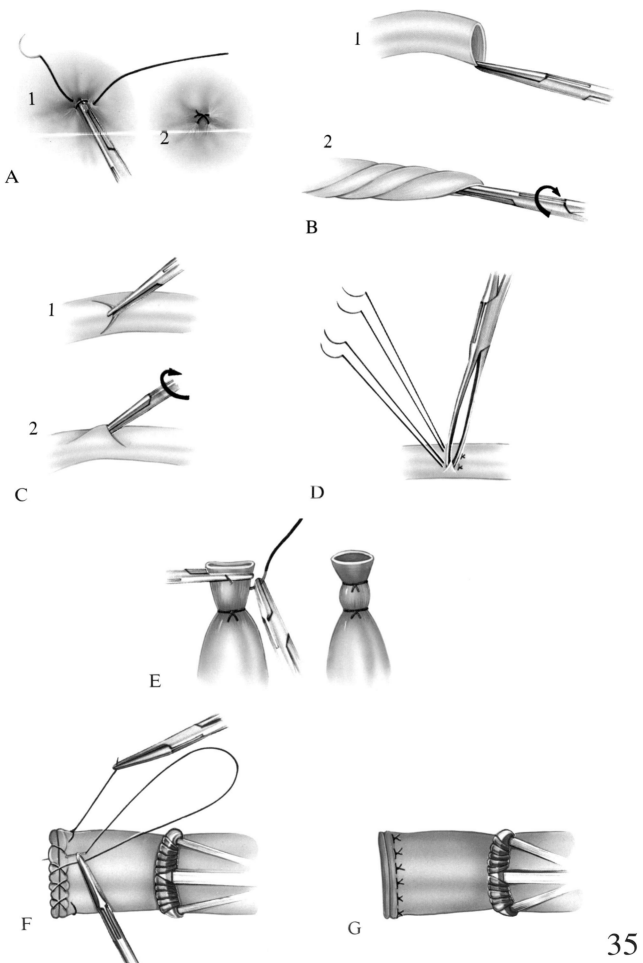

35

Plate 14

A TECHNIQUE OF VASCULAR
SUTURING

This illustration demonstrates the straight needle "push" technique of blood vessel suturing in the construction of an end-to-side anastomosis between a saphenous vein autograft and the distal popliteal artery. The two bulldog clamps control a segment of the artery. The vein graft has been sutured at each end of the anastomosis with mattress sutures (a) and (b), using fine, straight, cutting point needles with a No. 5-0 arterial Teflon-coated Dacron suture. The straight needles are bent in a ski shape to facilitate the placing of the mattress sutures and then they are straightened to continue the anastomotic suturing. This method is much more satisfactory than using a 3/8 or 1/2 curved needle because, after the placing of the first two mattress sutures, when it is best to straighten the needles. It is much more difficult to straighten a curved needle satisfactorily than to restraighten a straight needle that has been purposely bent.

The suturing has commenced with the suture (a) and is continued as a running over-and-over type of stitch. Note that the needle has been straightened so that it can be placed in the tip of the needle holder at an acute angle without the necessity of picking it up with the left hand, which is so necessary when a curved needle is used. It is pushed forward through the graft from the outside to the inside of the artery as shown by the direction of arrow (c). The tip of the needle is then readily grasped with the needle holder and pulled through. The needle is next repositioned in the needle holder without the necessity of picking it up with the left hand. The forward motion of the tip of the needle holder is greatly facilitated by using this instrument as a lever, with the fulcrum point (e) at the edge of the incision, exerting slight pressure downward as shown by the arrow (d). The placing of each stitch can also be done more accurately by this method since it can be accomplished simply by pointing the tip of the needle holder with the needle in it at the exact point that is desired for the next stitch. Constant tension is maintained on the vein anastomotic cuff during suturing with a fine forceps (f) held in the left hand to prevent wrinkling of the vein, which would destroy the streamlining characteristics of the anastomotic site. It is necessary that the first assistant maintain firm tension on the suture with his right hand as shown (g) after the placing of each stitch in order to make the suture line hemostatic.

The chief advantages of this method of suturing with a straight needle are as follows: (1) the needle need never be picked up with the left hand to place it in the needle holder; (2) this leaves the left hand free to maintain constant tension on the vein cuff during the suturing, a matter of extreme importance for success; (3) the needle holder can be used as a lever by exerting pressure against the incision edge, thereby greatly stabilizing the instrument and permitting more accurate placing of the sutures; (4) it is much easier to pass a straight needle through the tough, resistant vessels and grafts that are frequently encountered; and (5) the sutures can be placed more accurately by this technique than by any other method.

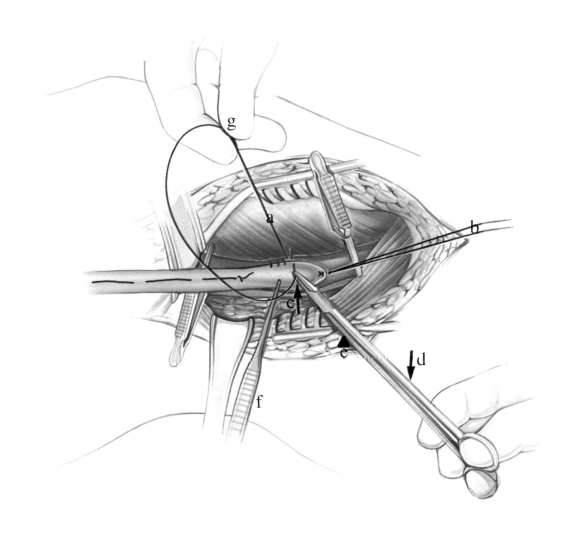

Plate 15

INSTRUMENTS

SCISSORS

General Purpose Scissors with Blunt-Pointed Blades

　　1. Straight scissors with narrow blades for cutting fine sutures.

　　2. Straight scissors, Mayo type, for cutting all other types of sutures.

　　3. Slightly curved scissors with shorter blades, Mayo type, for dissection of the more superficial vessels.

　　4. Scissors with long, slightly curved blades for dissection in deep operative fields.

Special Scissors

　　1. Scissors with long blunt-pointed blade curved at a right angle for use in deep operative fields.

　　2. Angled Potts' type scissors for making arteriotomies.

　　3. Short scissors with blunt-pointed blades for fine work and removing adventitia from vein grafts.

　　4. Scissors with slightly curved, sharp-pointed blades for the neat and accurate trimming of atherosclerotic intimal plaques so that suturing of distal edges is not necessary.

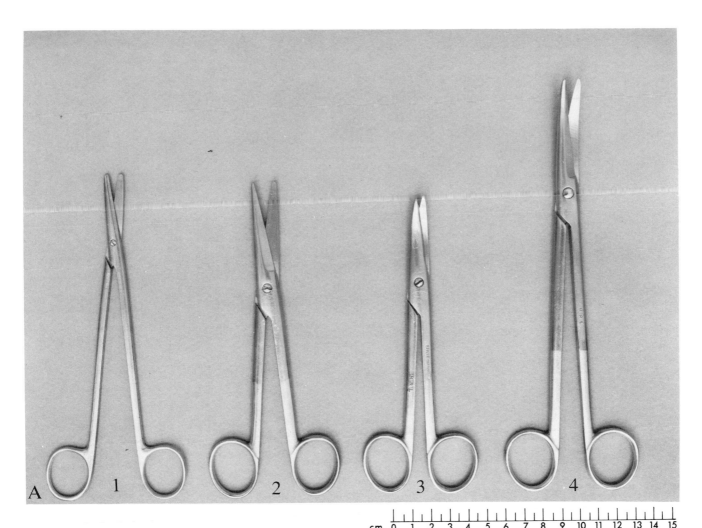

cm. 0 1 2 3 4 5 6 7 8 9 10 11 12 13 14 15

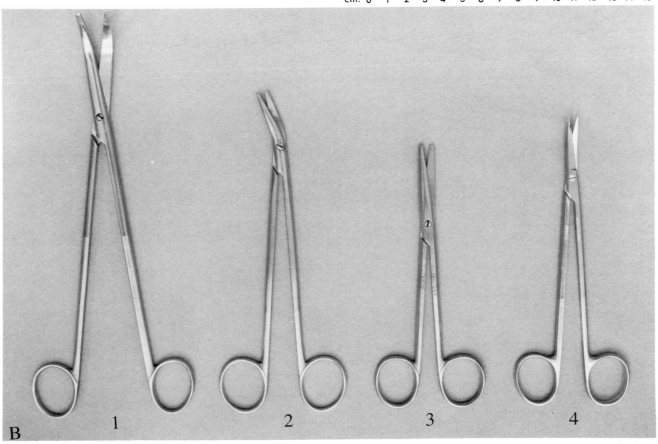

cm. 0 1 2 3 4 5 6 7 8 9 10 11 12 13 14 15

39

Plate 16

INSTRUMENTS *(Continued)*

FORCEPS

1. Long forceps with ring ends for use in the dissection of large blood vessels in deep operative fields.

2. Long, fine, smooth-ended forceps for use in blood vessel suturing in deep operative fields.

3. Long, wide, smooth-ended forceps for the dissection of blood vessels.

4. Fine-pointed forceps with special "atraugrip" tips for use in dissecting and suturing blood vessels.

5. Forceps with angled tips which are especially useful in deep operative fields.

6. Shorter fine-tipped forceps for use in suturing blood vessels and in the construction of vascular anastomoses in superficial operative fields.

7. Forceps with teeth in their tips for general use in making and closing incisions.

RETRACTORS

Note that these metal retractors are covered with cotton tubular webbing to aid in the retraction of the intestines without the need of packing them off with large gauze packs.

1. An extra large, wide, Deaver-type retractor for use in performing abdominal aortic surgery.

2. A large Harrington retractor for use in patients with deep abdominal cavities. These are available also with narrower blades.

3. A large, standard, Deaver-type retractor for abdominal use. This type comes in narrow, medium and wide sizes.

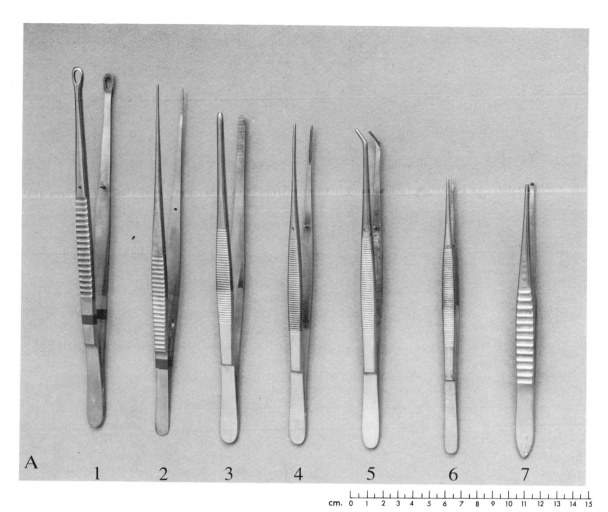

A 1 2 3 4 5 6 7

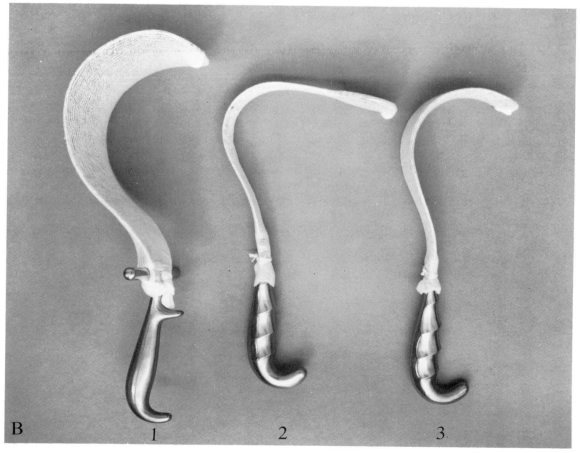

B 1 2 3

Plate 17

INSTRUMENTS *(Continued)*

ENDARTERECTOMY INSTRUMENTS

1. A long, curved, hysterectomy-type clamp with long, blunt-pointed blades for abdominal aortic endarterectomy.

2. A medium, curved Schnitt clamp with short, sharper-pointed blades to commence the endarterectomy of the aorta, the iliac and the common femoral arteries.

3. A small right-angle clamp with narrow, sharp-pointed blades.

4. A long, fine-tipped Allis clamp for the temporary control of lacerations in large veins and leaks in arterial anastomoses to aid in suture closing of them. The wider tipped ones are also useful for larger vein lacerations.

5. A ring-type stripper made from one piece of 18-gauge stainless steel wire. These are made with different sized rings. It is necessary that the long stem can be bent as shown to facilitate their passage, especially in the external and common iliac arteries.

6. A pin vise is placed on the long stem as a handle to aid in the passage and control of the stripper, especially when used in the external and common iliac arteries.

7. A Penfield dura elevator that is a useful instrument to commence endarterectomies.

MISCELLANEOUS INSTRUMENTS

1. A 50-cc. plastic syringe with a large nozzle for use in preclotting aortic bifurcation and tubular knitted Dacron prostheses.

2. A 35-cc. plastic syringe with a conical metal-type adapter for use in preclotting smaller knitted Dacron prostheses.

3. A 12-cc. plastic syringe with a small ball point needle for use in flushing out blood vessels at the site of an end-to-side vascular anastomosis and for tying into the distal end of a saphenous vein autograft to flush it during its removal and to distend it prior to its implantation. It is also useful to tie into the posterior tibial or radial arteries for retrograde flushing of the distal lower leg and forearm arterial system following femoral, popliteal or brachial embolisms with distal thrombosis that cannot be cleared with Fogarty catheters.

4. A 6-cc. syringe with a 22-gauge needle used for the intravenous injection of heparin solution during an operation and also to check arterial and anastomotic suture lines for leaks using dilute heparin-saline solution.

5. A 2-cc. syringe with a 25-gauge needle for the injection of dilute heparin-saline solution to dilate a portion of an artery isolated between occluding bulldog clamps that has gone into vasospasm from dissection. This is a very valuable procedure to perform at the site at which an anastomosis is to be constructed or an arteriotomy performed. Once the artery is dilated hydrostatically it remains dilated for several hours.

6. A Fraser-type metal suction tip for minor bleeding sources that is also used with the diathermy for the hemostatic control of oozing.

7. A glass drinking tube used for large bleeding sources and the cleaning out of vascular prostheses after preclotting them.

8. A polyvinyl tubing gauge with a blunt-ended Luer-Lok needle in one end for injecting dilute heparin-normal saline solution proximal and distal to occluding vascular clamps during reconstructive arterial and venous surgery.

9. Polyvinyl catheters of various sizes, 12- to 24-gauge French, for irrigation of blood vessels and for use (segments) as stents in reconstructing arteries to the correct size.

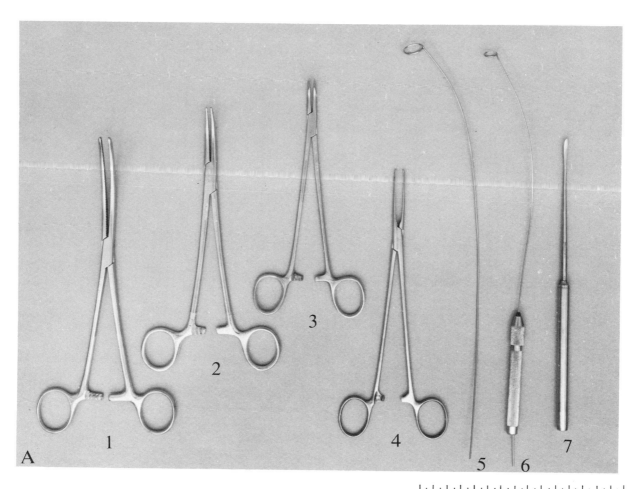

A

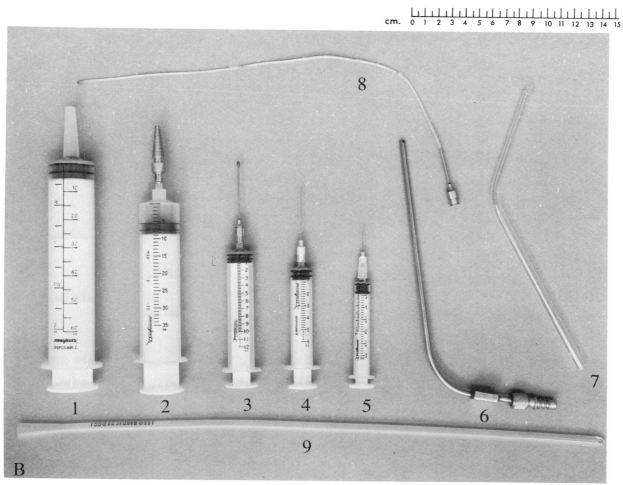

B

43

Plate 18

INSTRUMENTS *(Continued)*

SPECIAL CURVED CLAMPS

A. 1. A small, fine-tipped, right-angled clamp for passing fine ligatures around very small blood vessels.

2 and 3. Longer, right-angled clamps with blunt tips for passing ligatures around larger blood vessels.

4 and 5. Long, curved clamps with blunt ends to make tunnels for aortofemoral and femoropopliteal grafts.

B. Longer and larger right-angled, curved clamps of various sizes for passing umbilical tape or shoestrings used for the tourniquet clamps around the aorta and the inferior vena cava and, occasionally, for the temporary control of these large vessels when indicated.

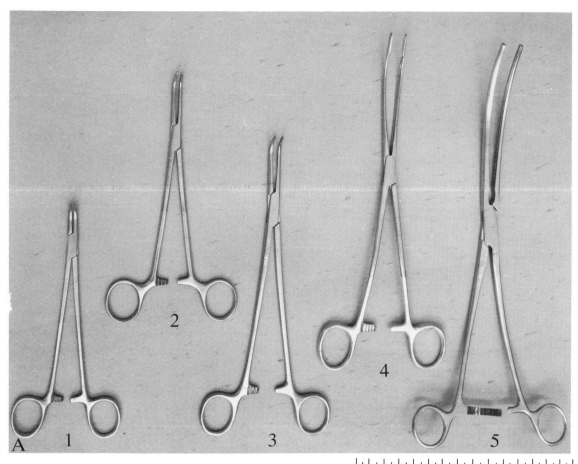

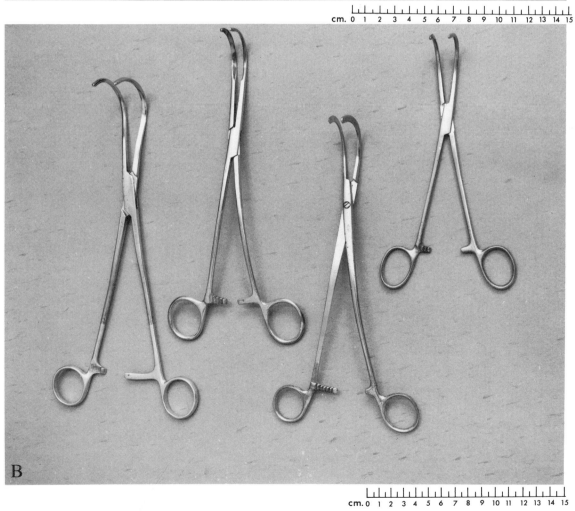

45

Plate 19

INSTRUMENTS *(Continued)*

CLAMPS FOR TEMPORARY CONTROL OF BLOOD VESSELS

A. 1. Small bulldog clamps of various sizes, shapes of blades and strengths of springs for the control of small arteries and veins.

2. Larger bulldog clamps, also of varying sizes, shapes and strengths of springs, with blades covered with short cloth shoestring segments tied on securely at each end of the blades.

TOURNIQUET CLAMPS (LINTON)

B. 1. A short tourniquet clamp for control of abdominal aortas 2 cm. or larger in diameter. Note the curved end piece that permits more effective control with less pressure. The two-ring ratchet handle moves up and down on the notched handle.

2. A longer, angled-handle tourniquet clamp for use on an abdominal aorta 2 cm. or less in diameter and the common iliac arteries. A shoestring has been passed through the distal end and the middle cross bar and to the hole in the two-ring ratchet handle. It has been tied in a square knot and the clamp closed on a rubber tubing that simulates a blood vessel. Note that the distal end has been covered by wrapping it with umbilical tape. This cushions the end of the clamp and also creates friction so that it does not slip so readily.

3. This shows the back side of the short aortic tourniquet clamp (1), demonstrating the cloth-covered wrap over the end of the clamp with the knot tied on the back side to keep it out of the way. The shoestring has also been placed and tied and the long ends removed.

4. A much smaller angled tourniquet clamp with a small tip for use on the common femoral artery.

The tourniquet clamp has the great advantage that once it is in place it may be opened and closed without even looking for the aorta or the blood vessel it is on. It always stays in place and is much less apt to damage the blood vessel wall than the metal crushing type of clamp. As a result, it gives the surgeon assurance that he has efficient and safe control of the aortic or arterial inflow tract at all times once the clamp has been placed.

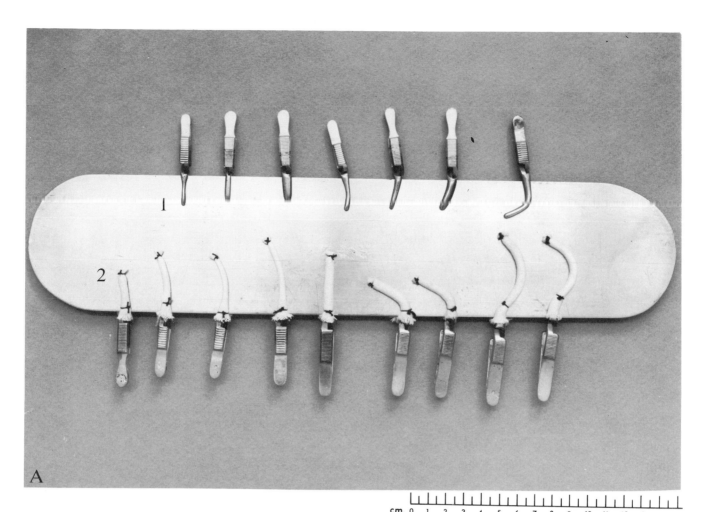

A

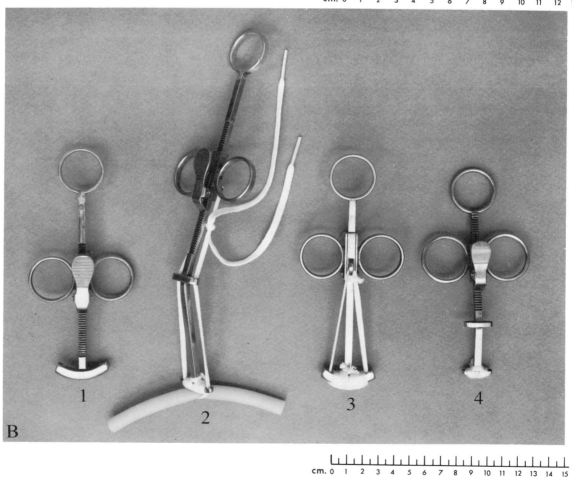

B

Plate 20

INSTRUMENTS *(Continued)*

Special Instruments

A. 1. A caliper for measuring the outside diameter of large blood vessels and aneurysms.

2. A direct reading caliper for measuring the outside diameter of small blood vessels.

3. A small hemostat with rubber-covered jaws for holding fine arterial sutures to prevent weakening and fracturing of the fine threads.

4. A small, double-ended retractor to pass underneath an artery and elevate it to facilitate its separation from its concomitant vein.

Needle Holders

B. 1. The preferred type of arterial suture — Teflon-coated Dacron with a straight needle or some of the newer monofilament synthetic sutures.

2. A short needle holder with short, fine-pointed jaws for use with fine arterial sutures during close work.

3. A standard-type, fine-tipped, longer needle holder for use with arterial sutures in shallow operative fields.

4. A longer, fine-tipped needle holder to use with arterial sutures in deep operative fields.

5. An extra long needle holder with short strong jaws for suturing in deep operative fields, especially when working with tough vessel walls and vascular prostheses.

For a running arterial suture it is best to have needle holders without diamond jaws because, as a result of the numerous applications of the holder to the single needle, they roughen the needle so that it becomes difficult to pass it through the delicate vascular tissues.

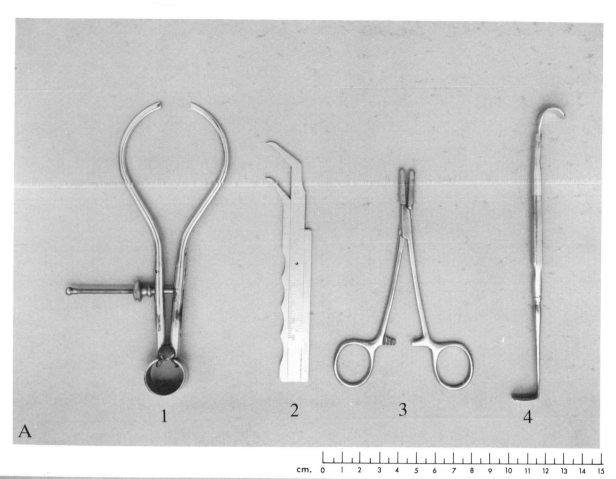

A

1   2   3   4

cm. 0 1 2 3 4 5 6 7 8 9 10 11 12 13 14 15

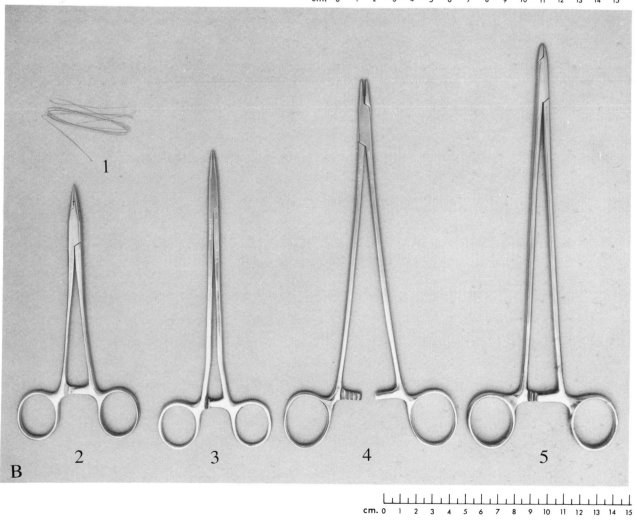

B

1

2   3   4   5

cm. 0 1 2 3 4 5 6 7 8 9 10 11 12 13 14 15

49

Plate 21

INSTRUMENTS *(Continued)*

CURVED CLAMPS FOR END-TO-SIDE ANASTOMOSIS

Venous Clamps

A.　1. A large curved clamp with blades that are covered with sections of shoe-strings for use on the inferior vena cava in performing large end-to-side anastomoses.

2. A small curved clamp with cloth-covered blades for the construction of end-to-side splenorenal anastomoses.

3. The same clamp without the cloth covering on the blades.

Arterial Clamps

B.　1, 2 and 3. Different sized Satinsky clamps for use on the aorta for end-to-side anastomoses. The jaws of these clamps have longitudinal ribbing to help to prevent the clamp from slipping.

4. A clamp with shorter curved blades but with multiple fine teeth to prevent slippage.

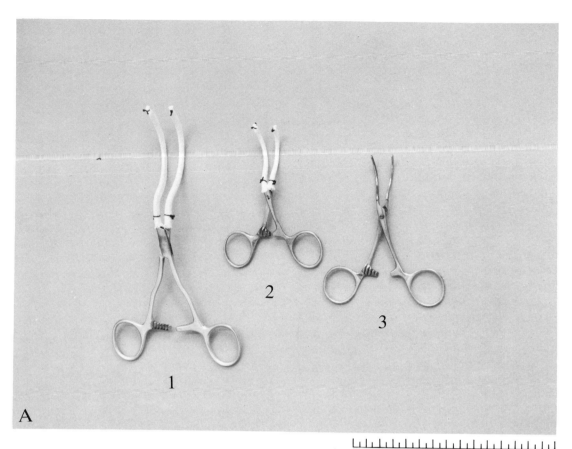

A

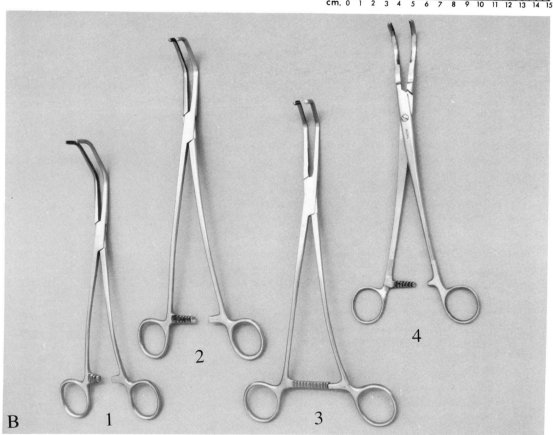

B

51

Plate 22

INSTRUMENTS *(Continued)*

LUMBAR SYMPATHECTOMY INSTRUMENTS

A. 1. Hartman forceps for use in isolating the lumbar sympathetic chain.
2. A long, Crile, blunt-tipped nerve hook.
3. A shorter and finer-tipped nerve hook.
4. The holder for silver dural clips.
5. A long dural clip applicator.

VARICOSE VEIN INSTRUMENTS

B. 1. Intraluminal vein strippers of different lengths and size of tips. The upper one has a metal washer on it to increase the size of the large end. Three sizes of washers are useful for the different sized veins. They are shown lying at the right end of the strippers. The strippers are made of 18-gauge stainless steel wire with different-sized small tips on one end to advance through the various-sized veins, and a larger tip on the other end to make the veins telescope on the stripper and to prevent the veins from turning inside out. The various-sized washers that are used for the different sizes of veins make this possible.
2. A medium-sized, self-retaining retractor.
3. A medium-sized, sharp-pointed rake retractor.
4. A small, sharp-pointed rake and smooth-ended retractor.

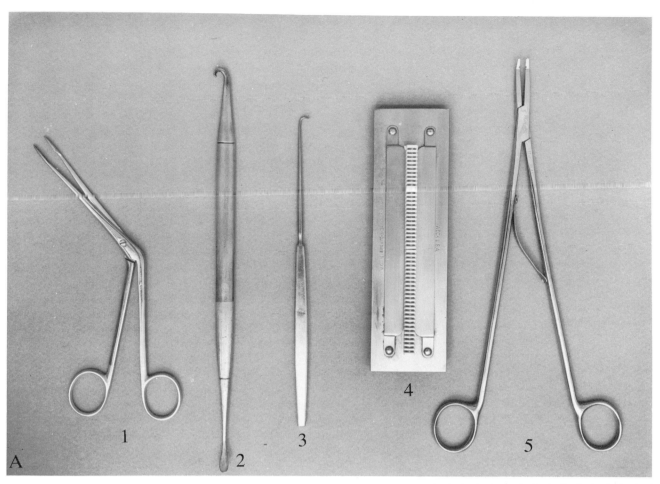

A

1   2   3   4   5

cm. 0 1 2 3 4 5 6 7 8 9 10 11 12 13 14 15

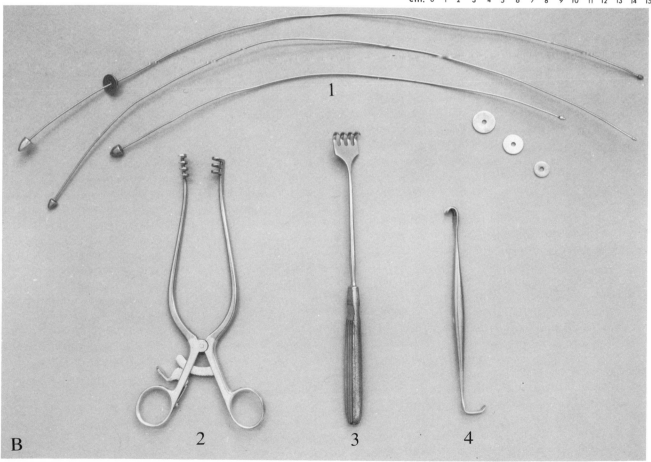

B

1

2   3   4

cm. 0 1 2 3 4 5 6 7 8 9 10 11 12 13 14 15

53

Part I

Diseases of the Veins

The diseases of the veins have never attracted the surgical attention that arterial diseases have for a number of reasons. The apparent lack of interest in this branch of vascular surgery, despite the frequency of disorders, especially of the veins of the lower extremity, may in part be because the results of treatment of some of the common conditions involving them have for the most part been unsatisfactory. Also, a number of the venous diseases do not endanger the limb or life of the patient as much as the arterial diseases more often do. In addition, because the anatomy and pathologic physiology of the veins is not well understood by the majority of surgeons, the surgical treatment is frequently inadequately performed, especially for the most common conditions, namely, the diseases of the veins of the lower extremity. Furthermore, few types of surgery require such meticulous, careful, nontraumatic and patient handling of tissues as the thin-walled venous channels. This may be especially true if a large venous channel is inadvertently incised or torn during dissection of it. The control of venous bleeding under these conditions, especially if the vein must be preserved (e.g., as is necessary in freeing up the splenic vein in order to do a splenorenal venous shunt), will often require the utmost care and ingenuity that a surgeon can muster. As a result, many surgeons unfamiliar with the technical difficulties of performing operative procedures for venous diseases become discouraged because of the poor results they obtain.

There is perhaps nothing more terrifying than the welling up of venous blood, especially in a deep wound, from injury to a large thin-walled venous structure such as the inferior vena cava, the common iliac, the external iliac, the hypogastric, the femoral, the popliteal, the subclavian or the axillary veins. This is because venous hemorrhage at a low pressure is much more difficult to control than arterial hemorrhage that spurts out at high pressure. Although the loss of blood may be large from these venous injuries, the most serious complication in obtaining control (of the large veins especially) is the damage that may be done to contiguous structures such as arteries, ureters and nerves. However, if the basic rules of venous surgery are understood, the bleeding can be readily controlled, frequently with salvage of the vein and preservation of adjacent structures. It is of some significance also that almost all veins in the human body with the exception of the superior vena cava, the inferior vena cava proximal to the renal veins and the portal vein are expendable in that they can be ligated without too serious consequences, which of course is not true of the aorta and many major arteries. These and other facts and methods of therapy will be demonstrated in the following pages.

VARICOSE VEINS OF THE LOWER EXTREMITY

Varicose veins of the lower extremity are one of the most common vascular diseases affecting the human race, and undoubtedly are the result of man's assuming the erect position as a biped, because this subjects the veins of the lower extremity at the ankle level to a high intravenous pressure that approaches arterial systolic pressure. This is especially true in the standing stationary position. The superficial veins which lie between the skin and the deep fascia in the subcutaneous tissues have little if any support and, as a result, they tend to become dilated and varicosed. There have been many theories advanced to explain the etiology of varicose veins, some of which seem far-fetched, such as constipation or sitting in chairs. These certainly do not explain why it is not unusual to find the condition in one leg and not the other in the same individual. It seems of significance that in obtaining a history from a patient with varicosities it is frequently found that the mother, father, aunts, uncles and siblings are or have been afflicted; in fact, it is rare that such a familial history is not encountered. There seems little doubt that the condition of varicose veins is an inherited characteristic, probably the result of incompetence of the venous bicuspid valves in the superficial and communicating system of veins in the lower extremity.

In order to understand the pathologic physiology of the lower extremity veins, it should be remembered that there are three venous systems: (1) The superficial veins lie between the skin and the deep fascia in the subcutaneous tissues. These consist of the internal or long saphenous vein and the external or short saphenous vein. They oscillate through their many branches so that frequently pathological conditions of one may involve the other. (2) The deep veins of the lower extremity lie between the muscles of the lower leg and the thigh and are protected from dilatation by the deep fascia, a tough fibrous envelope surrounding all the musculature of the extremity. These consist of the common, the superficial and the deep femoral veins in the thigh; the popliteal vein at the knee; the anterior tibial, the posterior tibial and the peroneal veins in the lower leg. (3) The third system is made up of the communicating veins that connect the deep and superficial systems. Most surgeons call these vessels "the perforators," which indicates only that they perforate the deep fascia. It is my opinion that the term "communicating veins" denotes their true function, and so for this reason it would be best to drop the former and maintain the latter. These are most numerous in the lower leg, but they also are present in the thigh. They play an extremely important role in the etiology of varicose veins of the superficial system and are even more important in the postthrombotic extremity.

These three systems of veins with their bicuspid valves, the muscles of the leg, and the deep fascia surrounding them constitute what is known as the venous heart of the lower extremity. By muscular action blood is pumped back to the heart through these vessels. A knowledge of this basic physiology of the lower extremity is extremely important in understanding the pathological diseases that result from a derangement of these venous systems with decompensation of the venous heart of varying degree in order that adequate therapy can be performed to correct any condition that develops.

Even though the deep veins are protected from dilatation, they may become diseased as a result of deep venous thrombosis. Recanalization of them invariably occurs with restoration of the venous lumen but with destruction and incompetence of the venous valves. This results in decompensation of the venous heart, with an increase in the venous pressure in the lower limb during muscular contraction so that a state of ambulatory venous hypertension develops in the lower limb.

This results in increased intravenous pressure in the communicating veins, especially of the lower leg, and causes dilatation of them so that their valves become incompetent. As a result, the increased pressure is transmitted to the superficial system of the saphenous veins so that they, in turn, become dilated and incompetent. These changes in the three systems of veins, if untreated, result in the postphlebitic or the postthrombotic state. The characteristics of this condition are capillary hemorrhages in the skin, with brownish pigmentation. A condition of stasis cellulitis develops later, as evidenced by fibrous replacement of the subcutaneous tissues most frequently seen on the medial side of the lower leg and ankle. The involved area is characteristically indurated, slightly swollen and exquisitely tender. An abrasion of the area usually results in a chronic ulcer which has been given various names, such as postphlebitic, postthrombotic or stasis ulcer, but which could more accurately be termed a "venous hypertensive ulceration," the result of decompensation of the venous heart of the lower extremity.

Many operative procedures have been described for centuries, even as far back as the time of Hippocrates, for eradication of varicose veins and cure of chronic ulcers of the lower extremity. It appears from the surgical literature that one method is in vogue for a short period of time, then is discarded for another. In fact, the treatment has apparently gone around in circles, coming back many years later to one of the earlier forms of treatment. For example, at the Massachusetts General Hospital in 1840 patients were admitted to the surgical wards for the injection of their varicose veins with a solution of ferric chloride solution. The results of this form of therapy were never published and presumably it was abandoned because of serious complications. The use of different sclerosing solutions and aseptic techniques was commenced again about 100 years later in the 1920's as an ambulatory form of treatment but again discontinued after a few years because of poor results.

The surgical treatment of varicose veins and the chronic postthrombotic syndrome with and without ulcerations of the lower leg still leaves much room for improvement, in part, it is believed, because of failure to understand the basic pathologic physiology and how these conditions can be corrected. Another reason for poor results is that the operative procedures are often turned over to the youngest members of the surgical house staff of the major hospitals for training surgeons. This has been going on for generations because the senior surgeons are not interested in the meticulous type of surgery that is required for the majority of these conditions. As a result, the training in this field is passed on from one young surgeon to another with such poor results that both patients and surgeons become discouraged with the surgical treatment of these conditions.

Plate 23

VARICOSE VEINS OF THE LOWER EXTREMITY

THE ANATOMY

A. The long, or greater, saphenous vein is shown from its origin on the dorsum of the foot to its termination where it joins the common femoral vein at the fossa ovalis. Note that there is a lateral and medial trunk to the main vein in the thigh; the medial vein even extends down the lower leg. Another important trunk is a posterior one in the lower leg that arises near the internal malleolus and terminates proximally with the main trunk at the knee level. In the majority of patients these blood vessels lie superficial to the deep fascia of the extremity, but in some the main trunk in the thigh may lie beneath it; in the lower leg they are always superficial to the fascia. The location of the communicating veins is also shown. Note that they are found in the foot and thigh as well as the lower leg, where they are most numerous. This system of vessels connects the superficial veins with the posterior tibial, anterior tibial and peroneal veins, so their distribution follows the course of these deep veins. The interruption of them when they are incompetent is essential if varicose veins are to be cured.

B. The short, or smaller, saphenous vein is shown from its origin on the lateral side of the dorsum of the foot, coursing up the posterolateral side of the ankle and lower leg. It goes through the deep fascia, usually in the upper third of the lower leg to terminate in the popliteal vein, most commonly in the mid portion of the popliteal space. Note the osculations with the branches of the long saphenous system and the venous tributary connecting the cephalad end with the main saphenous vein trunk. The location of the communicating veins is shown in the foot and the lateral side of the lower leg.

The goal of the surgeon treating varicose veins by surgery should be to cure the condition by performing the proper and adequate surgical procedure at the operating table, so that few if any postoperative injections of a sclerosing solution will be needed for residual veins. In order to attain the goal the surgical treatment should consist of (1) ligation and stripping of the long saphenous vein and any secondary trunks in the thigh and lower legs; (2) removal of the short saphenous vein, if incompetent, in a similar manner; (3) then, of great importance, interruption of all incompetent communicating veins by ligation and division; and (4) removal of all large tortuous varicosities that cannot be stripped through multiple short oblique and transverse incisions. The methods of performing these various procedures are demonstrated in the following illustrations and legends.

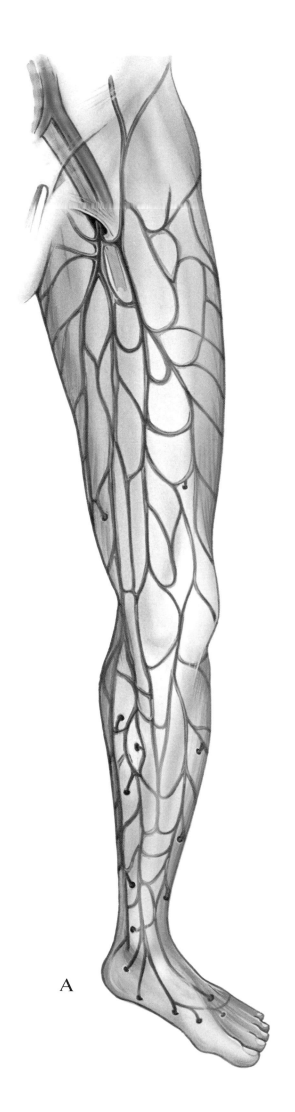

A

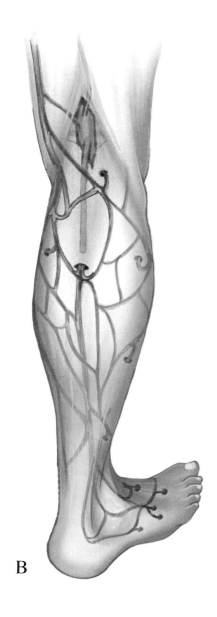

B

59

Plate 24

VARICOSE VEINS OF THE LOWER EXTREMITY *(Continued)*

THE PATHOPHYSIOLOGY

A. A drawing showing the normal condition of the three venous systems of the lower extremity. The long and the short saphenous veins of the superficial system, and the femoral and posterior tibial veins of the deep system are shown with their competent bicuspid valves that permit blood to flow only toward the heart. The communicating system of veins between these two systems, the superficial and the deep, are shown with their competent valves that permit blood to flow only from the former to the latter.

1. The venous pressure in a normal extremity with competent venous systems is demonstrated by cannulating a superficial vein at the ankle. Note that in the standing position it is equal to the pressure of a column of blood from the level of the heart to the point the venipuncture has been done, so that in a six-foot tall individual it almost equals the systolic arterial pressure.

2. The venous pressure in the same extremity is determined in the walking state. Note that it tends to approach zero. This indicates that the venous heart of the lower extremity is competent, with all the venous valves of the three systems functioning.

B. A drawing showing the abnormal condition of the superficial and communicating veins in the majority of patients with varicose veins. Note that the long saphenous vein has become dilated, resulting in incompetence of its valves. In addition, the communicating veins between it and the deep veins (most frequently just below the knee and at the ankle level) are likewise incompetent. The deep veins and the short saphenous veins are not affected, although they may be in the more extensive varicose conditions.

1. The venous pressure in an extremity with superficial varicose veins is shown. Note that the standing pressure is the same as in the normal extremity.

2. The pressure in the walking state, however, does not reduce but may even increase slightly. This is due to incompetence of the valves of the long saphenous vein and perhaps some of the communicating veins, resulting in mild decompensation of the venous heart of the lower extremity.

3. Note that if the long saphenous vein is occluded by finger pressure below the knee, the venous pressure falls. This determines that the valves of the deep venous and communicating system are competent, and that only the superficial system is diseased.

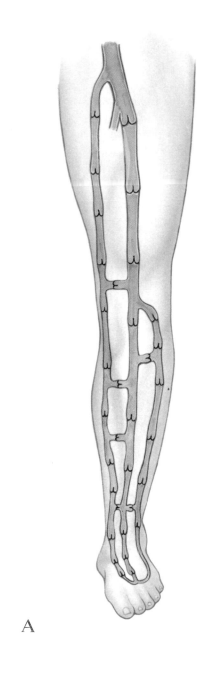

A

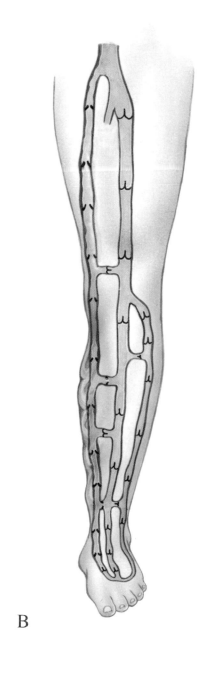

B

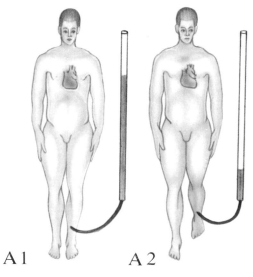

A 1   A 2

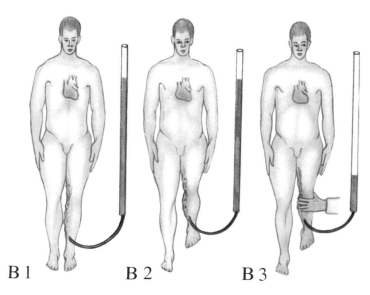

B 1   B 2   B 3

61

Plate 25

VARICOSE VEINS OF THE LOWER EXTREMITY *(Continued)*

THE ETIOLOGY

A. This shows the appearance of varicosities of the long saphenous system of the left lower extremity. In this case large varicose veins are seen in the groin, the medial aspect of the thigh and the lower leg. Note there is no edema of the lower leg and ankle since varicosities of this degree and location seldom are the cause of lymphedema.

B. The proximal close-up of the groin and medial thigh shows the common, superficial femoral and profunda femoris veins of the deep system and the proximal end of the long saphenous vein and its lateral trunk. The anterior walls of the veins have been cut away to show their valves. Note that in this case the valve in the proximal end of the superficial femoral vein is normal and competent, whereas those in the long saphenous vein and the lateral trunk are incompetent because of dilatation of these veins. It is believed that in many patients varicosities of these vessels develop because of incompetence of these valves stemming from some congenital defect. The dilatation of them continues in a retrograde fashion, with incompetence developing in each successive valve. It is frequently found also that incompetent communicating veins, especially in the lower leg, are a contributing factor in the development of varicose veins.

C. The distal inset shows one of the incompetent communicating veins in the lower leg and its osculation with the long saphenous vein and its tributaries. Note that the valve in the communicating vein is incompetent, as are those in the saphenous vein. It is believed that perhaps the communicating vein becomes incompetent first because of a congenital defect in it or in the deep veins. Then, as a result, a high pressure leak from the deep veins occurs, with resulting dilatation and incompetence of the saphenous vein and its tributaries.

An understanding of this basic pathologic anatomy clearly demonstrates that, in addition to removing the long saphenous vein in the treatment of varicosities of its system, one must also ligate and divide the incompetent veins in order to cure varicose veins of the lower extremity.

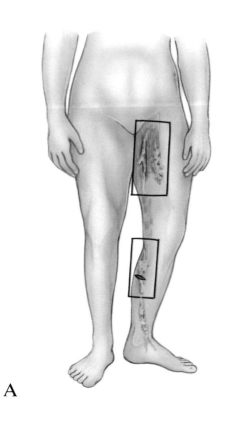

A

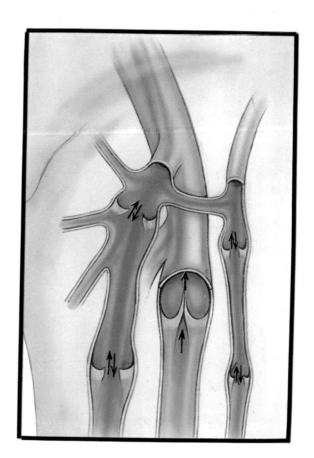

B

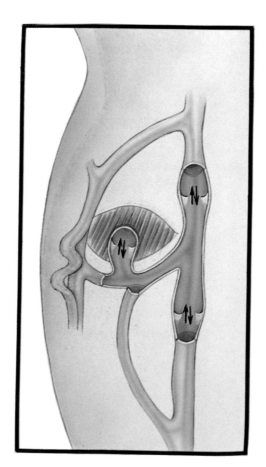

C

63

Plate 26

DIAGNOSTIC TESTS FOR VARICOSE VEINS OF THE LOWER EXTREMITY

THE TRENDELENBURG TEST

A. This test was described by F. Trendelenburg, a German surgeon, in the last century. It is useful chiefly to demonstrate the competence of the venous valves of the superficial and communicating systems of veins. This description of it is a modification of Trendelenburg's method. The patient first lies down on the examining table. The leg to be examined is elevated to a 30 to 45 degree angle for 10 to 15 seconds to drain the blood from the superficial veins.

B. A soft rubber venous tourniquet is placed around the leg just below the knee, instead of above it, and held by hand so that the long and short saphenous veins are occluded.

C. The patient then stands erect with the tourniquet still tight, and careful observation of the veins distal to the tourniquet is made. In the case of simple varicose veins, the veins will fill with blood very slowly, indicating competent valves in the deep and communicating systems. If on the other hand these veins are full of blood, almost as soon as the patient stands, it demonstrates that the valves in many of the communicating veins are incompetent and that the ones in the deep system of veins are also. If the veins fill more slowly but are full within one half to one minute, this indicates that deep veins are competent and that some, but not all, of the communicating veins are incompetent. If one suspects that the short saphenous vein is affected, the tourniquet should be placed above the knee and finger pressure exerted over the proximal end of the short saphenous vein in the distal part of the popliteal space. The patient then stands, and shortly afterward the finger pressure is released. If blood rapidly rushes down the vein on the posterior aspect of the lower leg, this proves that the short saphenous vein is incompetent.

D. The tourniquet has been released. Almost immediately one sees the blood cascade rapidly down from above in the large varicose veins of the lower leg. This demonstrates the incompetence of the valves in the long saphenous vein and its large varicosed tributaries. The large tortuous veins on the anterolateral aspect of the thigh are tributaries of the lateral saphenous thigh trunk which will be found to fill both proximally and distally. Since these veins will need to be excised because of their size and tortuosity, it is not essential to test them.

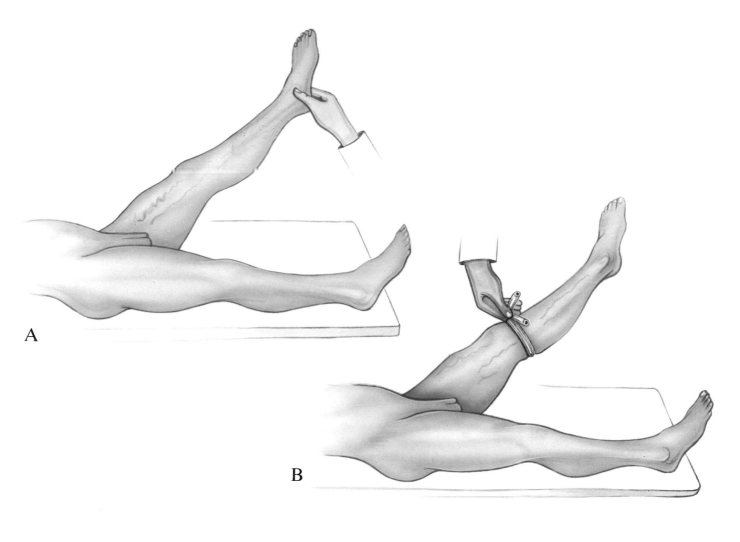

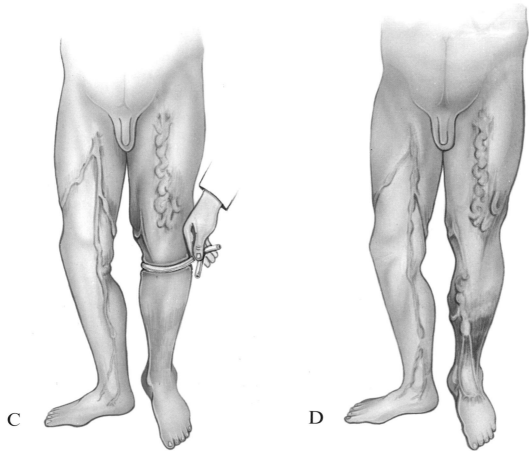

65

Plate 27

DIAGNOSTIC TESTS FOR VARICOSE VEINS OF THE LOWER EXTREMITY
(Continued)

THE SCHWARTZ TEST

This test was described by C. E. Schwartz, a French surgeon, in the latter part of the 19th century. It is helpful in outlining the course of the main saphenous trunks when they are not visible or readily palpable. It also helps to determine whether the main trunks of the long and short saphenous vein have competent valves.

A. This shows one method of performing the test. The fingers of the right hand are placed over the course of the long saphenous vein in the proximal thigh, then a large varix in the lower leg is tapped sharply with the fingers of the left hand. If an impulse is felt over the upper thigh with each tapping with the fingers, this means that the long saphenous trunk is varicosed and incompetent. This test also proves useful in detecting the location of the main trunk.

B. This demonstrates a more conclusive method of performing this test to determine the competence of the saphenous vein trunks. This is done by tapping the dilated veins in the proximal thigh, with the fingers of the other hand resting over the veins in the lower leg. If an impulse is detected in the lower leg veins with each tap, this demonstrates without doubt that the venous valves are incompetent. Were they competent, the impulse would travel only to the next competent valve, as the venous lumen is partitioned off between each set of valves. In some patients, however, it may be hard to find an enlarged vein in the proximal thigh to tap over, as the main trunk sometimes lies very deep, especially in obese persons.

THE PERTHES TEST

This test was described by G. C. Perthes, a German surgeon, in the latter part of the 19th century. It was devised to determine the patency and competence of the deep and communicating system of veins.

C. This shows the extremities of a patient with bilateral varicose veins of the lower extremity, most marked in the left one. While the patient is standing with the veins distended with blood, a venous tourniquet is placed around the upper part of the lower leg.

D. This demonstrates the same patient raising and lowering himself on the balls of his feet, thereby repeatedly contracting the flexor muscles in his lower leg, which results in a pumping action on the deep and communicating system of veins distal to the tourniquet. It should be noted that in this patient the blood leaves the superficial varicose veins, which demonstrates that the deep and communicating systems of veins are patent and competent. This indicates that the varicosities have developed because of dilatation and incompetence of the superficial system of veins. Theoretically, according to the test, treatment should be directed primarily to eradication of these. It has been learned, however, that with varicose veins as extensive as these there will usually be some incompetent communicating veins that will need interruption.

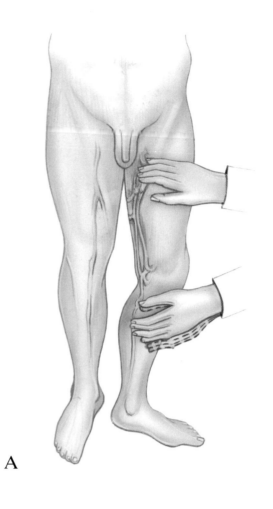

A

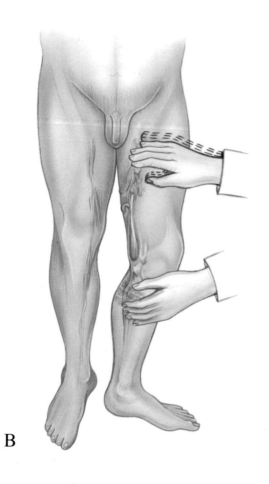

B

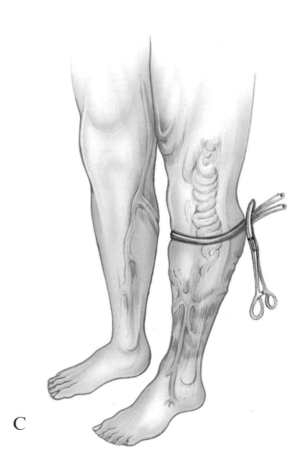

C

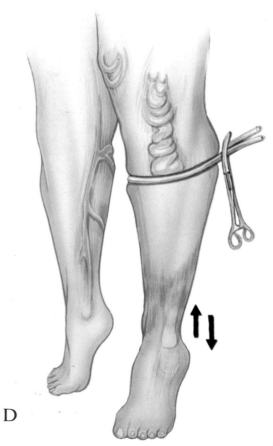

D

67

Plate 28

TYPES OF VARICOSE VEINS OF THE LOWER EXTREMITY

THE LONG SAPHENOUS SYSTEM

A. The distribution and patterns of varicose veins of the lower extremity have been found to be of greater help than the diagnostic tests to determine the type of operative procedure necessary to eradicate them.

This shows the long saphenous vein (1) from the lower left thigh to its origin on the inner aspect of the foot. The main trunk is readily recognized and should be removed from the groin to a level distal to the internal malleolus where it branches (2). The large group of varices seen on the inner side of the calf (3) is present in many patients with varicose veins. The presence of them always indicates that there are incompetent communicating veins, usually one to three, coming out through the gastrocnemius and soleus muscles and the deep fascia to join the superficial veins. Unless they are ligated and divided beneath the deep fascia, the patient will not be cured of his varicose veins. These vessels are not palpable, but large varices in this location will assure the surgeon of the presence of incompetent communicating veins at this location. Without these varicosities the communicating veins will be present but competent and so will not need to be interrupted.

Another common site for an incompetent communicating vein is at the ankle level 8 to 10 cm. above the internal malleolus. This location is shown by a star-shaped group of varices posterior to the main trunk (4), sometimes visible but most frequently palpable. Their presence here is also confirmatory evidence of an incompetent communicating vein that should be ligated as it comes out through the deep fascia. The varices frequently seen coming up from the plantar aspect of the foot (5) should be ligated and divided.

B. This shows a slightly different pattern on the inner side of the lower leg and ankle. The main long saphenous vein trunk (1) is seen. The large varices (2) that lie on either side of it in the proximal lower leg indicate the presence of incompetent communicating veins coming out through the deep fascia at the posterior edge of the tibia. These vessels should be ligated and divided beneath the deep fascia for the best results. It is not uncommon to find incompetent communicating veins at sites (3) and (4) as well. They should be ligated and divided through small incisions as they come out through the deep fascia. In addition to removing the main saphenous trunk by stripping, the distal branch at (5) should also be removed down as far as the lateral side of the foot.

C. This shows a chronic venous stasis ulcer of years' duration secondary to varicose veins of the long saphenous system and incompetent communicating veins, chiefly above, underneath and distal to the ulcer. The bluish discoloration of the surrounding skin is evidence of the chronicity of this lesion. It can be readily cured by healing the ulcer either with bed rest, elevation and 2 per cent boric acid solution dressings, or by keeping the patient ambulatory and using a Unna's paste or Elastoplast type of boot.

D. This demonstrates the venous pattern in the ankle and ulcer area after the ulcer has been healed. However, a cure can be obtained only by a radical procedure to remove all superficial varices and ligate and divide the incompetent communicating veins.

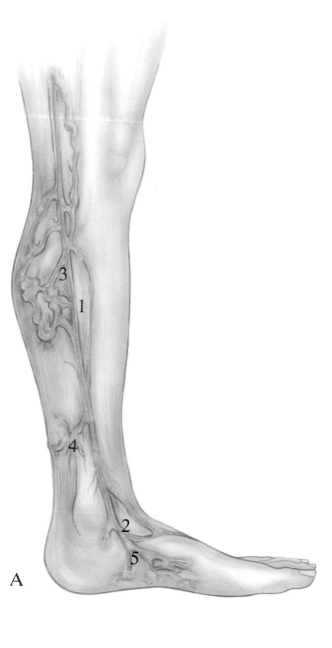

A

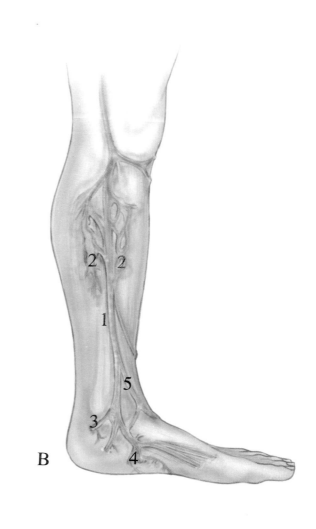

B

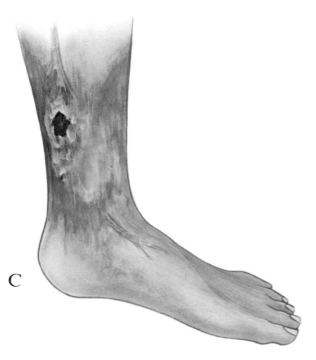

C

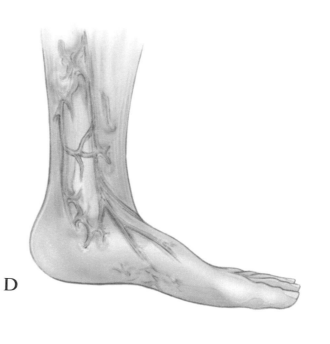

D

69

Plate 29

TYPES OF VARICOSE VEINS OF THE LOWER EXTREMITY *(Continued)*

THE SHORT SAPHENOUS SYSTEM

A. This shows the posterolateral side of the left lower leg, with varices involving the short saphenous vein system and some of the frequently observed incompetent communicating veins. The short saphenous vein (1) is seen from its origin distal to the external malleolus and extending proximally behind it, then a little lateral to the midline to terminate in the popliteal vein in the popliteal space beneath the deep fascia. It is important to remove this vein when it is varicosed. Usually the presence of varices on the outer side of the ankle, as shown, indicates that the vein is incompetent. Confirming evidence should be obtained by the Trendelenburg and Schwartz tests. The enlarged veins coming up from the lateral plantar surface of the foot (2) and some on the dorsum should be interrupted.

Another large varix is seen on the posterolateral side of the knee (3) that is best treated by multiple ligation and division through small incisions if the communicating vein cannot be found. Note that lower down at (4) the varix abruptly ends. This invariably indicates the presence of an incompetent communicating vein at this site, which should be ligated and divided.

B. This shows the anterolateral side of the left lower leg and the dorsum of the foot. Note that a portion of the short saphenous vein (1) is shown. The veins (2), (3) and (4) are tributaries of the long saphenous vein and frequently can be removed by stripping. The communicating veins shown on the dorsum of the foot (5) and (6) if ligated and divided will help to cure the prominent varicosities on the dorsum. Additional incisions should be made at (7) and (8) when the varices end abruptly in order to ligate the communicating veins in these locations. It may be possible to strip the other varices extending proximally; if not, multiple interruptions through small incisions should be used.

C. This demonstrates the varices around the external malleolus, in this patient requiring stripping of the short saphenous vein (1), interruption of communicating veins at sites (2) and stripping of varices (3).

It should be pointed out that varices of the short saphenous system are much less common than of the long saphenous system. As a result, short saphenous varicosities are frequently missed. It is believed this is because the examining surgeon does not turn the patient around so that he can examine the posterior aspect of the leg for the presence of such varicosities.

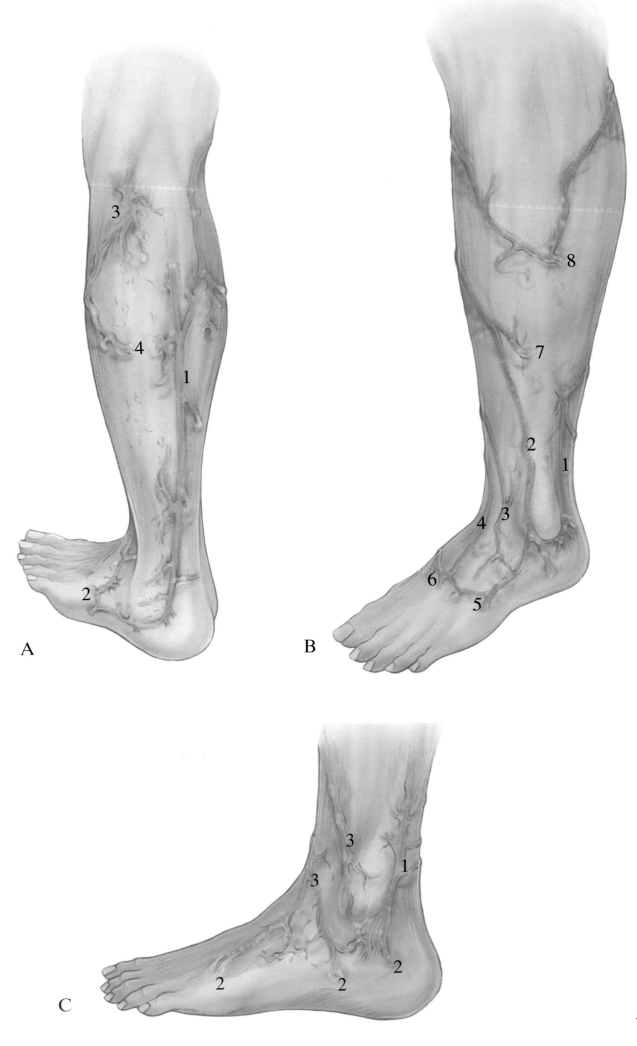

Plate 30

THE OPERATIVE TREATMENT OF VARICOSE VEINS OF THE LOWER EXTREMITY

The cure of varicose veins of the lower extremity can be accomplished by their surgical removal and the interruption of the incompetent communicating veins that are so important in the etiology. The percentage of cures depends on how radical these surgical procedures are. The best results cannot be accomplished unless the surgeon has personally made a thorough examination of the extremities when the patient was first seen in his office. At this time a drawing of the varices should be made, tracing in the largest ones and noting the location of the incompetent communicating veins. The reason for this is that the varices will be more prominent when the patient is ambulatory than they will be the morning of operation after the patient has been in bed overnight.

A. This shows the varicose veins and the location of the incompetent communicating veins of the long saphenous system of the lower extremities being marked with a black waterproof ink brush-type pen. Various other means have been tried, but this method has been found the most satisfactory. The marking is done while the patient stands, just before anesthesia is commenced, with reference to the drawing made in the office. It is recommended that the surgeon who is to perform the operative procedure be the individual to mark the veins. Special attention should be given to marking the course of the largest tortuous varices. The locations of the communicating veins to be interrupted are marked with X's. In addition, other X marks are placed where multiple transverse incisions will be required to excise the large tortuous varices that cannot be stripped.

B. This is a posterior view of the lower legs. The X marks on the left calf demonstrate the location of the incompetent communicating veins; the ones at the ankle indicate the location of others. The ones on the right calf indicate that there are incompetent communicating veins in this region. In addition, the large tortuous varices are marked so that they can be excised through multiple transverse incisions to obtain the best results; they are too tortuous for stripping.

C. General anesthesia consisting of intravenous pentothal, a muscle relaxant and nitrous oxide administered through an endotracheal tube is the preferred method. Spinal anesthesia works well, but because of the high percentage of postoperative spinal headaches, it is not recommended. The patient is shown lying supine. The skin of the lower abdomen, groins, legs and feet is cleansed with ether, then with an alcohol solution of hexachlorophene, care being taken not to rub away the previously placed ink marks. The toes and part of the feet are covered with rubber gloves. Sterile towels and sheets are used to drape the patient, leaving the groins and legs exposed.

The groin incision is made first about 1.5 cm. below and parallel with the groin crease. The location of the femoral artery pulsation is ascertained in order to make the incision so that at least three quarters of it lies medial to this artery and only one quarter lateral to it. This is because the saphenous vein courses slightly posterior to the femoral vessels after its takeoff; this makes for an easier and safer exposure of its proximal portion.

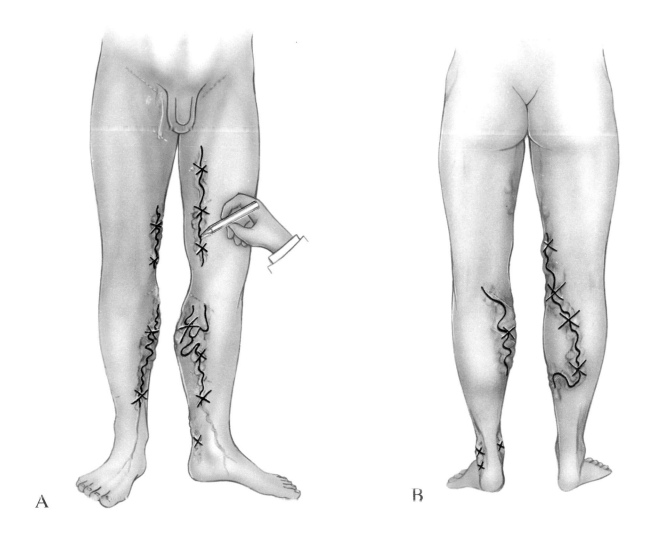

A

B

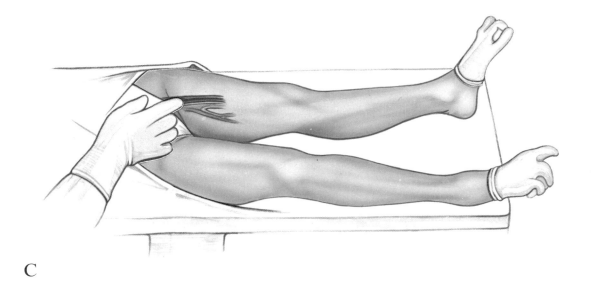

C

73

Plate 31

THE OPERATIVE TECHNIQUE FOR LIGATION AND STRIPPING OF THE LONG SAPHENOUS VEIN

A.   This depicts exposure of the cephalad portion of the left long saphenous vein. To avoid inadvertently lacerating it, it is exposed most safely by scissor dissection with upward traction on the skin and the subcutaneous tissues with tooth forceps. The advantage of this method is that it does not retract the vein upward with the fatty tissue surrounding it. The dissection is accomplished most satisfactorily with curved Mayo type scissors.

B.   After exposure of the blood vessel that is thought to be the saphenous vein, it should be carefully examined with the end of one's finger or by pinching it between two fingers to make sure it is not a pulsating artery before dividing it between clamps. It does not seem possible that the femoral artery could be mistaken for the saphenous vein, but this accident has occurred too often; in a few instances the artery has even been stripped, with disastrous results. Another error has been interruption of the femoral vein instead of the saphenous vein. It also should be remembered that the long saphenous vein lies superficial to the deep fascia of Scarpa's triangle, whereas the femoral artery and vein lie deep to it. Since the above mistakes may mean the loss of a limb, every precaution should be taken to avoid them.

C.   The main saphenous vein trunk is doubly clamped and then divided after assurance that this is the long saphenous vein and not some other blood vessel. The dissection is carried proximally to interrupt and ligate the proximal branches. This greatly facilitates the exposure of the fossa ovalis through which the saphenous veins go to join the common femoral vein. As a rule, three or four branches will be found. The lateral one is sometimes moderately large and is the cephalad end of a lateral trunk, which should be stripped.

D.   The distal clamped ends of the main trunk (1) and the lateral trunk (2) are shown. Three other branches are visible (one in a hemostat) and should be divided.

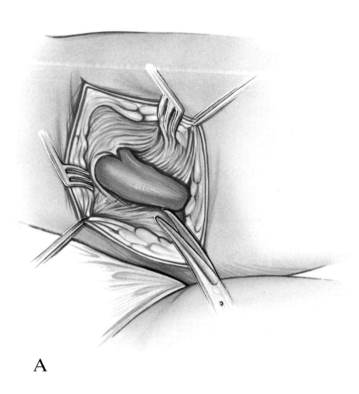

A

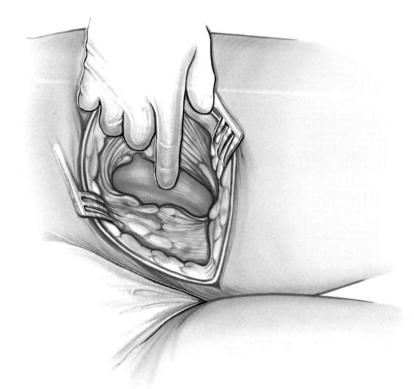

B

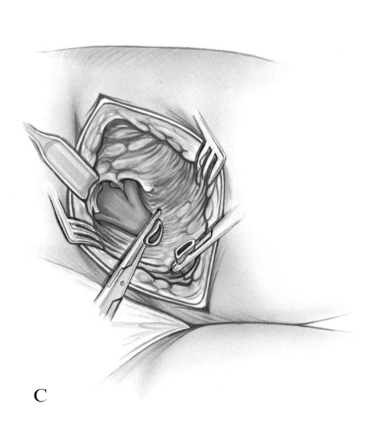

C

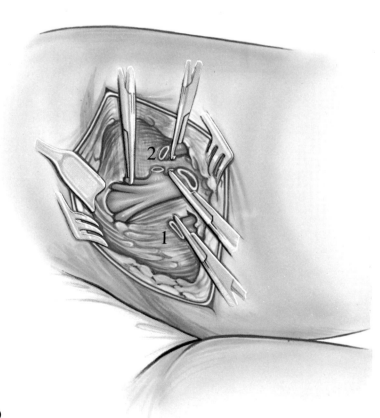

D

75

Plate 32

THE OPERATIVE TECHNIQUE FOR LIGATION AND STRIPPING OF THE LONG SAPHENOUS VEIN *(Continued)*

A.   Additional proximal branches to be ligated are revealed by raising the proximal end of the saphenous vein trunk upward. This also demonstrates the lower border of the fossa ovalis and the superficial external pudendal artery (1), a branch of the femoral artery. Not infrequently this small artery crosses anterior to the proximal end of the base of the saphenous vein, in which case it is necessary to ligate and divide it so that the proximal branches of the saphenous vein can be interrupted.

B.   After ligating the distal ends of the proximal branches, usually with fine linen or cotton ligatures, the main saphenous vein is also ligated flush with the common femoral vein with the same material to eliminate a nidus for thrombus formation in the proximal portion of the stump. Distal to this ligature a transfixion ligature is placed to ensure against postoperative hemorrhage from the vein stump.

C.   The completed proximal high interruption of the long saphenous vein and its branches is shown. In addition, a constant posteromedial branch is shown with a curved clamp on its distal end (1). Occasionally this vessel may go all the way down to the knee and can be stripped; however, it more often goes more posteriorly and does not need to be removed, but should be ligated to prevent it from bleeding postoperatively and causing an incisional hematoma. Its exposure is facilitated by pulling the main trunk cephalad and retracting the lower end of the incision distally.

D.   There are two types of vein strippers, the intraluminal and the extraluminal. The latter too often results in rupture of the veins and so is not recommended. The most satisfactory is the intraluminal type, of which there are many varieties. Those made of 18-gauge stainless steel wire are preferable to the ones of malleable metal or the very flexible ones, because they can be more easily passed in the desired direction and, with care, will follow the lumen of the vein to be stripped. Note that one end of the stripper is small, 2 or 3 mm. in diameter, and the other end about 8 mm. The smaller end is the one that is advanced in the vein lumen and the larger one follows, causing the vein to telescope on the wire portion of the stripper so that it comes out in one piece and is less likely to break. Breakage may occur if the large end is too small and the vein turns inside out. The size of the veins to be stripped will vary, so metal washers, which are available in sizes 1.0, 1.5, and 2.0 cm., are used to increase the size of the larger end of the strippers by slipping them over the small end as shown. It is important also to have a number of strippers with even smaller ends to use for the veins with very small lumens. It is recommended that the strippers be of various lengths, preferably 20, 30 and 50 cm. long. Longer ones are not necessary because the best results are obtained by stripping the long saphenous vein in two sections—from the ankle to the knee and from the knee to the groin, or from the groin to the knee—instead of in one piece. The principal reason for this is that secondary trunks that should be stripped are frequently found extending from the knee distally, and these would be missed if the knee incision were not made.

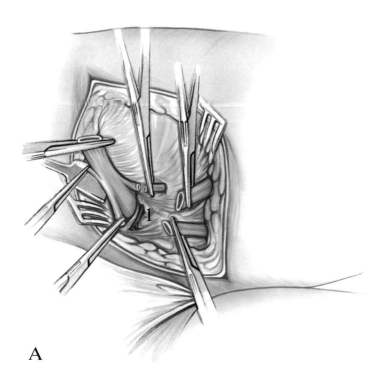

A

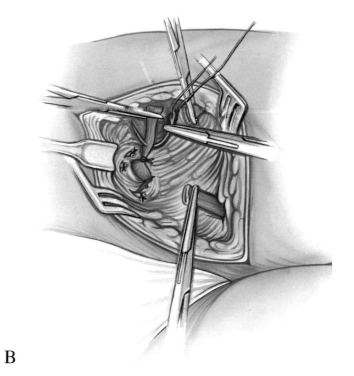

B

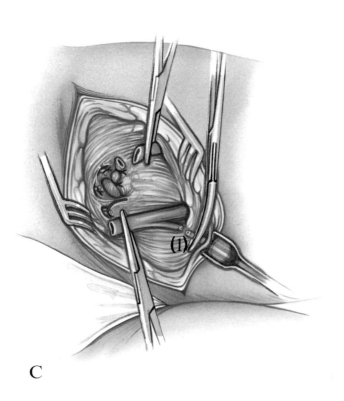

C

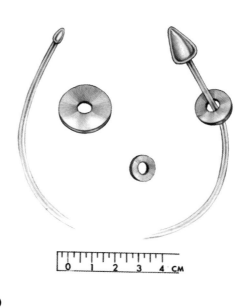

D

77

Plate 33

THE OPERATIVE TECHNIQUE FOR LIGATION AND STRIPPING OF THE LONG SAPHENOUS VEIN *(Continued)*

A.   This shows the method of inserting the stripper down the long saphenous vein trunk through a small opening made in it with scissors. Pressure exerted upward with the forefinger facilitates insertion of the small end of the stripper. Note that the larger end that is protruding has a metal washer on it to enlarge its diameter and make the vein telescope on the stripper as it is pulled out at the knee level later. Another stripper has already been passed down the lateral trunk to the knee level.

B.   This drawing demonstrates the position of the operating table during the remainder of the operation. Note that the table has been put in moderate Trendelenburg position and flexed at the hip so that the feet and lower legs are above the level of the heart. This reduces the venous pressure greatly, so that there is little blood loss even though many of the tributaries of the saphenous vein are not ligated at the time of stripping. This position also drains the blood out of the varices, so that it is difficult to remember their location if they have not been marked prior to the operation.

C.   After the operating table has been repositioned the distal end of the long saphenous vein is exposed through a short transverse incision distal to the internal malleolus, which is indicated at the tip of the forefinger. The advantages of an incision of this type and location are that it heals more cosmetically than a longitudinal one, and the distal branches of the saphenous vein can be individually divided and ligated, which frequently helps to eradicate varices in this area. The small rake retractor facilitates the exposure.

D.   After division of the main trunk and ligation of the distal ends and the branches, an opening is made in the trunk through which the stripper is passed cephalad. It has been found important to use fine catgut, size 3-0, for ligatures and fascial and subcutaneous sutures in all incisions below the knee instead of nonabsorbable materials such as silk, cotton or linen, because with the latter some of these ligatures and sutures too often become infected even months after the incisions have healed, resulting in unpleasant complications until the sutures are extruded or removed.

E.   The stripper is being passed cephalad again with a washer on it because of the large size of the vein. It usually goes readily up to the knee level, where another transverse slightly oblique incision is made.

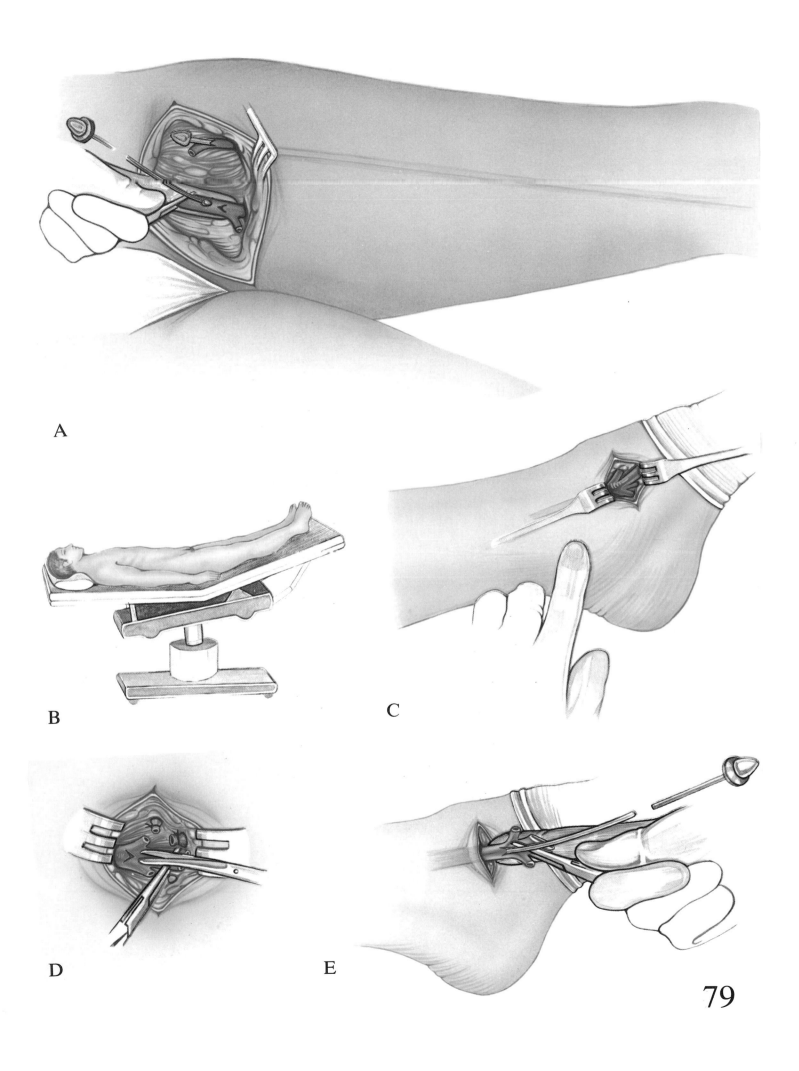

A

B

C

D

E

79

Plate 34

THE OPERATIVE TECHNIQUE FOR LIGATION AND STRIPPING OF THE LONG SAPHENOUS VEIN *(Continued)*

A. The incision at the junction of the lower leg and knee is shown at the left. It is made after passing the stripper to the knee level. The main trunk is readily isolated with the metal stripper in it. The other trunk should be searched for, as it is frequently present. This patient had these two trunks in the lower leg and so demonstrates the advantage of an incision at this level; otherwise, the lesser of them would not have been found and removed. This trunk usually remains posterior to the main one but in some, as in this patient, it crosses from behind proximally to become anterior at the level of the internal malleolus. The stripper in the main trunk is passed cephalad and the other is more readily passed distalward.

B. This shows the left lower extremity from the groin to the foot. Note the three incisions—one in the groin, the second just distal to the knee and the third distal to the internal malleolus. This extremity has two trunks in the thigh and in the lower leg. The secondary ones (3) and (4) are separate veins and are not in continuity as the main trunk was. The strippers in (3) and (4), and the main thigh trunk (1) have been passed distalward. If the surgeon prefers, the stripper may be passed cephalad in the latter, as it has been in the distal main trunk in the lower leg.

C. A strong curved clamp is used to grasp the small-tipped end of the stripper. With a slow, steady pull the vein is telescoped on the stripper as it is withdrawn. The other trunk stripper is removed in a similar manner, but pulled distalward. One of the commonest complications of this procedure is that some of the fibers of the saphenous nerve may be removed, with a resulting area of hypoesthesia on the inner side of the ankle. As time goes on, the normal sensation usually returns, although in some patients this may constitute a permanent but not serious complication.

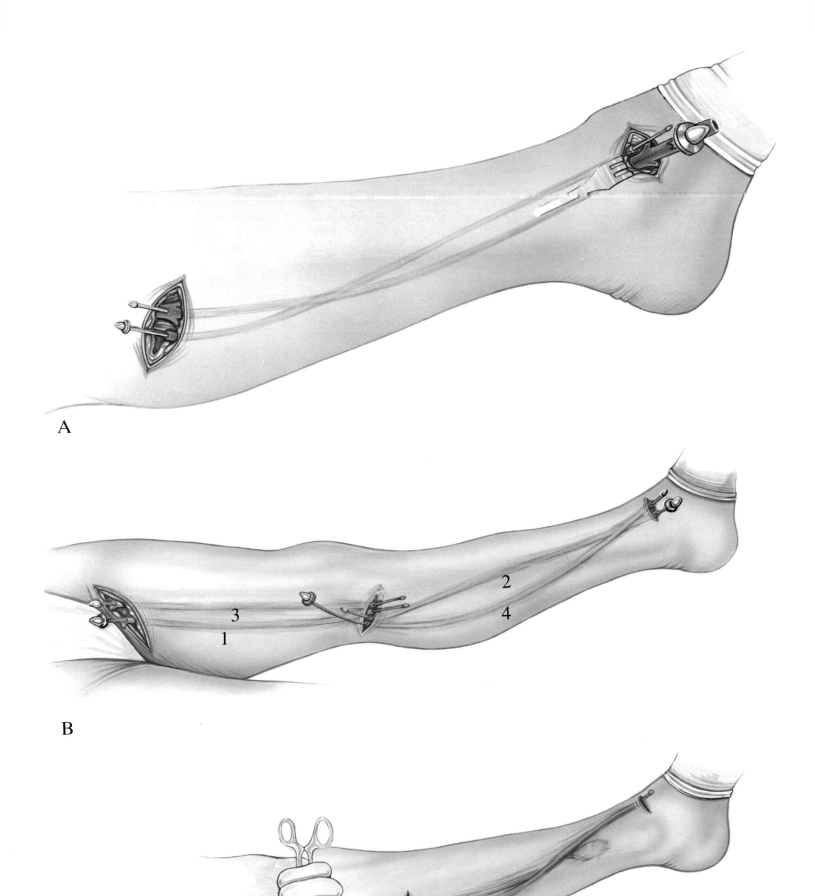

A

B

3

1

2

4

C

81

Plate 35

THE OPERATIVE TECHNIQUE FOR LIGATION AND STRIPPING OF THE LONG SAPHENOUS VEIN *(Continued)*

A. The stripping of the two trunks in the thigh is next performed. The main trunk may be stripped either up or down, but the smaller one is always stripped down. Sometimes this vein does not go all the way to the lower incision, but with the stiff wire stripper it is possible to readily push it through the vein wall and then through the subcutaneous tissues to the incision where it is grasped and brought out, thus avoiding the necessity of another incision.

B. This shows the thigh (1) and the lower leg (2) segments of the main long saphenous vein trunk telescoped on the large ends of the strippers, each with a washer to increase the diameter of the end of the stripper to prevent the veins from turning inside out.

THE SUBFASCIAL INTERRUPTION OF INCOMPETENT MEDIAL CALF COMMUNICATING VEINS

C. This shows the lower leg with a group of large varicosities in the posteromedial aspect of the calf and an intraluminal stripper in the long saphenous vein. If only the long saphenous vein is removed, these varicosities will persist because they have developed as a result of the incompetence of the communicating veins in this region and not primarily because the main saphenous vein is incompetent. For this reason, an oblique incision is made as shown. It is impossible to pinpoint the exact location of the communicating veins or to know for certain how many will be found. The keynote to success is to find all the incompetent veins and to interrupt them beneath the deep fascia. The subfascial approach and interruption make it possible to perform this much more effectively and completely than ligation superficial to the deep fascia; in fact, it would be impossible to find all those superficial to the fascia.

D. Blunt dissection with the forefinger of the left hand between the deep fascia and the calf muscles is readily carried out because there is only loose areolar tissue and the communicating veins between them. As this cleavage plane is developed, the enlarged incompetent communicating veins are readily located. The dissection can easily be carried to the midline posteriorly. The only structure to be avoided is the sural nerve, or the median component of it. Many surgeons persist in calling these perforating veins, presumably because they pass through the deep fascia. The term is otherwise meaningless, and the term "communicating vein" is much more significant since it indicates that the veins connect the deep and superficial systems. When the communicating veins become incompetent they play an exceedingly important role in the etiology of varicose veins and the pathological changes that develop in the leg. Furthermore, without the eradication of these veins the varicosities and the stasis dermatitis and ulcers will persist. Instead of diagnosing them as recurrent varicose veins, they should be called persistent when they are observed a year or longer postoperatively. Their presence under these conditions is evidence that an incomplete operation had been performed

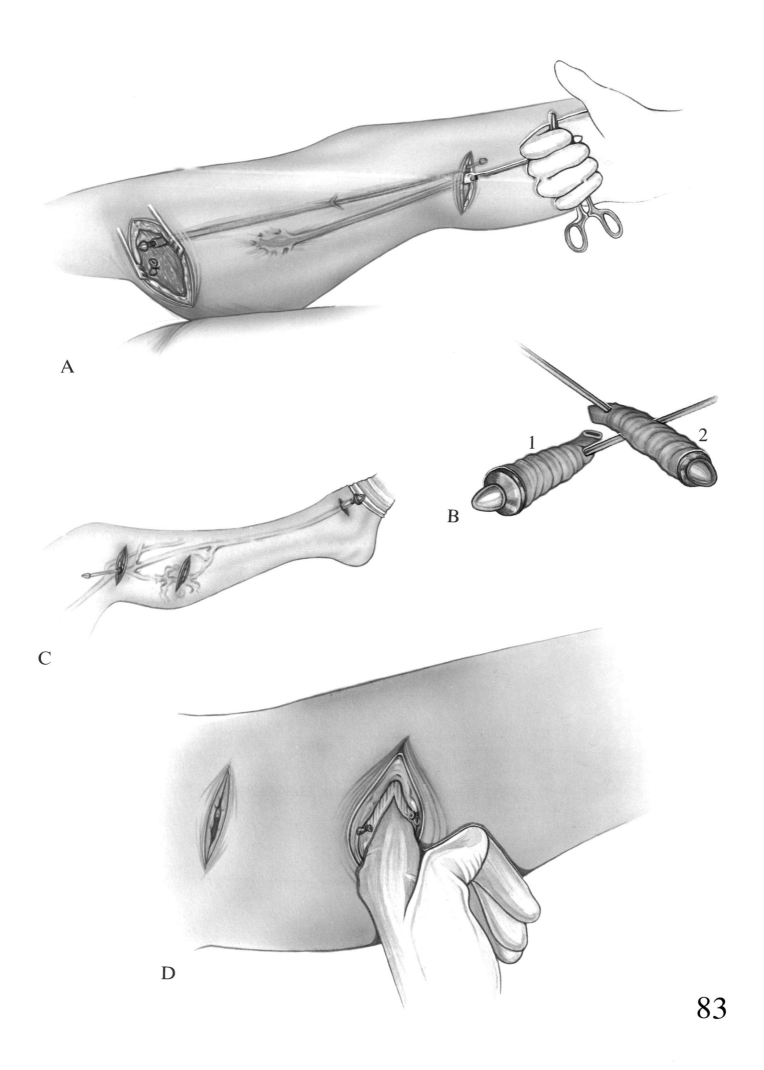

A

B

C

D

83

Plate 36

THE SUBFASCIAL INTERRUPTION OF INCOMPETENT MEDIAL CALF COMMUNICATING VEINS *(Continued)*

A. This demonstrates the forefinger dissecting through the areolar tissue between the deep fascia and the muscles and hooking one of the communicating veins with the end of the finger. Traction on a structure in this location, where it passes through the deep fascia, if it is a communicating vein, will always cause the skin to dimple as shown. Because these vessels are often hidden from view some distance from the incision, this dimpling of the skin is important confirmatory evidence that the subfascial structure encountered is a communicating vein, since no other structure beneath the deep fascia with tension on it will cause this.

B. After the communicating vein has been located by this maneuver, it is brought into view with retractors so that its point of emergence from the gastrocnemius and soleus muscles is clearly visualized.

C. The vessel is then doubly clamped and divided between the clamps. Each end is ligated separately with 3-0 plain catgut ligatures. It is important to make certain that the proximal end coming out of the muscle is tied adequately because, if not, subfascial hemorrhage may occur. This is really the "high pressure" end of the vein, whereas the other end going through the deep fascia, although also better ligated, probably would not bleed postoperatively since it is the "low pressure" end. After completion of the ligatures, further exploration is carried out with the forefinger because there may frequently be several incompetent communicating veins; as many as four have been found on occasion. The complete eradication of these veins by ligation and division is necessary if a complete cure of the varicosities is to be obtained, since if one is left intact it is certain there will be residual superficial varicosities.

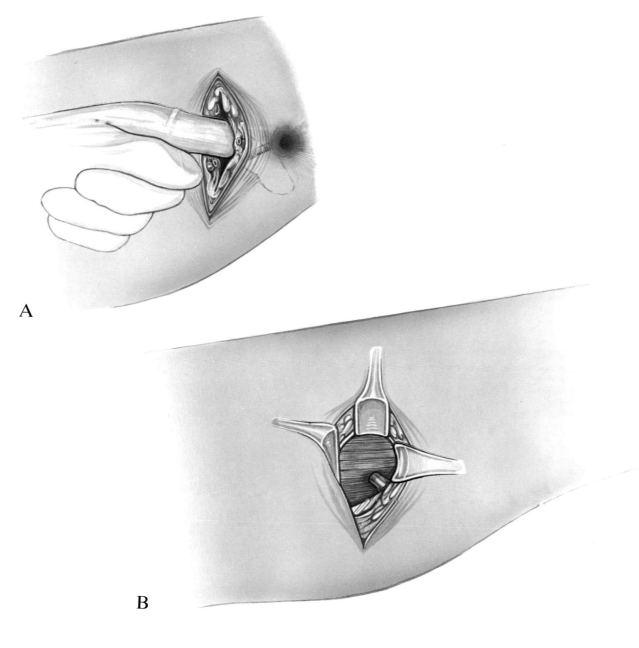

A

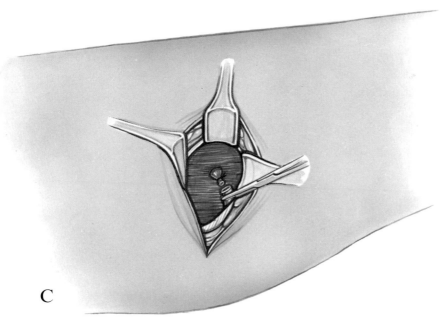

B

C

Plate 37

THE SUBFASCIAL INTERRUPTION OF INCOMPETENT PROXIMAL POSTERIOR TIBIAL COMMUNICATING VEINS

A. This shows the left lower leg with an intraluminal stripper in the long saphenous vein from the ankle to the knee. Note that the superficial network of varices that lies on either side of it is more extensive lateral to it over the tibia. This location of varices indicates that there are incompetent communicating veins piercing the deep fascia at the posteromedial edge of the tibia. In order to cure the varices in this location, in addition to stripping the long saphenous vein, the surgeon should interrupt these incompetent communicating veins that connect with the superficial varices. Note that the location of the calf incision is the same as for the calf communicating veins but is extended a little further toward the edge of the tibia.

B. The deep fascia must be incised. With good retraction with rakes on the incision edges it is often possible to readily find one, two or three of these incompetent communicating veins coming out between the muscles and the edge of the tibia.

C. Each vein is doubly clamped, divided and each end ligated with a plain 3-0 catgut ligature.

D. After satisfactory hemostasis has been established the incision is closed with interrupted sutures of plain 3-0 catgut to the deep fascia. The ends of the varices shown in the subcutaneous tissues are sometimes stripped or dissected out for several centimeters if they are large and tortuous. This is a safe procedure with the oblique type of incision in the cleavage planes of the skin but should never be done with longitudinal incisions because of the danger of skin sloughs.

E. The skin is closed neatly with vertical mattress sutures.

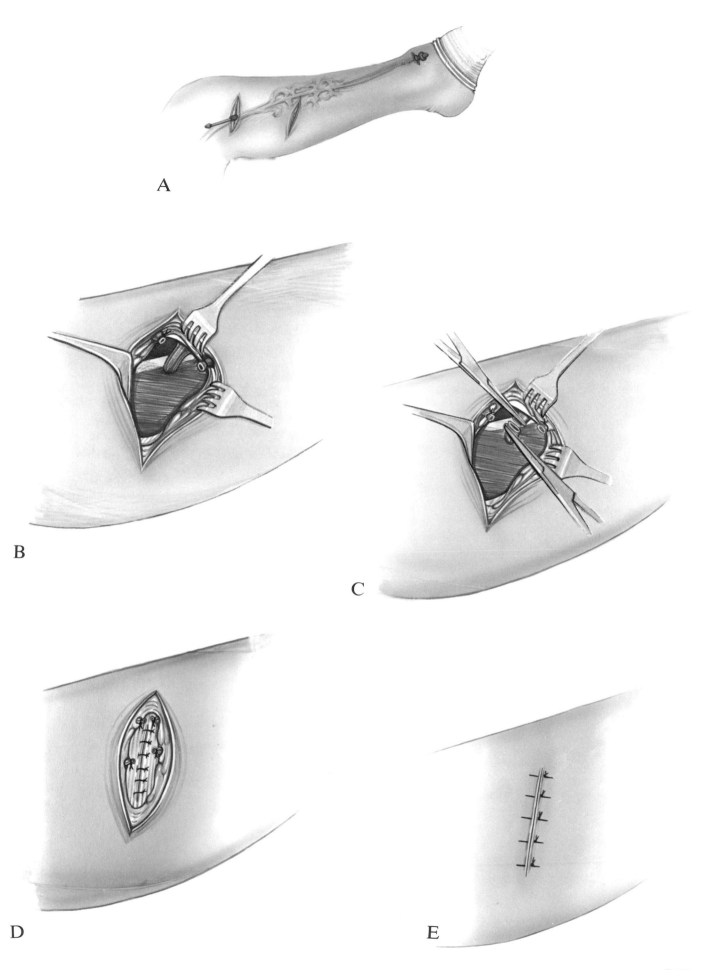

A

B

C

D

E

87

Plate 38

INTERRUPTION OF INCOMPETENT DISTAL POSTERIOR TIBIAL COMMUNICATING VEINS OF LEFT ANKLE

A. The inner aspect of the left lower leg is shown with intraluminal strippers in the main and accessory saphenous vein trunks. The location of the incisions to interrupt the calf communicating veins (1) and the distal ankle communicating veins (2) and (3) are shown. Note the superficial varices in these three areas that tell the surgeon that there are incompetent communicating veins at these locations.

B. Note that the proximal incision (1) is oblique and the distal ones (2) and (3) are a little more longitudinal. The reason for this is that it is not possible to ascertain the exact location of the communicating veins, so it is necessary to utilize incisions that permit exploration of them from a longitudinal aspect. It has been found that these oblique incisions heal with a much better cosmetic type of scar. Note that a large communicating vein is shown in incision (1) coming out through the deep fascia. There are two in incision (2), the proximal one coming out through the deep fascia; the distal one, after incision of the deep fascia, can be seen to be arising from the posterior tibial vein. The saphenous vein trunks have also been removed by stripping.

C. This shows the double ligation and division of the communicating veins. This is done just at the level of the deep fascia for the two proximal veins. The distal one is ligated beneath the deep fascia since in this case it was necessary to incise the deep fascia to expose the posterior tibial vein to make sure it was a communicating vein. It is obvious that at this level of the ankle it is not possible to do the extensive subfascial finger exploration that is carried out in the calf region.

D. This shows the skin closure with interrupted vertical mattress sutures of silk. The only subcutaneous closure is by interrupted sutures of 3-0 plain catgut to the deep fascia.

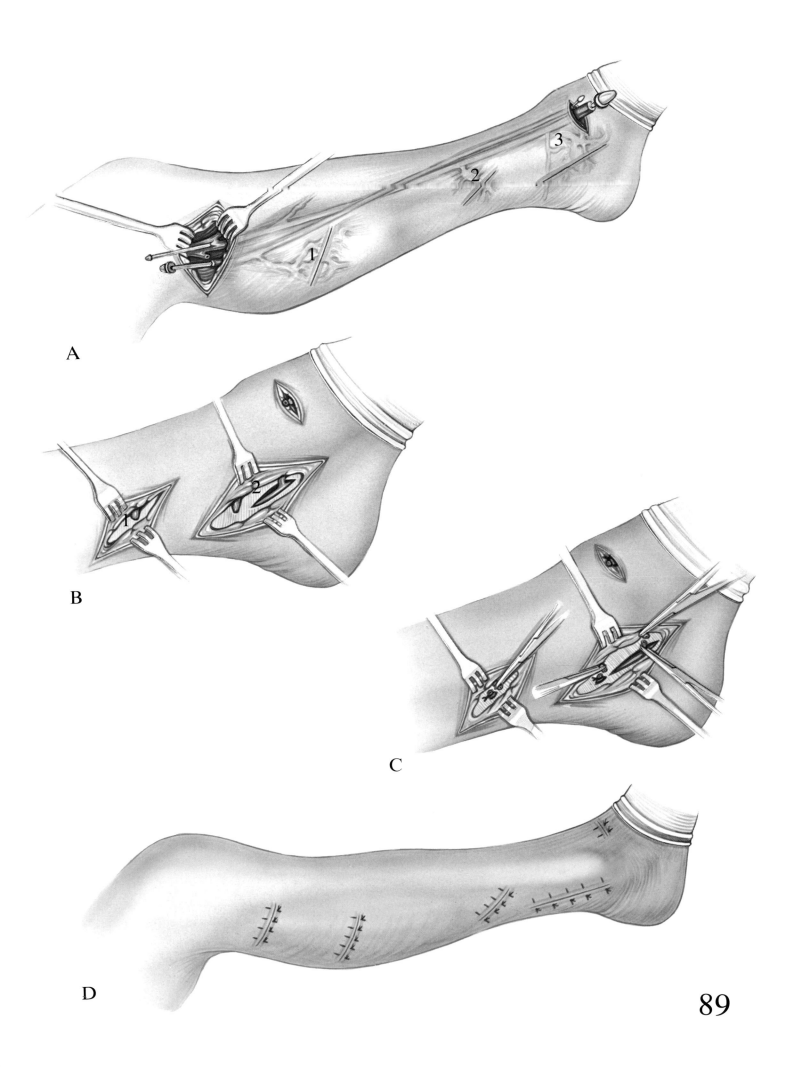

A

B

C

D

89

Plate 39

PHLEBECTOMY AND INTERRUPTION OF INCOMPETENT LATERAL LEG AND FOOT COMMUNICATING VEINS FOR LARGE TORTUOUS VARICOSE VEINS

A. The lateral side of the right lower thigh and the lower leg are shown with large superficial varicose veins. They are so tortuous it is not possible to strip them; for that reason they must be excised through multiple, small, slightly oblique incisions. In addition, the location of two incompetent communicating veins should be noted at (1) and (2). These may be identified by the abrupt ending of the varices at these sites. It is important to interrupt them as they emerge from the deep fascia.

B. This is inset (a) on the lower part of the thigh to demonstrate the method of removal of the tortuous varix. The incision crosses it at almost a right angle. If the incision is made directly over and parallel to the varix the skin edges may slough because the skin is so thin. As shown in the diagram, with a small rake retractor and with steady traction on the severed end of the vein it is possible, using sharp scissor dissection, to unravel and extract the varix subcutaneously halfway to the next incision. The remainder of it is removed in a similar manner through the adjacent incision. The complete removal of such varices is accomplished by use of multiple incisions.

C. This is inset (b) on the lower leg and shows the proximal ligated end of a communicating vein as it emerges from the deep fascia. The other end, which is the varix, may be partially removed as shown in *B*, or stripped if it is not too tortuous. Sometimes simple ligation may be all that can be done. It is surprising how frequently these communicating veins are relatively small in caliber, yet are such an important factor in the etiology and persistence of lateral leg varices.

D. This shows some of the communicating vein sites on the lateral and dorsal aspect of the right ankle and foot and the short incisions made to interrupt them. The most lateral ones feed the distal end of the short saphenous vein and so should be interrupted. In addition, the long varix (1) should be stripped. As a rule, this is most readily done from the lower leg to the foot. It usually is a tributary of the long saphenous vein.

E. Similar communicating veins will frequently be found on the dorsum and inner side of the foot, feeding the distal end of the long saphenous vein. In addition to stripping the saphenous to just below the internal malleolus, it is worthwhile to continue down to the distal incision. The other incisions are used to interrupt the communicating veins where the varix ends abruptly.

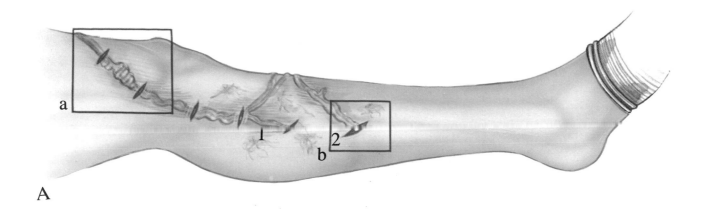

A

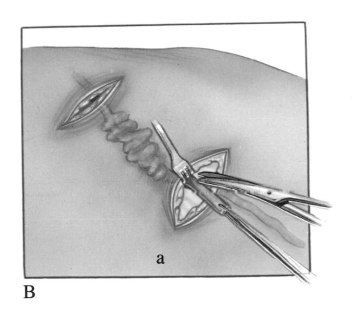

B

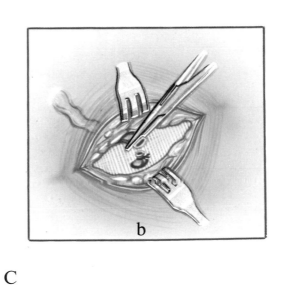

C

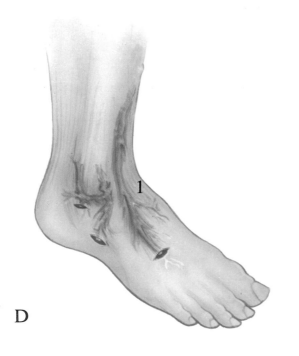

D

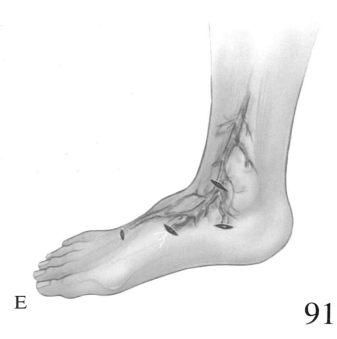

E

91

Plate 40

THE OPERATIVE TECHNIQUE OF LIGATION AND STRIPPING OF THE SHORT SAPHENOUS VEIN

The short saphenous vein in a few patients may be the only one that needs to be removed. More frequently, however, both long and short saphenous veins are incompetent and should be stripped, although only about 15 per cent of all operative cases require this.

A. After completion of the operative procedure on the long saphenous vein and the incompetent communicating veins and closure of the incisions, the patient is turned prone on the operating table with the feet projecting beyond it. The anesthetic should be administered through an endotracheal tube to provide good aeration of the lungs and to prevent stridor with an increase in venous pressure that may lead to bleeding and subsequent hematomas. The operating table should be placed in moderate Trendelenburg position to reduce venous pressure in the legs, thereby also preventing bleeding from the unligated branches of the stripped short saphenous vein.

B. This shows the extent of the operative field that gives the most adequate exposure of the distribution of the short saphenous vein. It facilitates a much more adequate removal of the vein than attempting to do the procedure with all the acrobatics necessary when the patient is in the supine position. The vein is first exposed posterior to the external malleolus through a short transverse incision as shown on the left leg.

C. With good retraction and sharp scissor dissection the trunk of the short saphenous vein (1) is readily exposed. The sural nerve (2) lies parallel and often adherent to it. It is important to isolate this nerve to prevent interrupting it when dividing the vein trunk, even though it is entirely a sensory nerve. This is because the nerve supplies the skin of the outer side of the foot, and it would become anesthetic, which would be troublesome to the patient, especially when wearing a shoe.

D. This shows the distal end of the short saphenous trunk after division and beginning insertion of the small end of the stripper into it. In a few instances when the distal end of the vein is large, it may be stripped down to its termination on the anterolateral side of the foot.

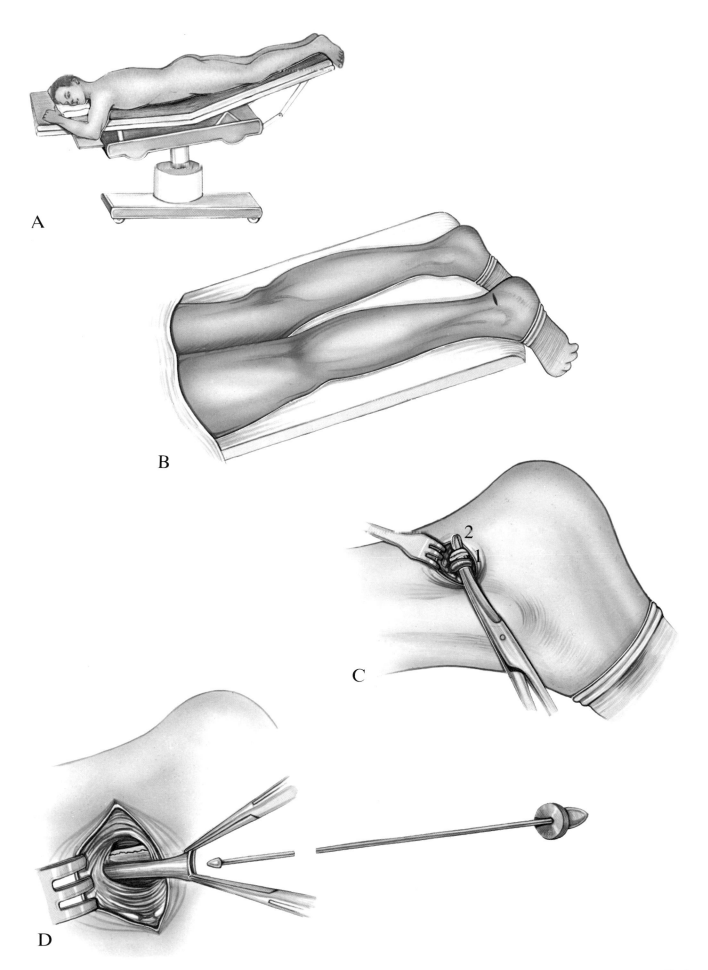

A

B

C

D

93

Plate 41

THE OPERATIVE TECHNIQUE OF LIGATION AND STRIPPING OF THE SHORT SAPHENOUS VEIN *(Continued)*

A.   This shows an intraluminal stripper that has been inserted into the vein at the ankle and passed proximally in it to the popliteal space. The tip of the stripper can be readily palpated at the level at which the short saphenous vein turns acutely to go deeper to join the popliteal vein, so that exposure of the proximal end of the vein is greatly facilitated through a properly placed small transverse incision. Care should be taken not to attempt to pass the stripper higher unless it stays relatively superficial, because sometimes the junction of these two veins is at an acute angle and the stripper may pass up into the popliteal vein. Under these conditions the tip of the stripper is lost to palpation. It should be immediately withdrawn in order to place the incision at the correct level, since the location of the junction of the two veins does vary considerably. The exposure has been carried down to the deep fascia of the popliteal space. The proximal portion of the short saphenous vein is shown beneath it because, at this level, it is always subfascial.

B.   This shows that the popliteal fascia has been incised trasversely to expose the short saphenous vein. The small end of the stripper has been forced through the wall of the vein and grasped with a hemostat.

C.   This shows the enlarged and incompetent short saphenous vein telescoped on the stripper against the metal washer and the large end of the stripper. The proximal end of the vein is held with a hemostat. Moderate tension is applied so that a linen or cotton ligature can be placed more proximally on it. Exposure of the exact junction of the short saphenous and popliteal veins is not advisable routinely because it lies relatively deep in the popliteal space; injury to the peroneal and/or the posterior tibial nerves has occurred from the use of retractors in attempting to do this.

D.   This shows the closure of the distal small incision with vertical mattress silk sutures. The proximal incision is being closed with interrupted sutures to the fascia. It is important that this be done carefully with nonabsorbable sutures, preferably linen or cotton, to prevent disruption. All the sutures should be placed and then tied, with the lower leg flexed at the knee to prevent tension on the fascia until all are tied. If this method of closure is not used, patients develop a herniation of the popliteal fat at this location which results in a very ugly and unnatural appearing popliteal space that women, especially, complain of bitterly because it is so unsightly. Even men are disturbed about it, although other than cosmetically it causes no complications. It should be emphasized again that operative details such as these can be performed better with the patient in the prone position than in any other position. Occasionally one will find incompetent communicating veins lateral and distal to the main trunk of the short saphenous vein. It is important to interrupt these also, and again this positioning is of great help.

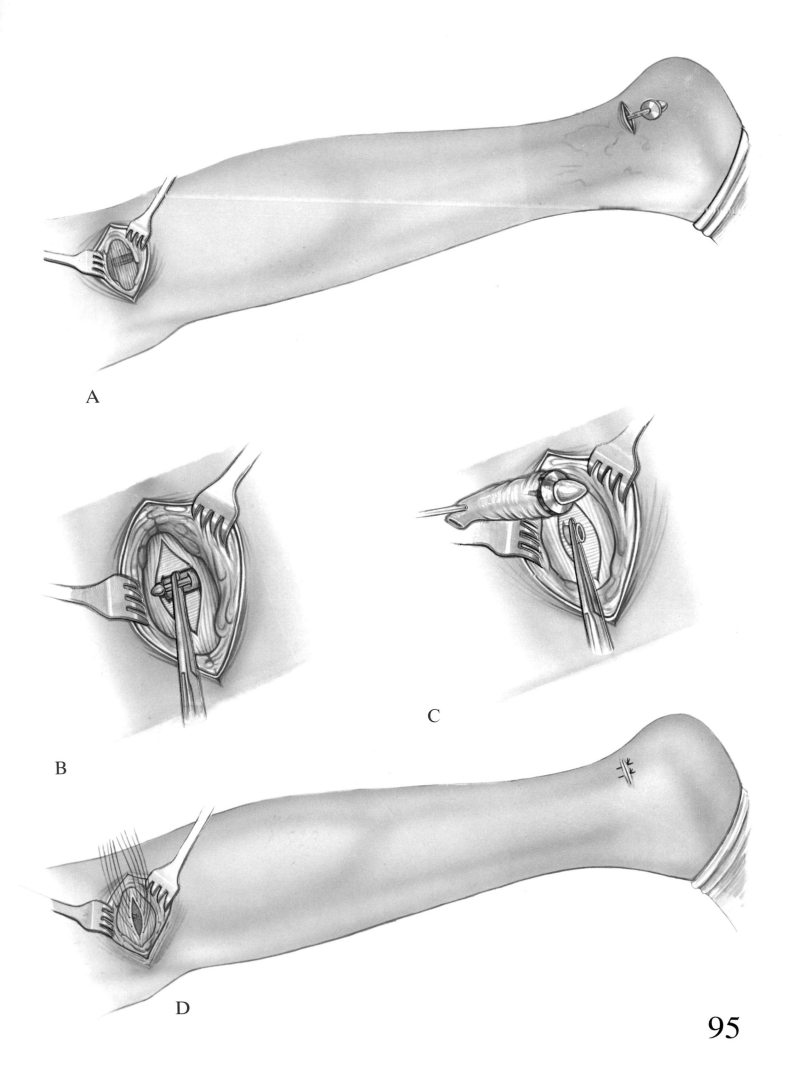

A

B

C

D

95

Plate 42

POSTOPERATIVE CARE OF EXTREMITIES AFTER RADICAL OPERATION FOR VARICOSE VEINS OF THE LOWER EXTREMITY

A. This shows the location of the incisions, all of which have been closed with vertical mattress sutures of silk. The long saphenous vein has been removed from distal to the malleolus to the saphenofemoral junction. A lateral trunk was stripped to the small anterior low thigh incision. Through the oblique calf incision incompetent communicating veins were interrupted beneath the deep fascia, and through the two incisions at the ankle other communicating veins were interrupted at the point of their emergence through the deep fascia.

B. Small gauze dressings held in place with Elastoplast adhesive tape are applied to the incisions. A large soft gauze roll about 5 cm. in diameter is held in place with a few strips of adhesive tape over the course of the stripped long saphenous vein.

C. The leg is then bandaged with two 4-inch Ace bandages from the base of the toes to the groin. The wrapping should be performed by coming around the leg from inside out, putting a little extra pressure over the large gauze roll to prevent postoperative subcutaneous bleeding.

For the first 24 hours slight Trendelenburg position is maintained by elevating the foot of the bed six inches. The next morning the dressings on the lower leg are replaced by new ones; any incisions on the thigh and groin are left uncovered. The long gauze roll is removed; only the lower leg is rewrapped with a rubberized type of Ace bandage. The patient is ordered to commence walking for five minutes every two hours the first postoperative day. The patient may be discharged home on the fifth postoperative day after removal of all skin sutures. He is instructed to keep the ankles and lower legs bandaged with the rubberized Ace bandages during the day, and for two months to wear heavyweight, two-way stretch, knee length elastic stockings with a heel. The first postoperative checkup is between two and three weeks to see if any varicosities persist. If any do, these are injected with a small amount of sclerosing solution. The majority of patients, however, do not need this. A final checkup is usually done in another two to three months.

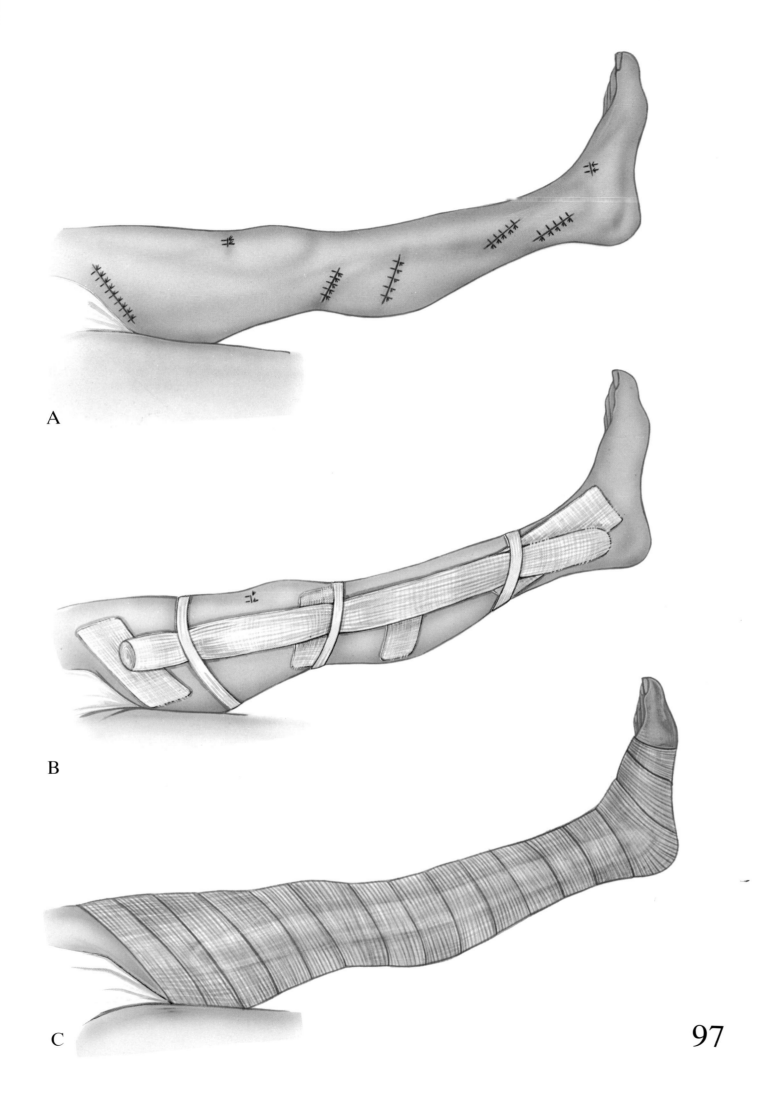

A

B

C

97

Plate 43

RESULTS OF RADICAL OPERATIVE PROCEDURES FOR VARICOSE VEINS OF THE LOWER EXTREMITIES

A. This drawing demonstrates how extensive superficial tortuous varices can be. It shows the numerous transverse incisions necessary to excise them, with stripping of short segments between some of the incisions where possible. In addition, the long saphenous veins are stripped through the usual groin, below the knee and the ankle incisions, and communicating veins through oblique calf incisions and one ankle incision on the left. This method will obviate the necessity for the postoperative injection of sclerosing solution. In addition, the patient will obtain a pleasing cosmetic result as well as relief of symptoms. Sclerosing therapy, especially with this type of extensive thigh and lower leg involvement, has not proved too satisfactory. The veins are so large it is difficult to accomplish, painful and not so cosmetically pleasing as this surgical method.

B. This shows the same extremities two years later without evidence of persistent varicose veins. Note the good cosmetic result from the utilization of multiple small transverse incisions. Such results require as complete as possible removal of the tortuous varices, ligation and stripping of the long saphenous veins and interruption of the communicating veins.

C. This drawing shows extensive varices on the inner side of the right calf and an incompetent long saphenous vein. The pattern of the varices in the lower leg indicates that there were incompetent communicating veins in the calf and the ankle regions which would require multiple incisions for ligation and division.

D. This shows the same extremity one year after the operative procedure of ligation and stripping of the long saphenous vein and interruption of the communicating veins on the inner side of the leg. Note the location of the incisions and the neatness of the scars. A moderate amount of edema of the lower leg follows this radical type of operative procedure for varicose veins. This is limited to the lower leg and foot. It is important to have the patient wear during the day a heavyweight, two-way stretch, knee length elastic stocking with a heel for two to three months to prevent the edema from forming. If this is done religiously, use of the elastic support can usually be discontinued at the end of that time. It must be commenced immediately postoperatively to prevent edema from forming; otherwise, it may be extremely difficult to cure it even if it has been present for only a few weeks.

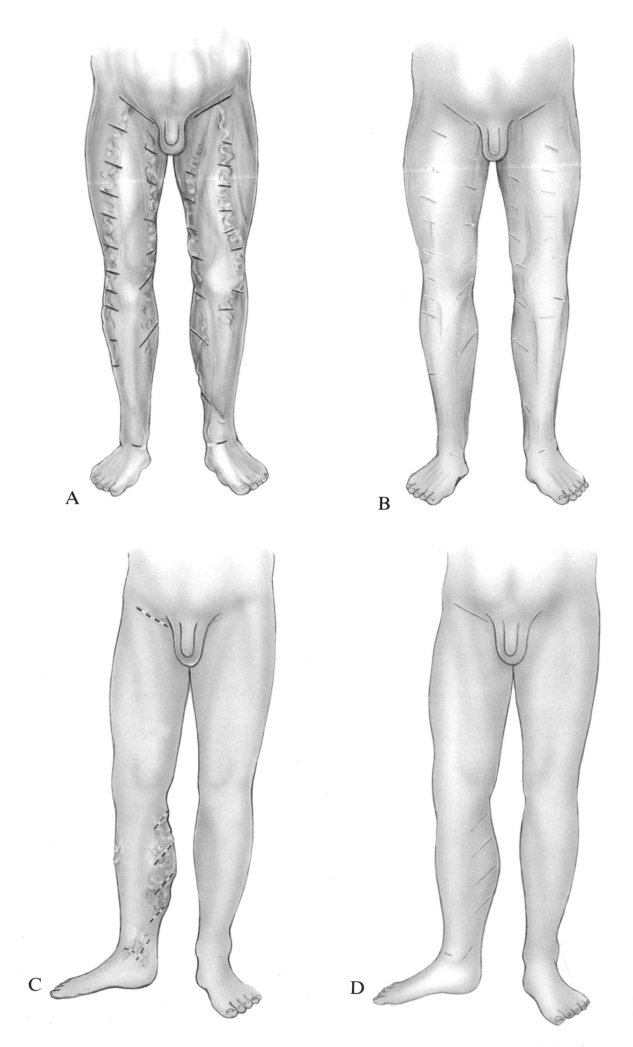

A

B

C

D

99

THROMBOEMBOLIC DISEASE

Introduction

Prophylaxis of Postoperative Deep Venous Thrombosis and Pulmonary Embolism

Many attempts have and are being made to discover the etiology of postoperative deep venous thrombosis in an attempt to determine how it can be prevented in order to save patients' lives from massive fatal pulmonary embolism following successful surgical operative procedures. Some progress has been made in the last three decades, since deaths from this dreaded complication have diminished. It has never been proved that there are changes in the blood clotting mechanism that might be a cause of the condition, but the use of anticoagulants, especially of the warfarin group, in adequate amounts does have a beneficial effect in controlling the condition when administered in the early stages of the disease. Its value as a routine prophylactic measure in all patients has not proved to be a panacea. Also, anticoagulation does carry some risk in the postoperative patient because of the danger of hemorrhage. In elderly patients, who are the patients most frequently afflicted with thromboembolism, it may cause bleeding from unsuspected lesions. It is recommended, however, that any patient who has had a previous episode of deep venous thrombosis, with or without pulmonary embolism, and who requires further surgery be given the protection of postoperative anticoagulation provided by Coumadin therapy. The use of elastic stockings during the postoperative period has some advocates, but it is doubtful that they are of much value, and serious ischemic lesions of the feet have developed from their use in elderly patients.

There seems little question that early ambulation has contributed more to the prevention of thromboembolic disease in postoperative patients than any other form of therapy. It is well known that deep venous thrombosis rarely develops in an individual who is able to be up and walking about. This is confirmatory evidence that in the vast majority of patients the condition begins in the lower extremities and that most frequently it first involves the deep veins of the calf muscles. These facts have been known and reported for many years, first by the pathologists in the last century and later by surgeons.

Elevation of the foot of the bed to favor drainage of blood from the lower limbs is one of the more common so-called prophylactic measures that was recommended many years ago and is still adhered to by some. Other measures such as passive leg exercises and bicycle exercises with the legs elevated have proved to be of little or no value; one reason is that they usually require the assistance of someone at the bedside. This is difficult to provide today and, as a result, exercises are done too infrequently to be of any special value. Furthermore, they do not contract the calf muscles sufficiently actively to push blood along and to prevent it from stagnating. Fortunately the use of tight abdominal bandages and binders around the abdomen, which contribute to venous stasis in the lower limbs, has been discontinued.

There seems little question that stagnation of the blood in the veins of the lower extremities is an important etiological factor of deep venous thrombosis. This is increased in the elderly patient, in part because with increasing age the caliber of the deep veins of the lower extremities gradually becomes greater so that the blood flows through them at a slower rate. Another contributing factor in the elderly is the degenerative changes that develop in the venous endothelium as a result of phlebosclerosis, which can act as a nidus for thrombus formation, especially in the presence of a sluggish blood flow. With this rather simple plausible explanation of the cause of deep venous thrombosis, it seems obvious that some form of treatment should be instituted that will stimulate the flow of blood through the veins of the lower extremity and prevent it from stagnating. Without question this is what early ambulation does, since it has definitely reduced the incidence of the disease. Fortunately it is so generally practiced today that most postoperative patients are ambulating several times a day beginning usually on the first postoperative day. It is advised that the time out of bed be spent walking rather than sitting in a chair for an indefinite period of time, since sitting tends to favor stagnation and thrombosis of the blood in the lower extremities.

Unfortunately following some of the major vascular operative procedures this practice cannot be carried out the first postoperative day, so it is necessary to utilize some other method of ambulation while the patient is still in bed (see Plate 44). It is necessary to emphasize again and again that the postoperative care, especially in these patients, should include daily examination of the calf muscles to detect at the earliest possible time any evidence of tenderness which might indicate the presence of an early deep venous thrombosis. The development in a postoperative patient of a concomitant rise in temperature, pulse and respiration, irrespective of any positive signs of phlebitis in the extremities, should make one suspect the presence of deep venous thrombosis with a small nonfatal pulmonary embolism. Since most fatal pulmonary emboli are preceded by a small warning embolus, it is recommended that measures be taken to prevent the development of additional emboli, preferably by bilateral superficial femoral vein interruption followed by anticoagulant therapy with Coumadin for a period of at least two weeks. This method of therapy is also recommended if a definite diagnosis of deep thrombophlebitis limited to the calf veins is made even without preliminary pulmonary embolism. To wait after the diagnosis of an early localized deep phlebitis in the calf has been made until a patient develops an iliofemoral thrombophlebitis or a pulmonary embolus before carrying out definitive treatment shows a serious lack of judgment, since an inferior vena cava interruption may be necessary if the patient has not already succumbed to a massive pulmonary embolus.

A number of patients who have had massive pulmonary emboli have been saved by an emergency pulmonary artery embolectomy utilizing a cardiopulmonary bypass. Despite these successes, there are still patients who die so quickly from complete occlusion of the pulmonary artery that they cannot be moved to the operating room in time to perform this operation. It seems, therefore, that the prevention of deep venous thrombosis is the goal that we should aspire to. With more attention given postoperatively to the lower extremities and to the use of the available prophylactic measures, the incidence of this dreaded complication can be greatly reduced.

101

Plate 44

PROPHYLAXIS OF DEEP VENOUS THROMBOSIS BY AMBULATION IN BED

A. These drawings demonstrate the author's method for ambulating patients who must remain in bed longer than 24 hours postoperatively. Note that the bed is placed in slight reverse Trendelenburg position with the head higher than the feet. This is accomplished, if necessary, with blocks under the bedposts at the head of the bed. In most of the modern, electrically controlled hospital beds it can be done easily. The patient is also allowed a low to medium head rest. In this way the legs are made dependent. An overhead beam or Balkan frame is attached by uprights to the head and the foot of the bed. A trapeze hangs from this within reach of the patient's hands so that he can use it to help move himself about and to raise his body up and exercise his arms. At the foot of the bed is a right-angled footboard made of an aluminum alloy that is placed under the end of the mattress with the vertical portion extending 30 cm. above it. This serves two functions: One is that the bed coverings are placed over it, which prevents the bed from being made up with them tucked too tightly under the mattress, thereby providing the patient with freedom to move his legs and feet, an important factor in the prevention of deep venous thrombosis. The other function is for the performance of the foot and leg exercises.

B. This demonstrates the patient pushing against the footboard with the balls of his feet, keeping the knees in extension as if he were rising on his tiptoes by contracting the calf and anterior thigh muscles.

C. After maintaining this position for a few seconds, the patient relaxes his muscles and allows his heels to return to the footboard as in the inset.

He is instructed to perform this exercise at least one thousand times a day, spreading them out over his waking hours rather than trying to do them in a short period of time. The actual number is not so important, but this number gives him a high goal to work for and impresses on him the importance of the exercises. It is explained to him carefully just why these exercises are important, namely, to prevent "blood clots." The purpose of this type of exercise is to put into action the venous heart of the lower extremities to make the blood circulate and to prevent it from stagnating and clotting in the deep veins of the gastrocnemius, soleus and flexor muscles of the lower leg by pumping blood out of them toward the heart.

The method is also advocated for patients who are slow to return to normal ambulation, even though they are permitted out of bed. The exercises also have the great advantage that they are active and not passive, so the patient can do them by himself without bedside help from nurses or other hospital personnel. The slight reverse Trendelenburg position of the bed is maintained because it is believed better to keep the veins full of blood rather than empty, thereby avoiding intimal damage that might occur in the collapsed state, especially in the phlebosclerotic veins of the elderly. The slant of the bed tends to cause the patient to slide down, and pushing on the board and pulling on the trapeze to keep himself up provides additional exercise. Another advantage of this method of prophylaxis for the patient who must remain in bed is that the exercises keep his muscles in better condition so that when he does get up, walking is more easily accomplished. When possible, it is recommended that the patient be instructed in these exercises, simple as they seem, prior to operation. There can be no question in anybody's mind that anything that can be done to prevent deep venous thrombosis and pulmonary emboli is of extreme importance and far better than attempting to treat the condition after it develops, and this method of bed ambulation has been found to be very successful.

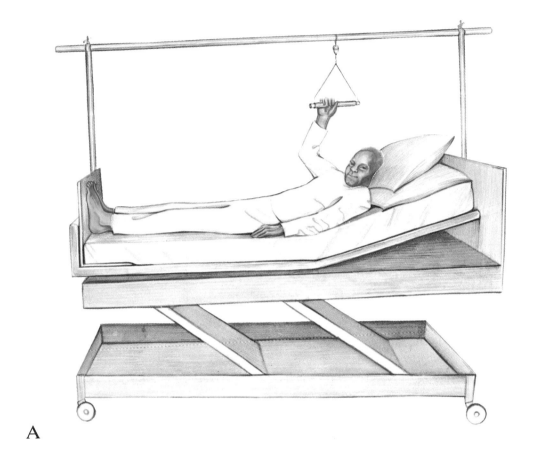

A

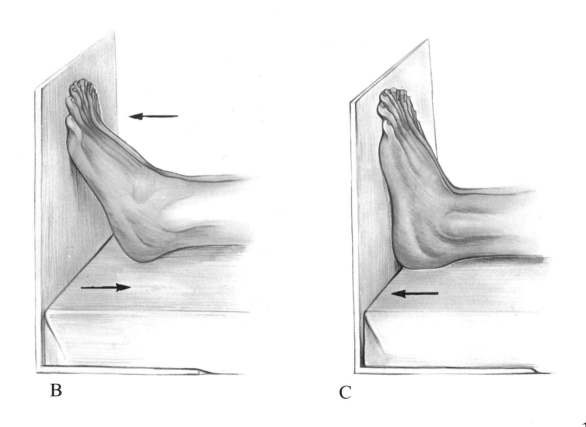

B

C

103

Plate 45

DEEP VENOUS THROMBOSIS OF THE LOWER EXTREMITY WITH MASSIVE PULMONARY EMBOLISM

A. The commonest site of venous thrombosis is in the deep veins of the muscles, shown here diagrammatically. The observation of local tenderness deep in the calf muscles to finger pressure and pain in the calf muscles on forceful dorsiflexion of the foot, a positive Homans' sign, is the earliest signal of this condition. Other signs such as edema and dilatation of the superficial veins are seen later. The observation of tenderness usually indicates an inflammatory process; under these conditions it is termed thrombophlebitis. The local condition in the calf is seldom serious, but the clot that propagates from a calf vein nidus into the popliteal and femoral veins is a threat to life because it often is nonadherent to the venous intima except at its origin, as shown. This floating type of clot has been termed "silent venous thrombosis" because there are no signs or symptoms of it. It is in this stage, however, that proximal vein ligation can be life-saving therapy, as the clot may result in a fatal pulmonary embolism if it breaks loose.

B. This shows a massive pulmonary embolus occluding both the right and left pulmonary arteries that has arisen from the floating thrombus in the popliteal and femoral veins. Pulmonary emboli of this magnitude result in sudden death unless they are removed. Fortunately few are so massive, so that the pulmonary arteries are not so completely occluded. This allows time to move the patient to the operating room to remove the thrombi from the pulmonary arteries with use of a cardiopulmonary bypass. It should be pointed out that, with careful attention to the postoperative examination of the legs, proximal vein interruption when early leg signs are detected is a much better method of treatment by localization of the process to the extremity. In addition, it is recommended that anticoagulant therapy with Coumadin be used after the venous interruption.

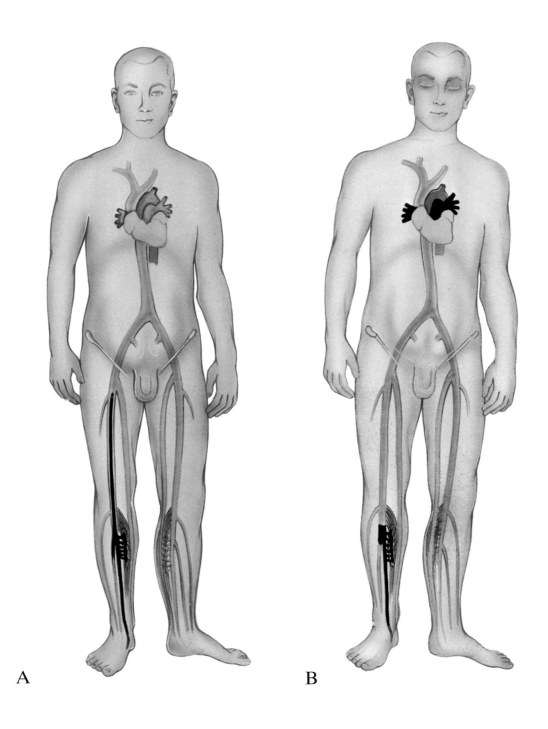

A   B

105

Plate 46

PROXIMAL SUPERFICIAL FEMORAL VEIN INTERRUPTION

A positive diagnosis of deep calf venous thrombosis is sufficient indication to perform interruption of the superficial femoral vein at its junction with the profunda femoris vein. If a patient has had a warning, nonlethal pulmonary embolus, it is a good rule that the femoral veins in both extremities be interrupted irrespective of whether there are positive signs of venous thrombosis in the extremities. It is believed that this is a better operation for the patient than interruption or clipping of the inferior vena cava. The operative procedure may be performed under local infiltration anesthesia or light general anesthesia.

A. This shows the operating table in slight reversed Trendelenburg position. It is important that the patient's body be elevated 10 degrees to produce positive pressure in the femoral vein to prevent thrombi from being dislodged and sucked proximally to result in pulmonary embolism.

B. This shows the location of the incision for femoral vein interruptions. The incision should be made longitudinally directly over and parallel with the femoral artery pulsations. It extends up to the groin crease for the superficial femoral vein interruption as shown in the left groin; for the common femoral it should extend proximal to the groin crease as seen in the right groin for a more proximal exposure which is necessary.

C. The superficial femoral artery and vein are isolated by opening the Scarpa's fascia. The dissection should be commenced distally and worked proximally to prevent injury to the common femoral vein. At the same time the surgeon should look for the bulge in the superficial femoral vein which indicates accurately the location of the profunda femoris vein just proximal to it. The femoral vein should be carefully palpated to make sure it does not have a thrombus in it because, if it does, the interruption should be of the common femoral vein instead of the superficial femoral vein.

Note the proximal portion of the saphenous vein (1), which should not be injured. The superficial femoral artery (2), with a small sensory branch of the femoral nerve coursing along it, lies lateral to the common femoral (3) and the superficial femoral (4) veins. The profunda femoris vein (5) terminates at the junction of these two veins, just proximal to a bulge in the superficial femoral vein, the site of a venous valve. This is a constant anatomical landmark and is an aid in locating the profunda femoris vein.

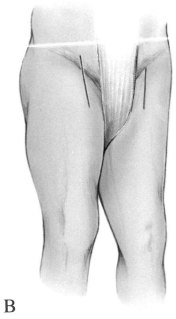

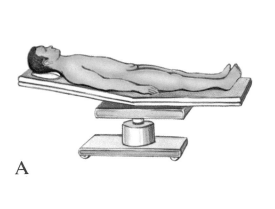

A

B

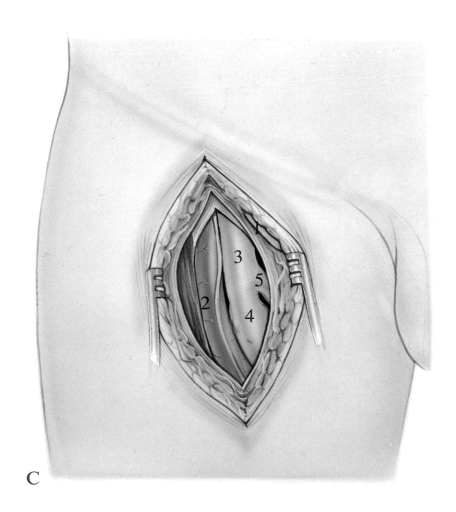

C

107

Plate 47

PROXIMAL SUPERFICIAL FEMORAL VEIN INTERRUPTION *(Continued)*

A. The femoral artery must be treated with great care to prevent injury to it. Under no conditions should it be retracted with a rubber tube or catheter around it because of the danger of fracturing its wall, with resulting thrombosis and occlusion. (See Introduction, Plate 12 *A.*) Instead, it is best retracted by grasping its adventitia to dissect it free from the femoral vein with scissors. This may cause it to go into spasm, but it will not become thrombosed and occluded if treated in this manner. Two ligatures of linen or cotton are passed around the proximal end of the superficial femoral vein approximately a centimeter apart. These are held loosely while a transverse incision is made in the vein between them. Bleeding usually occurs from both the proximal and distal ends if there is no thrombus present. Sometimes the bleeding from the distal end is not very vigorous because of a more distal thrombus that cannot be seen.

B. The bleeding is readily controlled by grasping the edge of the venotomy with a hemostat as shown, then twisting the instrument about 360 degrees, which gives immediate control of the bleeding.

C. The proximal and distal edges of the venotomy are both grasped with hemostats for better control of the vessel. It is important to make sure there is active bleeding, especially from the proximal end, to rule out a thrombus in the common femoral vein. This is ascertained by twisting the hemostat on the distal venotomy cuff to control the bleeding from this end, or by tightening the previously placed distal ligature. If the back flow from the proximal end is sluggish, it may be because of a proximal thrombus that should be removed. If this is found, the common femoral vein should be interrupted proximal to the profunda femoris branch after removing any thrombi in it. In most cases gentle palpation of the common femoral vein will help to determine the presence of a thrombus in this location before making the venotomy in the superficial femoral vein. If this is made and the common femoral vein needs to be interrupted in addition, the superficial femoral vein can likewise be interrupted without serious consequences, or the venotomy may be closed with a fine arterial suture.

D. Double ligation with division of the superficial femoral vein is recommended. This is accomplished most readily by placing two hemostats across the superficial femoral vein on either side of the venotomy.

E. The vein is then divided between them and each end is secured with a proximal ligature and a distal transfixion ligature of linen or cotton. The profunda femoris and saphenous veins are the main outflow vessels of the extremity. The incision is closed meticulously in layers with fine interrupted sutures of linen or cotton to prevent wound hematomas, which tend to interfere with lymph flow and cause lymphedema of the extremity. Great care is taken not to catch the branch of the femoral nerve, shown on the femoral artery in *A,* in one of the sutures; the nerve may also be found adherent to Scarpa's fascia, and catching it may result in severe neuralgia. The skin is closed with interrupted vertical mattress sutures of silk. Unless the patient needs to remain in bed for other reasons, he should be ambulatory the following day, a definite advantage of this form of therapy. It is recommended also that postoperative anticoagulation with Coumadin be carried out while the patient is still hospitalized and then discontinued. For control of lymphedema an elastic stocking to the knee, or two elastic 4-inch Ace bandages, are used during the day but removed at night.

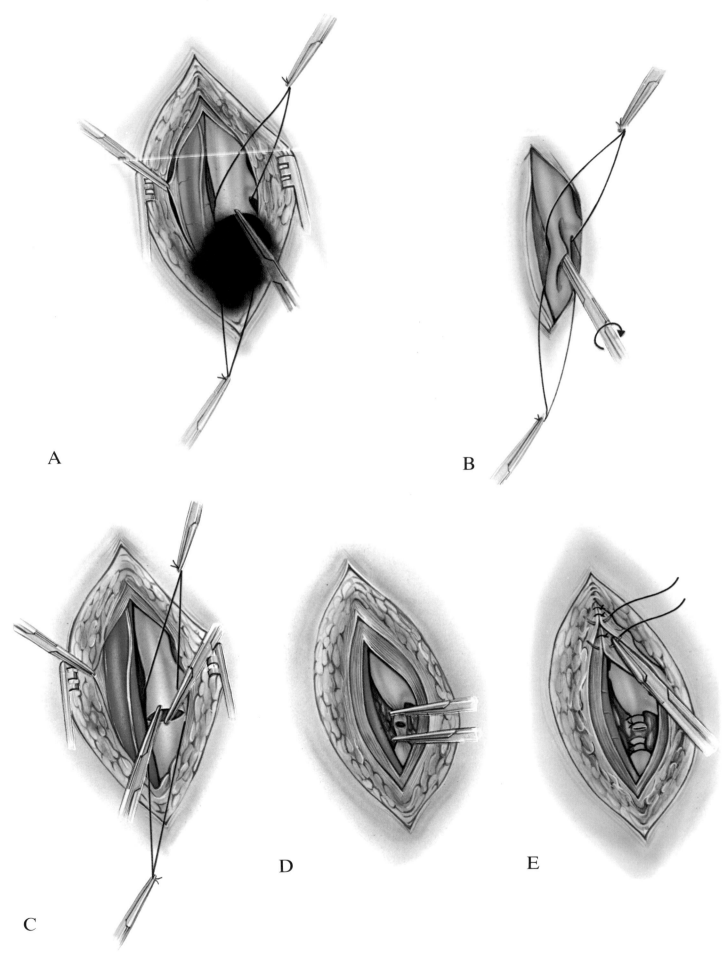

A

B

C

D

E

109

Plate 48

THE MODE OF PRODUCTION OF ILIOFEMORAL THROMBOPHLEBITIS

A. Fortunately not all silent deep venous thrombi in the popliteal and femoral veins lodge in the pulmonary artery when they break off from their distal attachment; some lodge in the common femoral vein. It is significant that some patients have been known to complain of pain in the calf without much attention being paid to this complaint. Others may have had an unexplained concomitant rise in temperature, pulse and respirations, a complication not infrequently caused by deep venous thrombosis of one of the lower extremities and a minor pulmonary embolus.

B. Suddenly the patient experiences severe pain in the thigh. The leg often becomes pale in color and later cyanotic; the entire extremity to the groin becomes swollen in a matter of hours. It is believed that the long venous thrombus becomes impinged in the common femoral vein because in some patients the lumen of this vessel is uneven in outline, tending to entrap the thrombus at this site. Proximal thrombosis quickly develops to involve the external iliac vein, so that the outflow tract is markedly occluded. Temporarily at least, massive pulmonary embolism does not occur, but may develop from proximal propagating thrombi. In some patients after 72 hours a sterile inflammatory reaction develops between the thrombus and the venous endothelium, which causes it to become adherent in the iliofemoral region and results in the condition termed "occlusive thrombophlebitis."

C. The above sequence of events should not occur if early surgical intervention by phlebotomy and thrombectomy is performed as soon as the diagnosis of an obstructing thrombus in the femoral vein is made. Phlebography may be resorted to, but too often it may produce more thrombosis from the irritating effect of the radiopaque dye. From experience it has been observed that if the thrombus has been lodged in the femoral vein for less than 72 hours it can be extracted readily through a venotomy, similarly to an arterial embolus through an arteriotomy. The venous intima will still be smooth and shiny without adherent blood clot. Some surgeons favor closure of the venotomy to restore the continuity of the common femoral vein. It is my opinion, however, that interruption of it, as shown in this illustration, is preferable. Not only does this give immediate protection from a massive pulmonary embolus, but it also is the best insurance against emboli should phlebitis recur in the extremity. It also has the advantage that it helps to prevent the sequelae of the thrombotic state seen so commonly in the postthrombotic limb with the uninterrupted femoral vein.

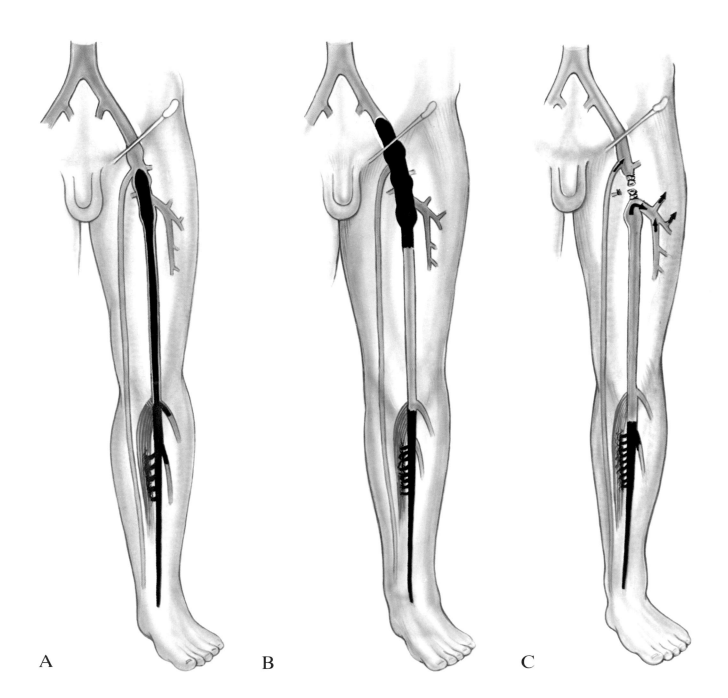

A

B

C

111

Plate 49

INTERRUPTION OF COMMON FEMORAL VEIN WITH THROMBECTOMY

A. Interruption of the common femoral vein is indicated when a thrombus is found in it, or if a patient has had a minor pulmonary embolus, irrespective of whether there are signs of venous thrombosis in the lower extremities. This level is chosen in order to perform the venous interruption proximal to the profunda femoris vein. The procedure should be performed in both extremities; it is recommended if a patient is seen within 48 to 72 hours after the onset of tenderness in the groin and edema of the extremity. The presence of a thrombus is readily detected by gentle palpation of the common femoral vein over a small right angle clamp passed behind it. Loose ligatures are placed around it, the distal one just proximal to the profunda femoris vein (1). The proximal one is placed proximal to the lateral circumflex vein (2), which should be ligated and divided, and distal to the medial circumflex vein (3). The rule is that there must be sufficient common femoral vein between the two ligatures so that later in the procedure it can be safely divided and both ends securely ligated. The proximal ligature should also be just distal to a tributary so that blood will continue to flow through the proximal end of the vein, in this case the medial circumflex vein. The long saphenous vein is not interrupted unless it is also thrombosed, in which case it is at the saphenofemoral junction. A transverse incision is made midway between the ligatures. A dark fresh thrombus can be seen being extruded through it.

B. This shows the thrombectomy being performed by strong suction through a glass drinking tube. The glass permits the surgeon to see the thrombus being sucked out and avoid the necessity of pushing the tube up the vein, which might loosen the thrombus and cause a pulmonary embolus. If the patient is operated on early, the thrombus comes out with surprising ease and is followed by a gush of venous blood, indicating that the proximal vein has been cleared of blood clots. If it is impossible to get adequate back bleeding and the patient has had a minor pulmonary embolus, inferior vena cava interruption should be performed immediately. The distal thrombus can usually be partially aspirated and more of it expressed out by pressure on the thigh.

C. Another effective way of removing the proximal thrombus is with a large, venous-type Fogarty catheter. This is readily passed up through the thrombus. If the thrombus is recent and nonadherent, it is brought out with ease. It is important to have the body of the patient elevated during this procedure also, so that the blood in the iliac and femoral veins is under positive pressure and will flush out small thrombi through the venotomy. Distal passage of the catheter has been recommended, but this probably results in damage to the venous valves, so its use in this manner is questionable.

D. Some surgeons prefer to maintain the venous continuity after thrombectomy by closure of the venotomy. However, since attacks may recur and because permanent interruption of the common femoral vein does not result in irreparable damage to an extremity, and furthermore since the postthrombotic syndrome develops because the femoral vein recanalizes, it seems justifiable to interrupt the common femoral vein by ligation and division. As shown, the vein is divided completely and both ends controlled with a ligature and transfixion suture of linen or cotton. One of the lateral branches of the vein had to be ligated to give sufficient length of vein to safely ligate and divide. The venous blood from the extremity returns through the profunda femoris and long saphenous veins as shown by the arrows. The incision is closed meticulously in layers.

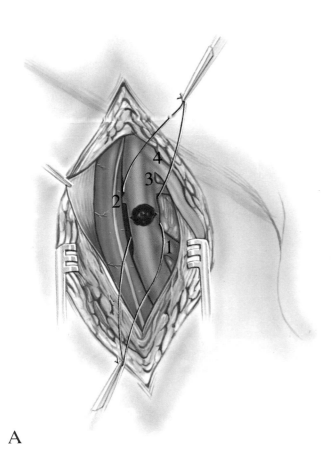

A

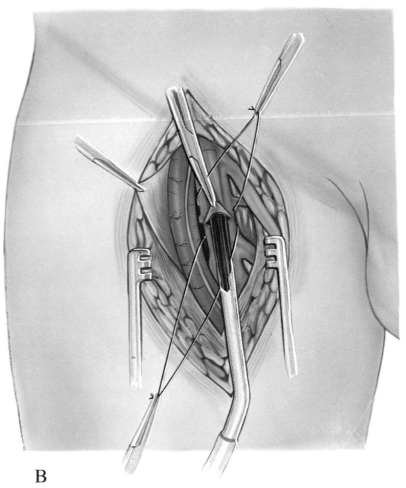

B

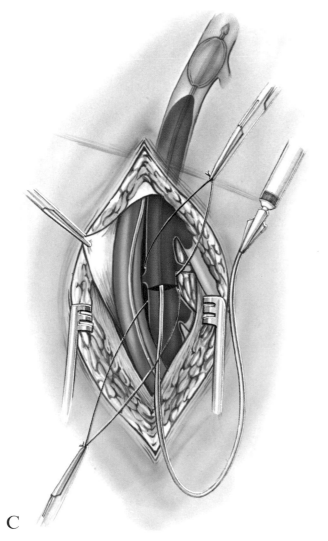

C

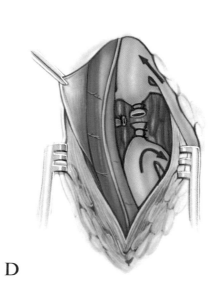

D

113

Plate 50

INTERRUPTION OF THE INFERIOR VENA CAVA

A. This shows the position of the patient on the operating table for the extraperitoneal exposure of the infrarenal portion of the inferior vena cava through a right flank incision. The patient lies supine with the right side elevated approximately 15 degrees by blanket rolls under the right chest, hip and thigh.

B. The inferior vena cava has been exposed through a right flank incision. In some cases the procedure is made easier by partial excision of the twelfth rib. The external and internal oblique muscles are partially divided. The transversalis muscle and lumbodorsal fascia are next divided in the line of their fibers to expose the retroperitoneal area. The retroperitoneal tissues, the kidney and the ureter are displaced forward and medialward with a large Deaver retractor over gauze packs. The psoas muscle is retracted posteriorly. These steps expose the inferior vena cava distal to the renal veins shown at the level of the proximal edge of the incision. Distal to them two sets of lumbar veins are seen with two ligatures being placed around the inferior vena cava with a right-angle clamp.

C. There is some difference of opinion in regard to which type of inferior vena cava interruption is the best and results in the fewest postoperative complications. It is believed the most effective method for prevention of further pulmonary emboli is to interrupt the inferior vena cava completely with two nonabsorbable ligatures a centimeter apart placed just distal and flush with a set of lumbar veins. This will permit blood to flow into the proximal end of the inferior vena cava to help to prevent the formation of a secondary thrombus that might result in a pulmonary embolism. Some surgeons prefer to place the ligatures just distal to the renal veins to permit blood to flow into the proximal end of the inferior vena cava and prevent a secondary thrombus. This site of interruption also permits more outflow channels from the distal vena cava through the lumbar veins, but from experience it does not seem to make a great deal of difference. Anticoagulant therapy should be started following the operation as an additional measure to help in prevention of proximal thrombosis in the inferior vena cava. One of the criticisms of ligation is that it results in sequelae that are not so frequently seen with partial occlusion. It has been observed that with adequate elastic support to the lower leg these sequelae are not too serious and usually can be controlled, so that for the additional safety from secondary embolism the complete interruption is the preferred method.

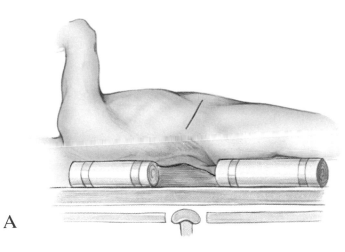

A

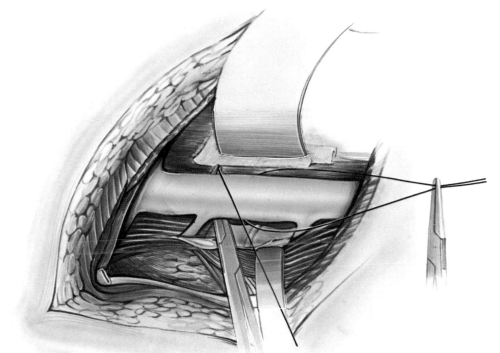

B

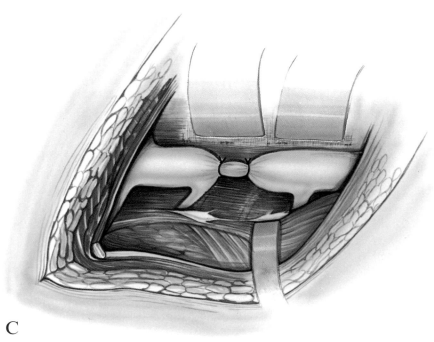

C

115

Plate 51

INFERIOR VENA CAVA INTERRUPTION
AND PLICATION

A. The inferior vena cava may also be exposed retroperitoneally with relative ease through a right paramedian right rectus muscle-retracting incision. The incision should extend from the pubis to 3 or 4 cm. above the umbilicus. The peritoneum is easily retracted at the distal part of the incision. The rectus muscle is retracted to expose the posterior rectus sheath. This is carefully dissected away from the peritoneum with wide, blunt-pointed scissors, then divided to permit further retraction of the peritoneum and the abdominal viscera.

B. The retroperitoneal area has been opened up to show the bifurcation of the aorta and the distal portion of the inferior vena cava with its bifurcation behind the aorta and right common iliac artery. The right ureter (1) is shown pulled to the right of the operative field by the large retractor. A small constant tributary of the vena cava is shown, care having been taken to ligate and divide it as it arises distal to the level at which the inferior vena cava is ligated. The inferior vena cava is ligated with two nonabsorbable ligatures placed approximately 1 cm. apart. The proximal one is placed close to but not occluding the lumbar veins just proximal to it. The incision can then be closed in the routine method used for a right paramedian rectus-retracting incision. In female patients who have developed septic pulmonary emboli from a source in the pelvis, this incision is recommended for performing the interruption of the vena cava transperitoneally rather than extraperitoneally so that at the same time interruption of the ovarian veins can be performed, a necessity under these conditions. This incision has the advantage that it interrupts fewer of the collateral veins in the abdominal wall for the return of venous blood from the limb than does the transverse flank incision.

C. Various methods of partial occlusion of the inferior vena cava have been devised. The one in favor at this time is some form of clip that is placed around the inferior vena cava, dividing its large lumen into four small ones after the clip is tied into place. This figure shows the plastic DeWeese type.

D. This shows the extraperitoneal exposure of the infrarenal portion of the inferior vena cava through a right flank incision and the application of a clip. This usually requires a little more adequate exposure than for ligation of the vein. It is recommended that the clip be placed close to the proximal lumbar veins in case thrombosis of the vena cava distal to the clip should occur; this will help to reduce the formation of a proximal thrombosis as a source of pulmonary embolism.

E. The clip has been applied and the two limbs of it tied together. It shows how the large caval lumen has been changed to four small lumina. This method may prevent a massive pulmonary embolus, but small emboli do occur in a higher percentage than when total occlusion by ligation has been performed. It is also not known what percentage of clipped inferior venae cavae become completely occluded. It seems therefore that each surgeon must decide for himself which method he wishes to use, then follow his patients closely so that he may take care of any late sequelae that develop.

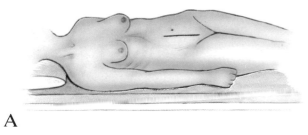

A

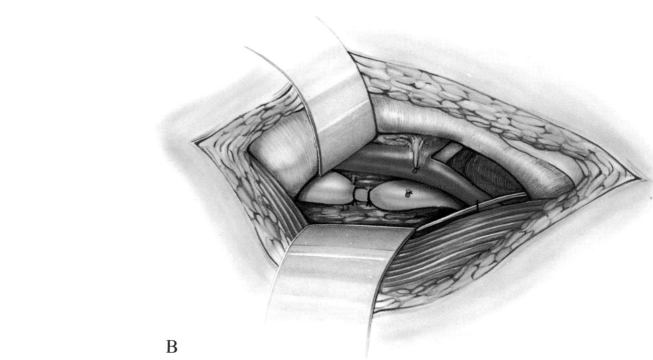

B

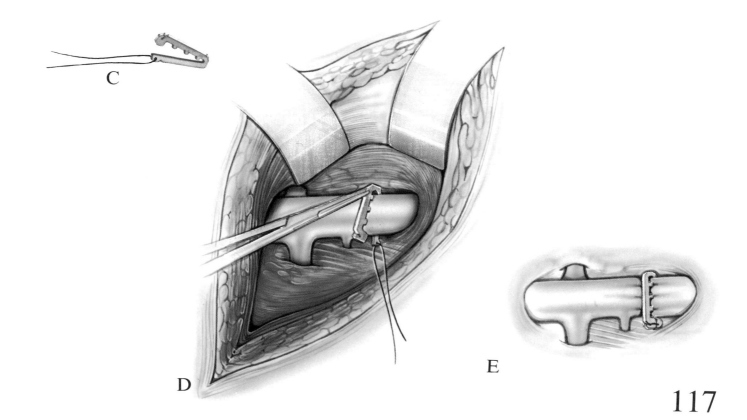

C

D

E

117

Plate 52

INTERRUPTION AND THROMBECTOMY OF INFERIOR VENA CAVA

A. It is important for a surgeon to learn how to determine the presence of a nonadherent thrombus in a large vein such as the inferior vena cava before clipping or tying it, because of the danger of causing a pulmonary embolus from the thrombus breaking off proximal to the clip or the ligature. To avoid this possible complication, after exposure the inferior vena cava should be palpated with extreme gentleness with the tip of the forefinger as shown. The presence of the thrombus partially occupying the lumen of the vena cava is readily detected by gentle pressure of the vein against the bodies of the lumbar vertebrae.

B. The inferior vena cava must be opened in order to perform a thrombectomy. Before doing this it is advisable to place controls proximal and distal to the venotomy to control the gush of venous blood after removal of the thrombus. The tourniquet clamp has been found most useful for this purpose; two are placed around the vena cava in the open position. A transverse venotomy is performed since this permits an adequate thrombectomy and interferes much less with ligation of the large vessel than if a longitudinal incision is used. The exploring forefinger palpates the vena cava carefully to find the proximal end of the thrombus, then milks it distalward and out through the venotomy. This will be followed by a gush of blood which is readily controlled by closing the proximal tourniquet clamp. The distal portion of the thrombus is then removed by milking it proximally and using a large size Fogarty catheter if necessary. As a rule, blood will then gush from the distal end, but is quickly controlled by closing the distal tourniquet clamp.

C. Two transfixion suture ligatures of linen or cotton are placed, one proximal and one distal to the venotomy. If possible they should be close to the nearest lumbar veins. It is believed that this type of venous thrombosis should always be treated by permanent interruption of the inferior vena cava after thrombectomy and that the venotomy should never be sutured to restore the caval continuity because of the danger of secondary thrombosis and pulmonary embolism. The flank incision through which these inferior vena caval procedures are accomplished is closed by suturing the divided muscles back together with interrupted linen or cotton sutures and careful closure of the skin with silk sutures. Drainage of the retroperitoneal area is rarely necessary. Postoperative anticoagulation with Coumadin for the period of hospitalization is recommended following any operative procedure for thromboembolism.

118

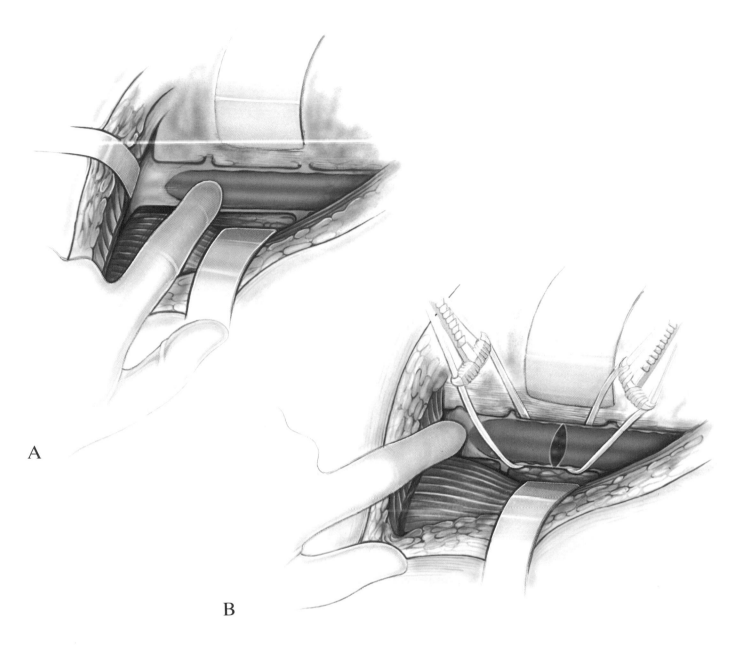

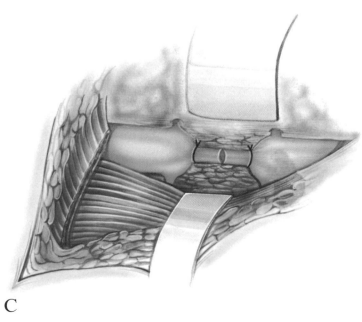

A

B

C

Plate 53

SUPERFICIAL THROMBOPHLEBITIS OF THE LOWER EXTREMITY

A. Superficial thrombophlebitis in the lower extremity is seen most frequently in middle-aged and elderly patients with longstanding varicose veins. It may result from minor trauma to the extremity, but it develops most frequently because of venous stasis in the large, dilated, tortuous phlebosclerotic veins that usually are tributaries of the long saphenous vein. The condition usually commences in the veins of the medial aspect of the upper part of the lower leg. It is characterized by tenderness over the involved veins, which are firm to hard on palpation. The skin overlying the involved veins becomes red, suggesting that there is underlying infection, but the condition is rarely septic. The thrombotic process may extend into the main saphenous trunk, then extend proximally in the common femoral vein if untreated. If seen early, the process may sometimes be limited to the tortuous varices by the use of elastic Ace bandages with a pad of cellucotton beneath for additional pressure over the involved veins. It is also important to keep the patient ambulatory instead of putting him at bed rest. If the process has extended up to the groin as shown, or even if it has extended only into the lower thigh, the patient should be treated surgically because of the danger that it may extend into the deep venous system, thereby resulting in pulmonary embolism.

B. In the case presented here the saphenous vein has been exposed through an oblique incision just below the inguinal crease with the patient under general anesthesia. The saphenofemoral junction is shown and a thrombus that originated in the varices of the lower leg is visible, extending in the saphenous vein almost to the femoral vein. Great care must be taken in dissecting it free, so that the proximal portion of the thrombus will not break off to produce a pulmonary embolus.

C. The saphenous vein has been interrupted by ligation and division at the saphenofemoral junction flush with the common femoral vein. It is usually safer to open the vein and remove the proximal portion of the thrombus before placing the ligatures to prevent breaking off the proximal end and causing a pulmonary embolus. An intraluminal stripper with a washer to enlarge the olive-tipped end has been passed down the trunk of the main saphenous vein to just below the knee, where a small incision is made so that the thrombosed vein can be removed. (See Plate 54 *A.*)

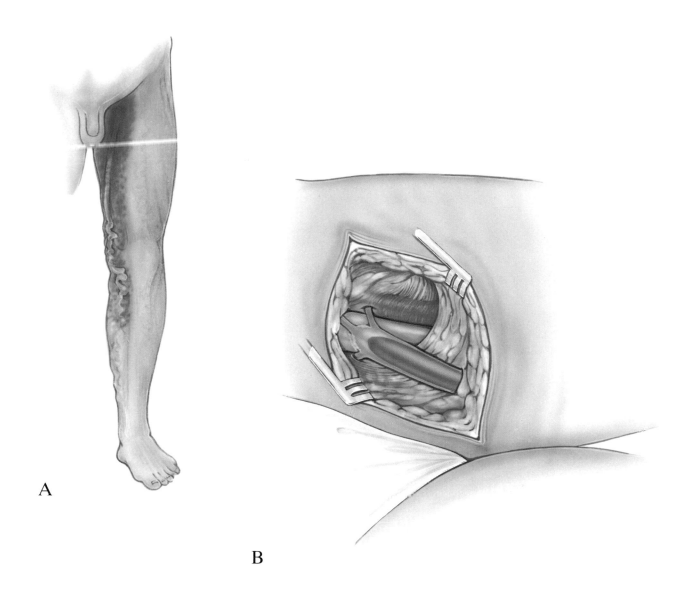

A

B

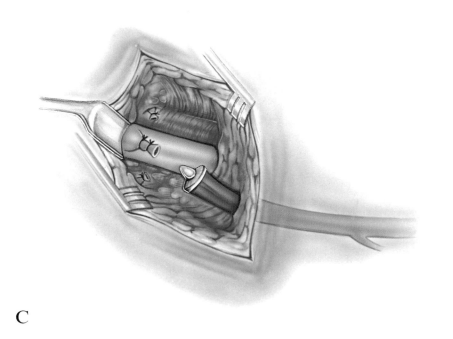

C

121

Plate 54

SUPERFICIAL THROMBOPHLEBITIS
OF THE LOWER EXTREMITY *(Continued)*

A. This shows the lower extremity of a patient with superficial phlebitis of the long saphenous vein and involvement of some large tortuous varices of the thigh and lower leg. The saphenous vein has been interrupted and ligated at the saphenofemoral junction. The intraluminal stripper has been passed down the long saphenous vein to below the knee, where another small oblique incision has been made and the saphenous vein exposed and divided. The distal end has been ligated, and the small end of the stripper is protruding from the proximal end. The main long saphenous trunk is next removed from the thigh by stripping. As a rule, the long saphenous vein in the lower leg does not need to be removed.

B. This is inset (1) and shows the excision of a large group of tortuous thrombosed varices in the thigh that are excised through an oblique incision because they cannot be stripped. It is important not to use a longitudinal incision to do this, because some portion of the skin that is dissected away from the veins will invariably slough. This rarely if ever happens with oblique or transverse incisions. Excision of these large thrombosed painful veins gives rapid relief compared to the method of allowing them to resolve by themselves under anticoagulant therapy.

C. This is inset (2) and shows another superficial group of large tortuous thrombosed veins on the inner aspect of the lower leg distal to the point at which the saphenous vein was removed. It demonstrates another simple method of treating them without excising them, especially very superficial thrombosed varices, because of the danger of skin slough. This consists of making several small incisions into the largest and most superficial varices. Then pressure is exerted on both sides of these incisions with thumb and forefinger to force the blood clots out. This method is most satisfactory if performed within a few days of the onset of the phlebitis before the thrombi become too adherent to the vein walls. It is surprising how little bleeding occurs after evacuation of the blood clots, and that secondary thrombi rarely develop.

D. This shows the extremity after completion of the operative procedure with closure of the larger incisions. The small ones do not need to be sutured. Gauze dressings are placed over the incisions and the leg is wrapped from toes to groin over a thick gauze roll placed along the course of the veins that were removed. Ambulation is commenced the same evening or the morning following the operation. Postoperative anticoagulants are not used routinely. This method of treatment cures the condition, shortens the convalescence and prevents the disease from involving the deep venous system with the potential danger of pulmonary embolism.

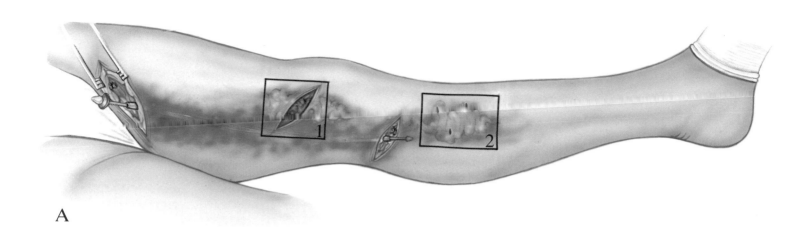

A

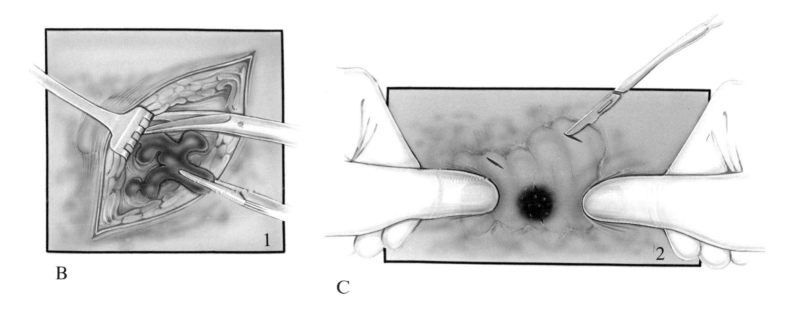

B

C

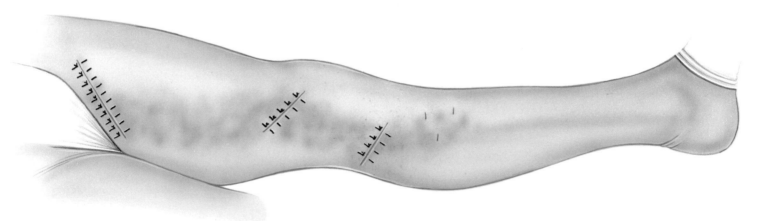

D

123

Plate 55

SUPERFICIAL THROMBOPHLEBITIS OF THE LOWER EXTREMITY *(Continued)*

A.   The propagation of a thrombus in the common femoral vein with extension of it proximally into the external iliac vein may occur with conservative treatment, especially when the patient is placed at bed rest. The extension of the thrombus is not always easily diagnosed, especially in an obese patient. If this is not detected it may result in serious pulmonary embolism. The proximal end of a thrombus is shown in the external iliac vein as an extension of the one in the long saphenous vein.

B.   The long saphenous vein is carefully divided near its junction with the common femoral vein, but a short stump is left for ligation after performance of the thrombectomy. Bleeding does not occur because of the occlusion by the thrombus both proximally and distally. The cut edges of the proximal cuff of vein are grasped with fine hemostats. The glass suction tube is placed against the thrombus; with suction, it usually comes out with ease and is followed by a gush of a large amount of venous blood. Finger pressure over the femoral vein distally will demonstrate retrograde bleeding from the iliac vein, indicating that the thombus has been removed. Pressure is then applied to determine that the distal flow is normal. Further bleeding is readily controlled by twisting the hemostats on the proximal saphenous vein cuff. This permits a satisfactory ligature and transfixion suture ligature. The operative procedure is completed as already described in Plates 53 and 54.

C.   The proximal propagated thrombus may also be removed with a large Fogarty catheter. This method is especially useful if it is not certain all the thrombus has been removed. If the thrombus should extend distally in the common femoral vein, which is extremely rare in patients with superficial phlebitis, the Fogarty catheter may be passed distally a short distance in an attempt to clear it and the profunda femoris vein. In such cases it is recommended that the common femoral vein be interrupted if the thrombus is adherent to the venous intima, rather than leave it in continuity with the danger of reclotting and causing pulmonary embolism. This may lead to edema of the limb, but immediate, adequate, heavyweight elastic stocking support will control the edema and prevent its becoming permanent. Under these conditions it probably will be better not to strip the long saphenous vein, but simply to close the groin incision carefully after proximal and distal ligation of the common femoral and the distal end of the saphenous vein. It is important that these patients be ambulated the day after operation. Anticoagulation with Coumadin is recommended while the patient is in the hospital but is discontinued at discharge. Adequate elastic support of these limbs from the base of the toes to just below the knee is very important and should be continued for at least three months, or longer if edema persists.

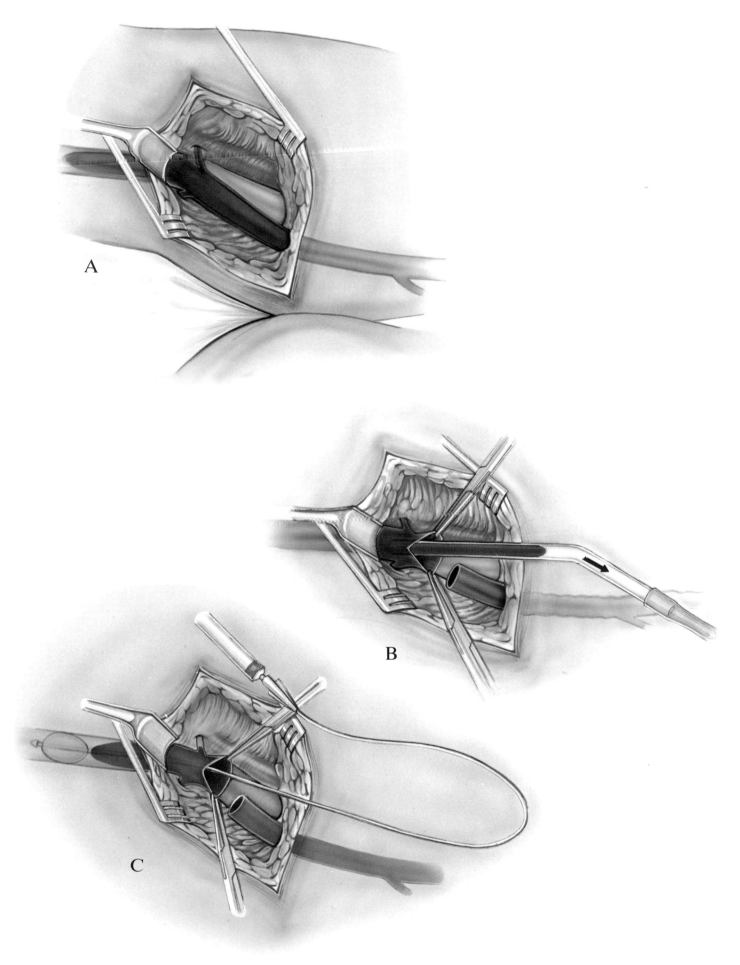

A

B

C

125

THE POSTTHROMBOTIC SYNDROME OF THE LOWER EXTREMITY WITH ULCERATION

Introduction

The postthrombotic syndrome of the lower leg with ulceration is a condition which has plagued the human race for many centuries. As a result of the better methods of preventing deep venous thrombosis in the lower extremity, especially the postpartum and postoperative forms, the incidence of the postthrombotic state has been considerably reduced. Many patients are still afflicted, however. Unfortunately too few surgeons know or are interested in the most effective surgical method of curing the condition. Even today there has not been a great change since Home wrote in 1801: "It has been unpropitious to the improvement of the treatment of ulcers on the leg, that they have been universally admitted to be the most unmanageable cases which become the object of surgery; that they are cases in which the most eminent surgeons are too often known to fail in performing a cure; and therefore, bring no imputation of want of skill on those practitioners who happen to prove unsuccessful. This has led the younger part of the profession in the army to be too diffident of their own ability; to despair of success where so many have failed, and to follow a beaten track, in which so little advance has been made, that ulcers on the leg are not unjustly considered as the opprobrium of surgery." One of the reasons for failure of most methods that have been advocated is that they do not correct the underlying pathologic physiology of the diseased venous systems of the lower extremity, undoubtedly because it is not widely understood.

It is of extreme importance to understand that this condition is a chronic disease. Furthermore, it is not possible to restore the limb to its normal prethrombotic state because of the irreparable damage to the valves of the deep, communicating and superficial systems of veins. On the other hand, it is possible to cure the chronic ulcer for which the patient comes to the surgeon. Furthermore, if the patient will follow directions explicitly after the proper surgical procedure has been performed and the ulcer has healed, he or she may return to a gainful occupation with assurance that the ulcer will not recur.

It is important to point out that the earlier treatment is carried out when the ulcer is small, the easier it will be to heal and to keep from recurring. The huge ulcers that almost encompass the leg are more difficult, but again it is possible to obtain good results with them. However, in addition to the adequate operative procedure, it is of utmost importance that these patients must cooperate fully and follow the aftercare directions precisely.

Plate 56

THE POSTTHROMBOTIC SYNDROME
OF THE LOWER EXTREMITY
WITH ULCERATION

A. This shows the lower extremities of a man 40 years of age and demonstrates the late typical thrombotic sequelae in the left leg five years following a femoro-iliac deep venous thrombosis complicating the postoperative recovery from acute appendicitis. The right leg shows only varicose veins.

These sequelae in the order of their appearance are (1) edema, (2) varicose veins, (3) stasis dermatitis, (4) pigmentation, (5) stasis cellulitis, a brawny induration of the subcutaneous tissues on the inner side of the leg and ankle, and (6) chronic stasis ulcer. It is important to understand that these do not develop because the deep venous system remains occluded; rather, because the veins of this system become recanalized and patent again. The venous valves in them, however, are irreparably damaged so they are incompetent, which leads to a decompensated venous heart in the lower extremity. The varicose veins in the groin area and the left lower quadrant are significant evidence of the recanalization of the deep veins and the incompetence of their valves, with secondary involvement of the proximal end of the long saphenous vein and its superficial epigastric branch. These varices are considered by some to represent collateral channels for the return of the blood from the lower extremity, but this is not true; they develop only as the result of an increased venous pressure secondary to the destruction of the valves of the deep venous system, so they should be ligated and partially removed as part of the surgical procedure for the treatment of the postthrombotic syndrome in this patient. Chronic lymphedema is the most common of the sequelae and unfortunately the one that cannot be relieved by any surgical procedure. It is believed to be secondary to scarring and fibrosis of the perivascular tissues in the groin with involvement of the lymphatic channels.

B. There has been a common belief, still held by many, that the thrombotic sequelae develop because the deep veins remain occluded after the deep venous thrombosis. As a result, surgeons have been afraid to eradicate the superficial varicosities because they have been considered to be necessary collateral channels for blood to return from the extremity. There have been a number of methods devised to determine whether the deep veins are patent or not. The reversed Trendelenburg test is the simplest and most reliable. It is performed by first having the patient stand to fill all the superficial veins, and then a venous tourniquet is placed around the thigh as shown.

C. The patient then lies down and elevates the leg to about a 40-degree angle, with attention being directed to the superficial veins that were distended in the erect position. As shown in the drawing, the prompt emptying of these veins with the tourniquet still in place demonstrates that the deep veins must be patent. The same result has been obtained in all postthrombotic extremities examined, thus proving that the deep veins of the lower extremity do recanalize following occlusion from deep venous thrombosis and that the sequelae, including the chronic ulcerations, are not the result of permanent occlusion of the deep venous system.

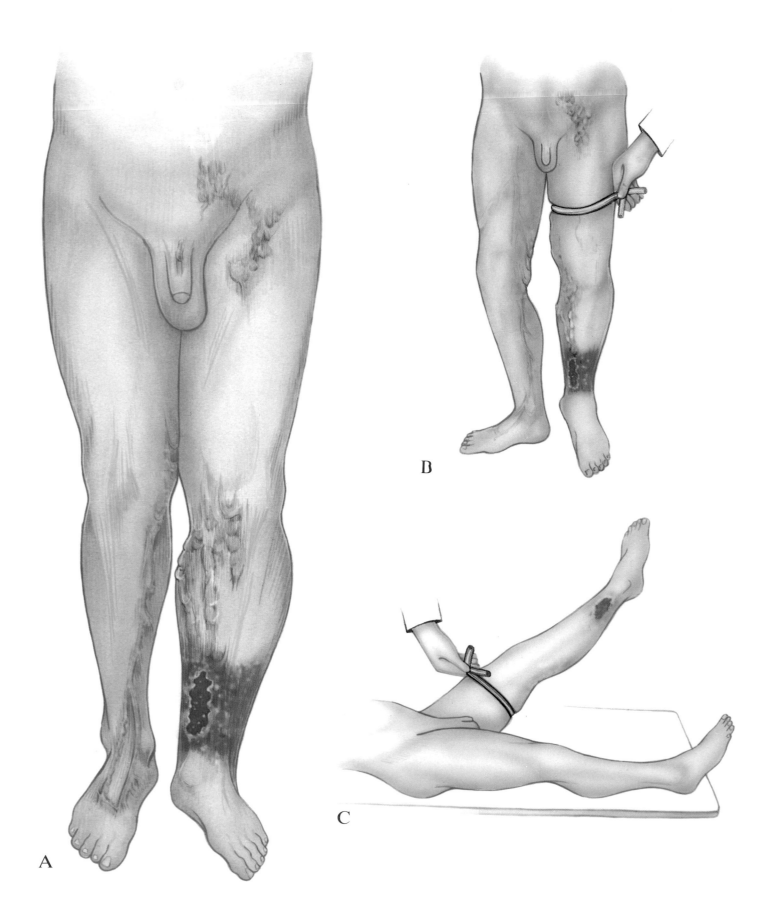

Plate 57

THE DEVELOPMENT OF THE POSTTHROMBOTIC SYNDROME

A. This shows the extent of the venous thrombosis in the deep major veins of the lower extremity. The thrombosis nearly always originates in the veins of the gastrocnemius and soleus muscles, then disseminates into the posterior tibial, popliteal, femoral and external iliac veins. It is frequently characterized by a sudden onset of pain and swelling of the entire leg, but often is preceded for several days by local pain and tenderness in the calf. In a few patients the condition may develop more slowly. Note that the entire lower extremity is swollen because lymphatic obstruction has occurred in addition to the venous occlusion. The valves of the veins that are still patent are shown to be competent. These are the classic pathological findings of the condition known as iliofemoral thrombophlebitis that develops within a short time into the so-called phlegmasia alba dolens, or milk leg, or in some patients, especially those with a poor arterial blood supply, phlegmasia cerulea dolens. Immediate operation with thrombectomy through the common femoral vein, usually with interruption of this vessel, is the best method of treatment (see Plate 49), followed by anticoagulation therapy.

B. The patients who are treated nonsurgically for iliofemoral venous thrombosis almost invariably develop the postthrombotic syndrome of the afflicted extremity in a relatively short period of time, one to three years postthrombophlebitis, and as the years go by may eventually develop chronic stasis or venous hypertensive ulceration of the lower leg. The reason for this is that the deep veins recanalize with extremely rare exception. This usually occurs within a year or two, the result of fibrinolysis of the occluding thrombus. Unfortunately even though venous patency does develop, the veins no longer act as an efficient conduit to return blood to the heart because the venous valves of the deep, communicating and superficial systems of the veins are incompetent, as shown. The lymphedema of the leg also persists, contributing to chronic skin and subcutaneous changes.

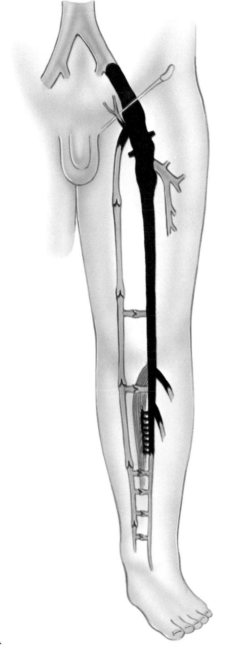

A

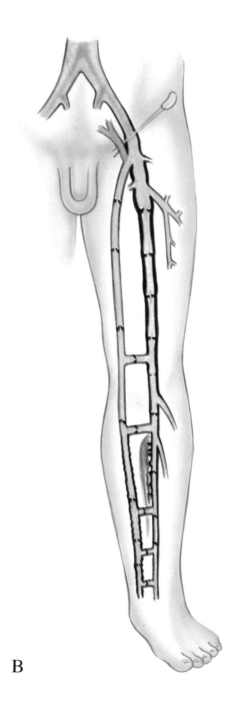

B

131

Plate 58

THE PATHOLOGIC ANATOMY AND PHYSIOLOGY OF THE POSTTHROMBOTIC SYNDROME

A. A drawing showing the gross changes in the deep, communicating and superficial systems of veins of the lower extremity that develop, in this order, in the postthrombotic syndrome. Note that the deep veins have all recanalized, but have thick walls that are incompetent because of destruction of their valves. The communicating veins have become dilated and, as a result, their valves are also incompetent. The superficial system, especially in the lower leg below the knee, has become incompetent for the same reasons.

The following sequence of changes, it is believed, occurs after an iliofemoral thrombophlebitis: First the deep veins that were occluded recanalize, often within a year. This results in an increase in the ambulatory venous pressure in the limb because of destruction of the venous valves. This is transmitted to the communicating system of veins which, because of inadequate support especially on the inner aspect of the lower leg, become dilated; as a result, their valves become incompetent. The increased pressure is then transmitted to the superficial system of veins of the lower leg, they in turn becoming dilated and incompetent. As a result of these changes, the state of ambulatory venous hypertension persists and is the cause of the chronic sequelae of stasis dermatitis, stasis pigmentation, stasis subcutaneous cellulitis and stasis ulcerations.

B. An enlargement of a microphotograph of a recanalized postthrombotic superficial femoral vein from the lower extremity that was removed 10 years after a deep iliofemoral thrombophlebitis. Note the extremely thick fibrous vein wall and the patent lumen. The venous valves were likewise stiff and fibrotic and, as a result, incompetent; even though patent, such a vein has lost its ability to effectively pump blood. For this reason experience has shown that it is better to interrupt such a diseased vein than to leave it in continuity, especially when a chronic ulcer has developed in the lower leg.

C. 1. The standing venous pressure in a postthrombotic extremity at the ankle is shown by cannulating a vein at this level. Note that the pressure is equal to a column of blood from the level of the heart to the point of venipuncture, the same as in a normal extremity.

2. The venous pressure in the same extremity is shown during ambulation. Note that it remains essentially unchanged; in some patients it has been noted to be slightly higher than the standing pressure.

3. The long saphenous vein is occluded at the knee level and, with the patient still ambulating, another pressure reading is taken. Again note there is no change. These studies clearly demonstrate the decompensation of the venous heart in the postthrombotic lower extremity that results in a state of ambulatory venous hypertension. It is these anatomical and physiological changes that have been observed that result in too much blood at too high a venous pressure, especially in the superficial and communicating veins, and are the main etiologic factor in the chronic ulceration of the postthrombotic syndrome. Since it is not possible to restore these venous systems to normal, it has been found that the best treatment for the condition is to perform a radical removal of the superficial veins, interrupt the communicating veins of the lower leg and, in addition, interrupt the deep system by ligation and division of the superficial femoral vein at its junction with the profunda femoris vein just distal to the common femoral vein, thereby forcing the blood to return through collateral venous channels.

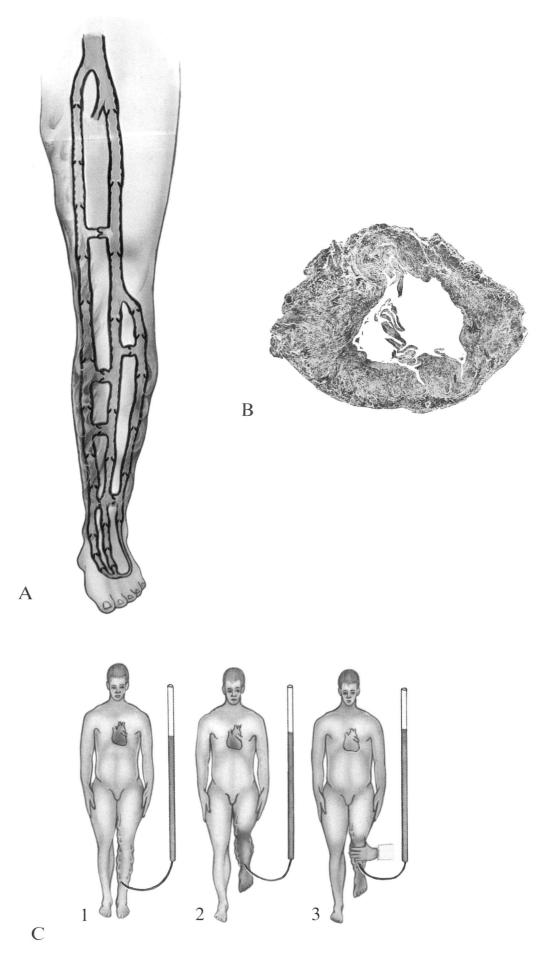

A

B

C

1   2   3

133

Plate 59

BED REST METHOD AND AMBULATORY METHOD OF HEALING POSTTHROMBOTIC CHRONIC ULCERATION OF THE LOWER LEG

A. The quickest method for healing a chronic postthrombotic ulceration of the lower leg is by bed rest, with the legs of the patient elevated and maintained above the level of the heart, as shown. The bed may be flattened for sleep at night. This is accomplished most easily with a hospital bed, but 6-inch blocks under the foot bedposts is a good method for home treatment. The ulcer is dressed daily at 8:00 A.M. with a large gauze dressing thoroughly wet with 2 per cent boric acid solution. The dressing is not changed until the following day but is wet again at 12:00 noon, at 6:00 P.M. and at bedtime. The patient is allowed lavatory privileges once a day, with the leg bandaged in a tight elastic 4-inch Ace bandage, and may have the head of the bed elevated to eat meals. With this treatment most ulcers will heal in two to three weeks; the larger ones will be clean enough so that they can be skin grafted.

B. This shows a typical recurrent chronic postthrombotic type of ulceration of the lower leg in a woman 42 years of age. She had seen many doctors and had had two operations performed on the veins of this extremity, but the ulceration had never remained healed. The great majority of chronic postthrombotic ulcerations of the lower extremity can be healed by ambulatory measures. This has the advantage of allowing the patient to continue at work. It is very important to determine to what materials and substances a patient's skin is allergic, because they have often used so many ointments and applications it is not uncommon to find they are allergic to some local applications. Many are sensitive to adhesive tape, and if so, cannot benefit from the following treatment. However, others are available. (See Plates 62 and 63.) One of the most satisfactory methods is to apply a tight Elastoplast boot from the toes to the knee. It is essential that the Elastoplast adhesive not come in contact with the skin even if the patient is not allergic to it. The first step is to apply a sticky substance to the skin which protects it and also prevents the gauze and Elastoplast boot from slipping about. It is absolutely essential that there be a firm bond between the skin, the ulcer dressing and the boot. One of the most satisfactory applications is to paint the entire skin of the lower leg and foot, except the ulcer area, with an alcoholic solution of resin which leaves the skin covered with a sticky film. Some patients are sensitive to this, and instead some of the spray materials available such as Vi-hesive may be used.

C. It is very difficult to remove this type of boot because it remains so adherent to the skin even two to three weeks after it has been applied. For this reason it is helpful to place a one-layer strip of gauze bandage up the lateral side of the foot and leg well away from the ulcer. This permits one to grasp the upper end of this strip to pull it away from the skin, allowing the insertion of the blade of a heavy pair of cutting shears beneath, thereby preventing injury to the leg.

D. A generous application of some form of ointment on the ulcer is recommended. One of the most satisfactory is bacitracin, but sometimes nitrofurazone (Furacin) in a water soluble base may prove more effective for a mixed infection, providing the patient is not allergic to it. A large gauze sponge dressing 1.5 to 2.0 cm. thick is applied to cover the ulcer area.

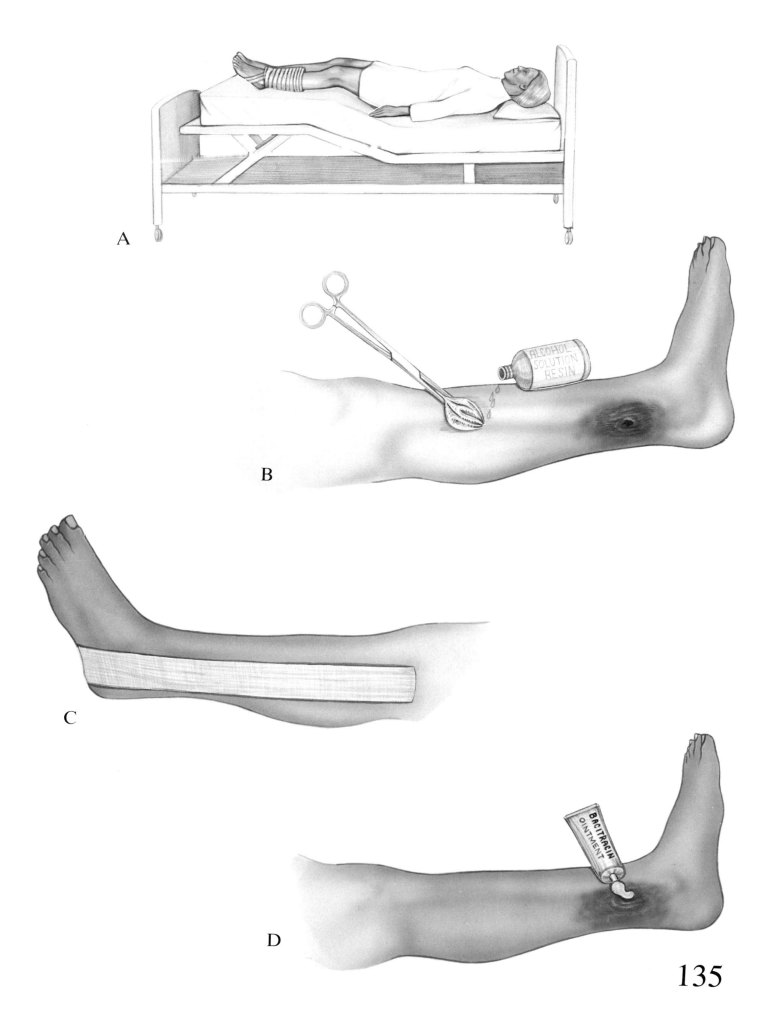

A

B

C

D

135

Plate 60

AMBULATORY METHOD OF HEALING POSTTHROMBOTIC CHRONIC ULCERATION OF THE LOWER LEG *(Continued)*

A. The next step is to wrap the leg from the toes to the knee with an entire roll of 4-inch gauze bandage, shown in white. It is applied loosely except over the gauze sponge dressing on the ulcer, where it is applied very snugly. The bandage becomes adherent to the resin that was applied to the skin. Sometimes, for extra pressure over the ulcer area, a ½-inch thick and 4- to 5-inch wide strip of cellu-cotton is wrapped around the leg one and a half times, with a double layer over the ulcer. This also is held in place with the gauze bandage. For some patients a large sanitary pad may be used for a pressure pad over the ulcer. This first layer of this type of boot gives the skin protection from the adhesive substance on the Elastoplast bandage. In addition, and of extreme importance, it permits the skin to breathe and some moisture to evaporate, thus preventing maceration.

B. The leg is then bandaged with a 4-inch wide 5-yard long Elastoplast bandage. This is commenced at the dorsum of the foot and carried from the inside to the outside around the foot nearly to the base of the toes. The bandage is then wound upward, making sure to cover the heel as shown. At the ankle level the bandage is wrapped tighter, especially over the thick dressing and any pads that have been used for extra pressure to obliterate all the superficial and communicating veins in that area. The bandaging continues up to just below the knee but is applied more loosely than in the distal area. This produces a pressure gradient from below upward on the extremity that helps to force the venous blood back toward the heart.

C. The Elastoplast bandage, having been carried as high as the gauze bandage, is then brought down the leg, reversing the diagonal application of the turns; this makes the boot much smoother, with fewer wrinkles. Note that the bandaging for an ulcer on the inner side of the leg should always be wrapped from the inside out, because this produces a much better pressure on the superficial and communicating veins to obliterate them than if it is applied the reverse way. The foot must be kept at 90 degrees of dorsiflexion during the bandaging to prevent wrinkling of the bandage over the instep.

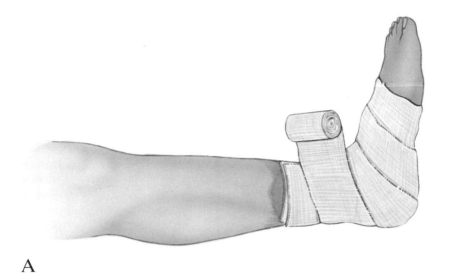

A

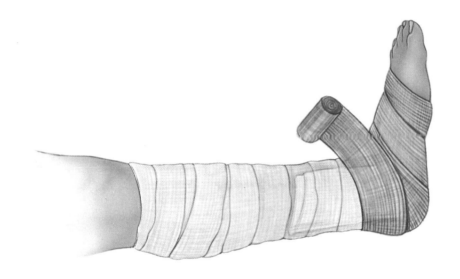

B

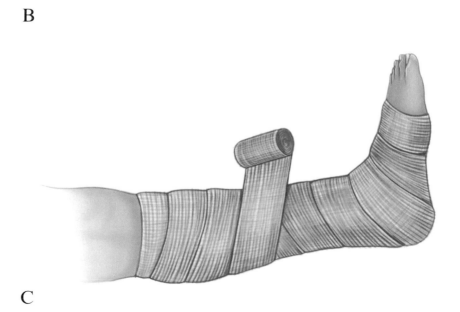

C

Plate 61

AMBULATORY METHOD OF HEALING POSTTHROMBOTIC CHRONIC ULCERATION OF THE LOWER LEG
(Continued)

A. This shows the completed Elastoplast boot, using the entire 5-yard length of the 4-inch bandage, which starts at the foot, is carried up to the knee and then down to end over the dorsum of the foot, with the end secured with 1-inch adhesive tape. It may be necessary to use a portion of another roll of Elastoplast bandage if a patient has an especially long, large leg. It is believed the complete double wrapping is important. It is important also to bring the second wrapping down from above so that each turn of the bandage overlaps the lower edge of the preceding turn. This prevents the turns from separating from each other and so keeps better even pressure on the leg. After the boot has been applied the patient is advised that walking will help to heal the ulcer quicker than sitting around, because the venous heart of the extremity has been compensated with this boot. It is very important that the bandage be kept dry, because if it gets wet maceration and infection of the skin develop; careful sponge baths are essential.

B. A diagrammatic drawing of the cross-section of the mid lower leg to show the location of the deep veins — posterior tibial, anterior tibial and peroneal. Extending from these are the dilated communicating veins joining with dilated superficial veins in the subcutaneous tissues exterior to the deep fascia. This abnormal dilatation of the communicating and superficial veins is the result of ambulatory venous hypertension and is believed to be the chief etiologic factor in producing the thrombotic sequelae, including chronic ulceration.

C. Another diagrammatic drawing to show the effect of a properly applied Elastoplast boot on these venous systems. Note the thick pads underneath the Elastoplast wrapping. The arrows denote the circumferential pressure that is applied by the boot all around the leg. A comparison of the size of the superficial and communicating veins shows that they are much smaller in caliber; some are practically obliterated.

D. These heavy cutting shears, that are closed by gripping them with the whole hand, are indispensable for removing the boot.

E. The boot is usually left on for a two-week period. If the ulcer is particularly large and has considerable discharge, it is best to change the first boot in one week and thereafter at two-week intervals. It is much easier to remove if the long strip of gauze bandage that was placed before putting on all bandages is picked up at the proximal end of the boot. By lifting the boot with the heavy cutting shears as shown, the shears are used to cut the boot without danger of injuring the underlying skin. Another similar type of dressing and boot are applied using the same technique. It usually requires four or five reapplications before the ulcer is healed. As soon as it is healed, the patient graduates to a two-way stretch, heavyweight, knee-length elastic stocking. A sanitary pad is placed on the inner side of the leg over the healed ulcer area and a mid leg length nylon stocking is worn to keep this pad in place while pulling on the heavyweight elastic stocking. This provides extra pressure to keep the veins obliterated in the ulcer area. The plan is to have the patient wear this stocking for six weeks, keeping ambulatory, before admitting him to the hospital for the more curative operative procedure.

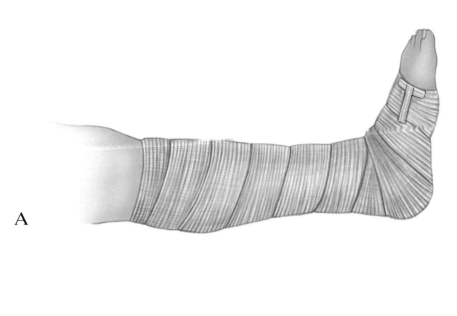

A

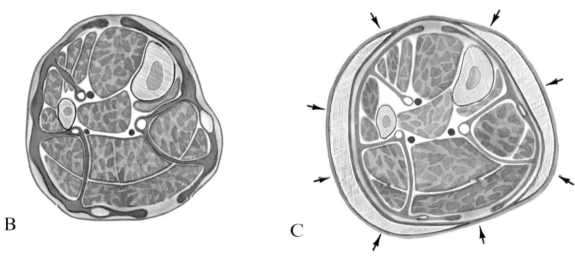

B

C

D

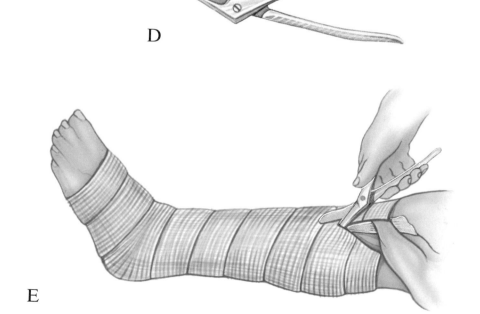

E

139

Plate 62

AMBULATORY METHOD OF HEALING POSTTHROMBOTIC CHRONIC ULCERATION OF THE LOWER LEG
(Continued)

A.   Some patients may be sensitive to the alcoholic resin solution, or the Elastoplast adhesive bandage, or both, and other methods should be available for them. The most useful one has proved to be some form of a Unna's paste type of boot. There are a number available on the market. My preference has been a Gelocast or an English primer type of impregnated 4-inch gauze bandage. These are moist and so do not adhere too well to the skin. Because of allergic reaction to resin, a spray type of application such as Vi-hesive is sprayed on the skin from the toes to the knee except over the ulcer.

B.   Several layers of the medicated bandage approximately 10 inches long are laid together and placed on the inner side of the foot, ankle and lower leg lengthways over the ulcer (1), usually after covering the ulcer with bacitracin ointment. The purpose of this is for more even application of pressure and to prevent the edges of the circular bandage wrappings from cutting into the skin. The circular bandages are next commenced just below the knee. The first few layers should be from a 4-inch white gauze roll bandage (2) which adheres to the compound sprayed on the skin. Then the medicated bandage (3) is started, and both bandages are continued as shown so that they interlock with each other. This method is used to prevent the bandage from slipping up and down on the leg, which might cause a new ulcer. Fixation of this type of boot to the skin is just as important as with the Elastoplast type. It should be noted that the heel must be completely covered with this type of boot also.

C.   The bandaging of the remainder of the leg, ankle and foot is completed with the medicated bandage. After several turns of the bandage have been completed, a thick pad of cellucotton or gauze or a large sanitary pad (1) is placed lengthways on the inner side of the lower leg and ankle over the ulcer area and incorporated into the remainder of the bandaging. This is for additional selective pressure on the ulcer area, in order to compress superficial and communicating veins.

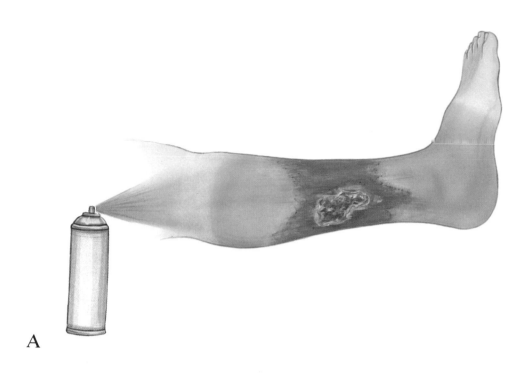

A

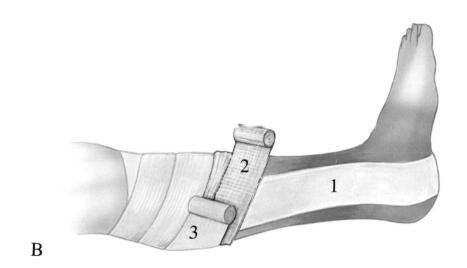

B

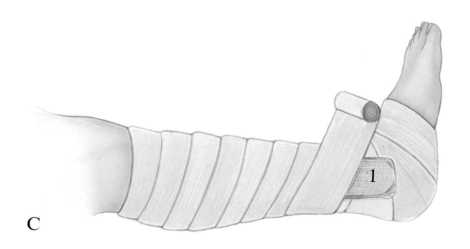

C

Plate 63

AMBULATORY METHOD OF HEALING POSTTHROMBOTIC CHRONIC ULCERATION OF THE LOWER LEG
(Continued)

A. The boot has been completed with the medicated bandage. Outside this another layer of white gauze bandage is applied and held in place with long adhesive strips. A final wrap is made with a 4-inch wide elastic gauze and rubber bandage that is applied very firmly. The patient removes this elastic bandage each night and reapplies it on arising in the morning. This helps to hold the medicated bandage against the skin more firmly.

B. The completed boot with the last wrapping is shown on the left leg. Note that this bandage starts at the foot and ends just below the knee. Some may prefer to do this the reverse way, which is equally effective and perhaps has the advantage that the individual turns of the bandage stay in place a little better, but it is more awkward for the patient to apply and to make neat at the ankle.

C. The same method is used to apply the bandages to the right leg, with the wrapping going from the inside to the outside anteriorly. The bandages are best applied to the right limb with one's back to the patient, whereas for the left limb one should be facing the patient. The only exception to this rule of bandaging is when the ulceration is on the outer side of the leg or ankle. Under these conditions it is better to apply the bandage with the wrapping from the outside to the inside anteriorly. This type of medicated boot should be changed at two- to three-week intervals. It has an advantage over the Elastoplast boot in that the drainage from the ulcer tends to dry, so that the skin does not often become macerated. The bandage does become quite rigid, which is troublesome if the ulcer is over or near the malleoli. It is also worth pointing out that ulcers between the malleoli and the os calcis, or just distal to the malleoli, are difficult to treat in this manner because motion at the ankle joint causes continual movement of the dressing over the ulcer. This type of ulcer is usually best treated with bed rest, elevation of the legs above the heart level, and application of a 2 per cent boric acid solution dressing in the morning that is moistened again at 12 noon, 6:00 P.M. and bedtime. Ambulation is limited to toilet privileges once a day. After the ulcers have been healed either with the medicated boots or the bed rest and elevation technique, heavyweight, knee-length, two-way stretch elastic stockings with a heel should be worn, with pads of cellucotton or sanitary pads over the ulcer area for one to two months, after which venous surgery is performed. (See Plate 59*A*.)

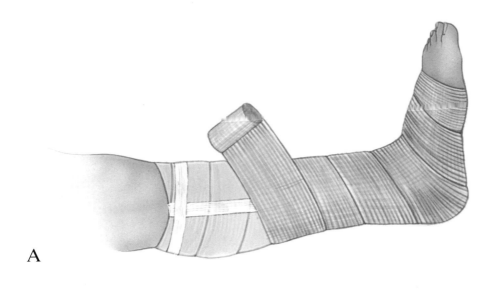

A

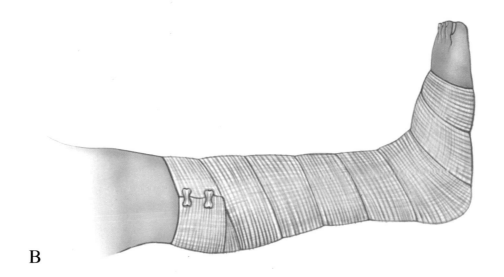

B

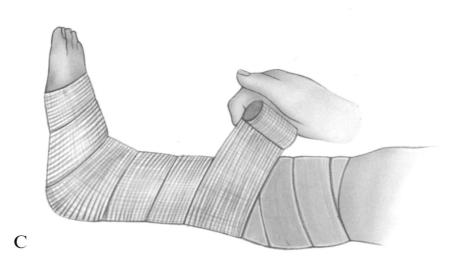

C

143

Plate 64

SURGICAL PROCEDURES FOR THE POSTTHROMBOTIC SYNDROME OF THE LOWER EXTREMITY WITH ULCERATION

LIGATION AND STRIPPING OF THE LONG SAPHENOUS VEIN AND INTERRUPTION OF THE SUPERFICIAL FEMORAL VEINS.

After the patient's ulcer has been healed for four to eight weeks and the stasis dermatitis has cleared up, an operative procedure known as the "Linton Flap Operation" is performed to interrupt the long saphenous and the superficial femoral veins, to remove the long and short saphenous veins, and to interrupt the communicating veins beneath the deep fascia of the lower leg.

A. The first step in the operative procedure is to expose the long saphenous (1), the common femoral (2), the superficial femoral (3), and the profunda femoris (4) veins at the groin through a longitudinal incision a little to the inner side of the femoral artery pulse. The saphenofemoral and the superficial femoral and profunda femoris junctions should be clearly visualized. If the patient has had a previous iliofemoral thrombophlebitis, the femoral vein may be adherent to the femoral artery by scar tissue so that care must be taken not to injure either, especially the artery. The safest method of dissecting it is to retract the adventitia as shown, which also helps the surgeon to separate the vein from it. The superficial femoral vein, except in the most rare instances, has always recanalized in the postthrombotic state. The wall will be very firm, thick and grayish in color if thrombophlebitis has pre-existed.

A ligature is passed around the long saphenous vein and the superficial femoral vein. A preocclusion venous pressure (5) is taken in the superficial femoral vein; then the saphenous and superficial femoral veins are occluded by tightly clamping the ligatures. A postocclusion pressure is taken distal to the ligature in the superficial femoral vein. Note that the preocclusion level (5) is 17 cm. of normal saline and the postocclusion (6) is 20 cm., an increase of only 3 cm. In some patients it may be even lower. If the venous pressure rises only a few centimeters, the surgeon is able to determine by this simple test whether the venous collaterals are competent to take care of the return blood flow of the saphenous vein and the superficial femoral veins and that it will be safe to permanently occlude them by ligation and division. On the other hand, if the pressure rises to three to four times the initial pressure, it is recommended that the superficial femoral vein not be interrupted.

B. The superficial femoral vein has been ligated and divided flush with the profunda femoris vein. Each end has been doubly ligated with a ligature and a transfixion suture of linen or cotton. The saphenous vein has also been interrupted and the trunk stripped distalward. The incision is closed meticulously in layers with interrupted sutures of fine linen or cotton.

C. An enlargement of a photomicrograph of a recanalized superficial femoral vein removed at the time the vein was interrupted nine years after a deep iliofemoral thrombophlebitis. Note the thick scarred fibrous walls, that are so stiff the muscles cannot compress them efficiently. For this reason it is believed better to interrupt these badly diseased veins than to leave them in continuity.

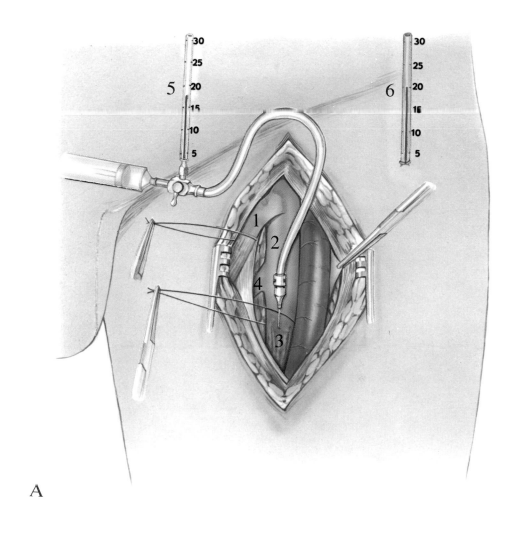

A

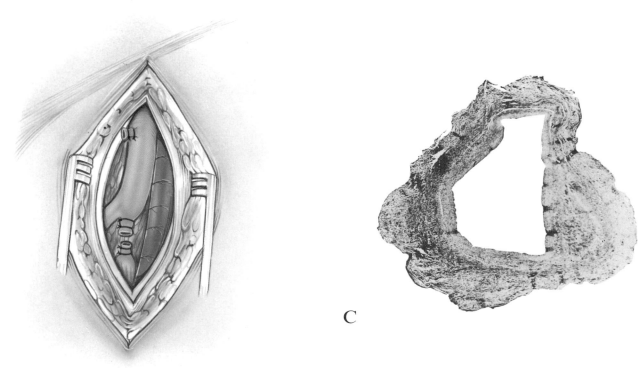

B

C

145

Plate 65

SURGICAL PROCEDURES FOR THE POSTTHROMBOTIC SYNDROME OF THE LOWER EXTREMITY WITH ULCERATION *(Continued)*

INTERRUPTION OF THE COMMUNICATING VEINS OF THE LEFT LOWER LEG

A.   With the patient lying supine and the operating table in 15 degree Trendelenburg position, the knee is bent at about a 15 degree angle. A long linear incision is made from the level of the tibial tubercle distal and posterior to the internal malleolus with a hockey stick curve at the distal end. This incision in the proximal three quarters of the lower leg is about 1 cm. posterior to the inner edge of the tibia. As it is necessary to keep it straight, there should be no hesitation about cutting directly through the healed ulcer bed. This is much safer than trying to circumvent it, which will too often result in a skin slough. The value of the straight incision cannot be overemphasized as a means of preventing wound edge skin sloughs.

B.   The incision is carried down through the deep fascia. In the ulcer area there will be very thick scar tissue, sometimes 5 to 10 mm. thick. This fibrous overgrowth that replaces the subcutaneous fat is still believed by some to be the chief etiologic factor of the chronic ulcers. This has proved not to be true, as it is never excised in this type of operative procedure that gives such excellent long-term results. The divided varicosities that are encountered in the subcutaneous tissues are secured with 3-0 plain catgut ligatures. The Trendelenburg position reduces the bleeding and, surprisingly, the interruption of the superficial femoral vein carried out as the first step also frequently reduces the bleeding. The edges of the deep fascia on the anterior skin flap are grasped with Kocher clamps which are used as retractors to expose the communicating veins as shown. The number varies greatly. They are readily exposed, as there is an easy cleavage plane of loose areolar tissue between the muscles and deep fascia that is bridged only by the communicating vessels since there is usually a small artery with each vein.

C.   The dissection is carried further forward, raising the anterior skin and deep fascia flap. This exposes incompetent communicating veins that lie immediately posterior to the tibia and communicate with the posterior tibial veins. The proximal ones (1) and (2) along with their concomitant arteries and the ones coming out through the gastrocnemius and soleus muscles (3) have been ligated and divided. The deep fascia is being incised with a knife near its insertion to the tibia. A small strip of deep fascia on the flap edge is not removed as this is needed for the closure of the incision. This exposes a portion of the long saphenous vein which will be excised. The distal portion extending further toward the foot will be stripped with an intraluminal stripper to avoid raising a skin flap over the internal malleolus that might cause a skin slough. The origins of four distal communicating veins arising from the posterior tibial vein are shown; these will also be ligated and divided. Note the most distal one near the small rake retractor; it is this one that is frequently overlooked because the incision is not carried sufficiently distalward to expose it.

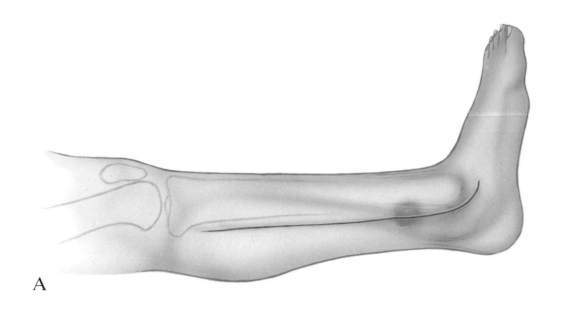

A

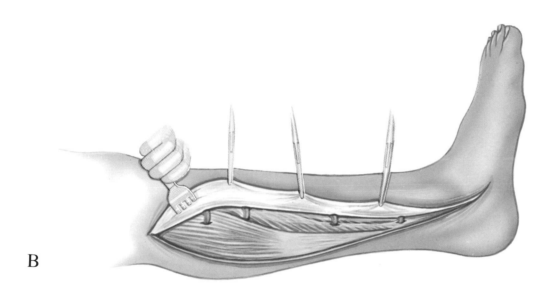

B

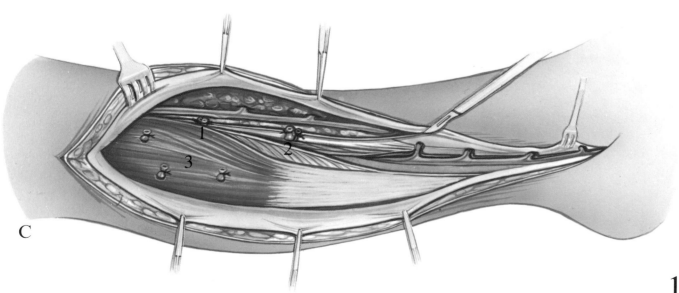

C

147

Plate 66

SURGICAL PROCEDURES FOR THE POSTTHROMBOTIC SYNDROME OF THE LOWER EXTREMITY WITH ULCERATION *(Continued)*

INTERRUPTION OF THE COMMUNICATING VEINS OF THE LEFT LOWER LEG *(Continued)*

A. The mid portion of the saphenous vein in the lower leg (1) held with the two hemostats has been excised. The proximal portion of it shown on the internal stripper has been removed up to the groin. The distal portion is shown with the stripper in it. The small end of the stripper can be seen coming out of another small incision made near the base of the great toe. This portion of the vein is then removed by pulling on the stripper. It is very important not to raise the skin flap over the medial malleolus because this may cause sloughing of the skin and another ulcer.

B. The anterior portion of the operative procedure has been completed with ligation and division of all the communicating veins and concomitant arteries. The success of the procedure depends in great measure on making sure that none have been left uninterrupted. The distal veins below the malleolus are the most often missed, so the dissection should be carried far enough distally to see the posterior tibial vessels disappear under the adductor hallucis muscle to make sure none have been missed, especially if there are stasis changes in the skin in this area.

C. The posterior part of the operative procedure is carried out by retracting the flexor muscles of the foot anteriorly in order to develop a large posterior skin and deep fascial flap. The short saphenous vein is usually visible through this at about the midline of the leg posteriorly. An incision is made in the deep fascia with a knife to expose the vein and the sural nerve that lies in close proximity to it. This is done carefully so as not to injure the latter.

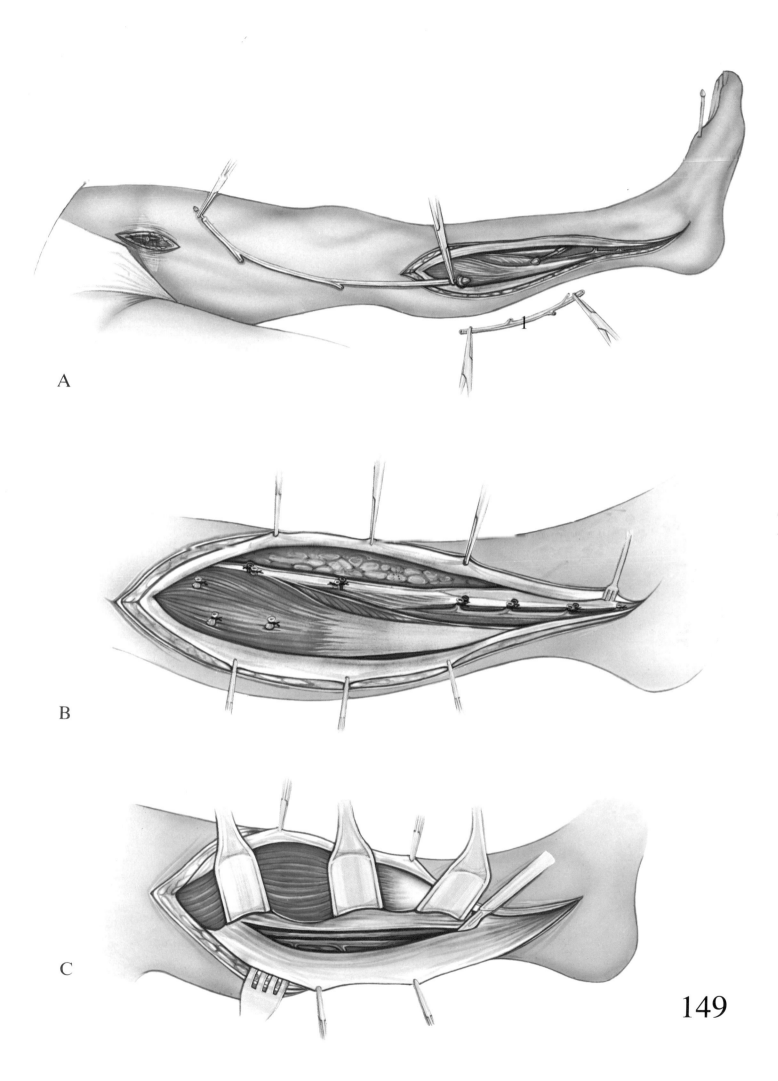

A

B

C

149

Plate 67

SURGICAL PROCEDURES FOR THE POSTTHROMBOTIC SYNDROME OF THE LOWER EXTREMITY WITH ULCERATION *(Continued)*

INTERRUPTION OF COMMUNICATING VEINS OF THE LEFT LOWER LEG *(Continued)*

A. The posterior flap is stretched out wide with the retractors still in place against the flexor muscles and Kocher clamps on the deep fascia of the main incision for countertraction. This permits removal of a large triangular piece of deep fascia to expose more of the sural nerve, the short saphenous vein and any subcutaneous varicosities. The chief reason for excising the fascia is that many varicosities can be uncovered and removed that otherwise would remain and probably cause stasis changes in the future. It should be remembered that the success rate of the procedure is directly proportional to the completeness with which one accomplishes removal of the superficial varicosities and interruption of the communicating veins. A second advantage is that this permits closure of the long incision without tension since the skin and subcutaneous tissues are relatively elastic. A third possible advantage is that it may allow lymph from the skin and superficial tissues to drain into the muscle lymphatics, similar to a Kondoleon procedure. Note that a centimeter-wide strip of the deep fascia has been left attached to the edge of the long incision. This is used for deep fascial closure but avoids suturing of the subcutaneous tissues, which if done would result in extensive wound edge sloughing.

B. The main trunk of the short saphenous vein is partially excised and the distal segment is removed with an intraluminal stripper that is passed distalward in it. The small end is brought out through a small incision just posterior and distal to the external malleolus, seen here projecting from the far side of the heel. The sural nerve is plainly visible so injury of it rarely occurs. The proximal and distal ends of the vein are ligated with 3-0 plain catgut ligatures. Any branches of the vein or varicosities are removed. The proximal ligation is not at the saphenopopliteal junction; but since the superficial femoral vein has been interrupted proximally in the groin, the danger of pulmonary embolism from this relatively long stump is prevented. Bleeding vessels are controlled with 3-0 plain catgut ligatures and the use of the diathermy.

C. The operative field is washed out thoroughly with normal saline solution. The incision is closed with interrupted sutures of 3-0 chromic catgut to approximate the narrow rims of deep fascia that were left on the edges of the incision. Note again that to avoid skin edge sloughs *no* sutures should be placed in the subcutaneous tissues. The skin is closed with simple sutures of No. 36 stainless steel wire. These are preferred to vertical mattress sutures since it may be helpful to leave them in place for two or three weeks to reduce the danger of skin sloughs.

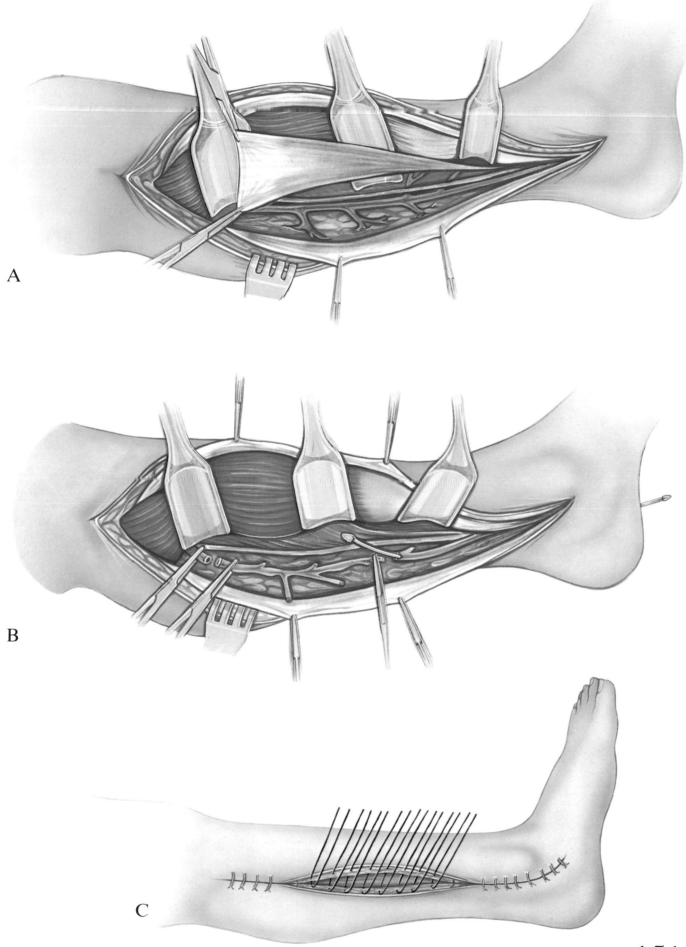

A

B

C

151

Plate 68

SURGICAL PROCEDURES FOR THE POSTTHROMBOTIC SYNDROME OF THE LOWER EXTREMITY WITH ULCERATION *(Continued)*

INTERRUPTION OF COMMUNICATING VEINS OF THE LEFT LOWER LEG *(Continued)*

A. A thick spongy gauze dressing should be placed over the incision and held in place with a 4-inch Ace bandage extending from the base of the toes to over the tibial tubercle, then a light plaster cast applied. Most patients with chronic ulcers have some degree of equinus because of pain. One of the purposes of the plaster cast is to place the foot back in a right angle position with the patient under anesthesia. The cast is removed in one week when the first dressing is done. Postural exercises are commenced if primary healing is observed, with the foot and leg snugly wrapped with two 4-inch elastic cotton bandages over a thick gauze dressing. These consist of three minutes of elevation of the leg to a 30 degree angle, then two minutes of dependency, followed by five minutes of horizontal rest. Three times a day this is repeated six times, for a total of three hours. After three or four days of this regimen the patient is permitted up to walk and is discharged home in a few days after removal of the wire skin sutures, with an Elastoplast boot for support. If healing is complete in two weeks, a heavyweight, two-way stretch elastic stocking with a heel is worn daily for at least a year. If skin sloughs do develop, the skin sutures at these sites should be removed. The sloughing area is exposed to the air to permit the development of dry gangrene with a clear line of demarcation. The blackened area is then excised with a sharp knife. The edges are pulled together with adhesive strips.

B. A color photograph of the right lower leg of a man aged 66 years shows a postthrombotic ulceration of the calf area that developed five years after a posttraumatic femoroiliac venous thrombosis. The location of the ulcer is higher on the limb than usual, but in the area of the calf communicating veins. Note the deep purplish color of the skin surrounding the ulcer from dilated and ruptured skin capillaries secondary to the postthrombotic ambulatory venous hypertension, and a much wider area of brownish discoloration, the late pigmentary changes due to hemosiderin that develop following capillary cutaneous hemorrhage.

C. A close-up view of the ulcer and the skin around it, showing numerous subepithelial petechial hemorrhages.

D. A color photograph of the same extremity one year following the operative procedure of interruption of the superficial femoral vein, the communicating veins in the lower leg, and ligation and stripping of the long and short saphenous veins. Note the well healed incision and ulcer, and especially the change in the color of the skin, which is the result of disconnection of the deep and superficial systems of veins, interruption of the valveless deep system and removal of the veins of the superficial system. The color of the skin has changed now to a light tan. Elastic support was still necessary because of persistent lymphedema, a small price to pay for a healed postthrombotic ulcer.

E. A close-up view of the healed ulcer and the skin surrounding it. Note the absence of capillary petechial hemorrhages seen in the preoperative photograph (*C*). The brownish tan pigment discoloration of the skin is permanent. It is less noticeable if the operative procedure described here is performed early in the development of the postthrombotic syndrome.

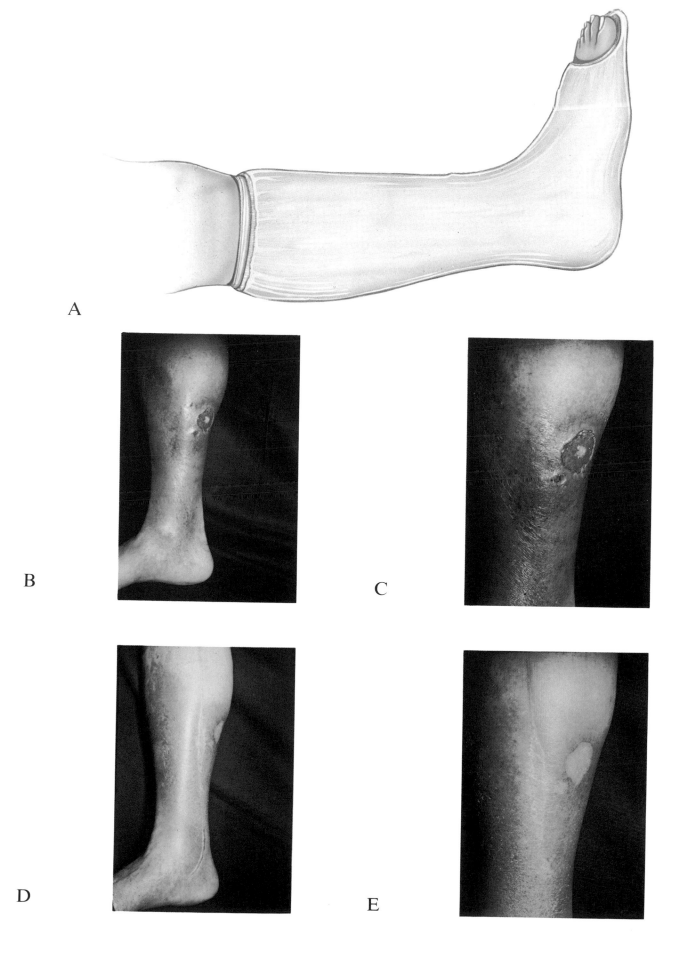

A

B

C

D

E

153

Plate 69

EXCISION OF A POSTTHROMBOTIC STASIS ULCER WITH PRIMARY SPLIT-THICKNESS SKIN GRAFT

A. In a few patients who have had a postthrombotic stasis ulcer for many years, as in the man aged 37 years who had this chronic ulceration for 19 years, the best form of treatment is wide excision of the ulcer and the surrounding diseased skin and subcutaneous tissues combined with an interruption of the superficial femoral vein and the communicating veins at the same operative procedure. The large ulcer is first cleaned up with topical application of an antibiotic solution to which the predominant bacteria are sensitive. Note the discolored skin around the large ulcer. The broken line at the periphery of the skin marks the area that is to be excised along with the ulcer.

B. The excision of the ulcer with careful beveling of the edges has been commenced, starting posteriorly then carrying the dissection anteriorly. The row of hemostats is on the deep fascia. It is of paramount importance that all the deep fascia and the subcutaneous scar tissue be excised to lay bare the muscles (1), the tendons with the peritendineum covering them (2), the periosteum of the tibia (3), and some of the tissue over the neurovascular bundle. It is essential for long-term success that the skin graft have normal tissues as a base. Most surgeons do not carry the dissection deep enough to excise the deep fascia and, as a result, their skin grafts are placed on scar tissue, which causes most of them to fail, with recurrent ulceration. Another advantage of the deeper excision is that the incompetent communicating veins beneath the ulcer area are divided and ligated near their origins. Anterior and posterior skin and fascia flaps are raised to interrupt the communicating veins in the calf area and also to facilitate the stripping of the long and short saphenous veins.

C. Complete hemostasis of the area for the skin graft is essential. Fine catgut ligatures for the larger vessels and diathermy for the small capillaries are used so that the area is absolutely "dry." The split-thickness skin grafts should be obtained before excising the ulcer in order to keep the donor site from bacterial contamination. Multiple small openings are made in the grafts to allow serum to leak out. It is better not to suture the grafts to the skin but rather to hold them in place by means of a large, firm, gauze dressing. It is helpful also to use a bacteriostatic preparation on the dressing, such as bacitracin ointment, which also aids absorption of the serous drainage into the dressing. A 4-inch elastic gauze Ace bandage is applied firmly. Penicillin and streptomycin are given intramuscularly for five to seven days.

It is essential that the ankle joint be immobilized by application of a plaster cast from the toes to the level of the tibial tubercle. (See Plate 68 *A*.) This is to prevent motion of the structures under the skin graft because if this occurs there will be a very poor take. The patient is kept at bed rest with slight elevation of the leg for one week. The cast is then removed and the graft inspected. As a rule, it will be found to have taken nearly 100 per cent. Moist dressings of normal saline are used for a few days and then the postural exercises are commenced. Ambulation with firm elastic support is started when the graft has cleaned up, usually not before two weeks after the operation. At the time of discharge from the hospital an Elastoplast boot is applied. (See Plates 59 to 61.) This is changed in two weeks and a new one applied. Following removal of this in two weeks, the patient is graduated to a heavyweight elastic stocking that must be worn for a year or longer.

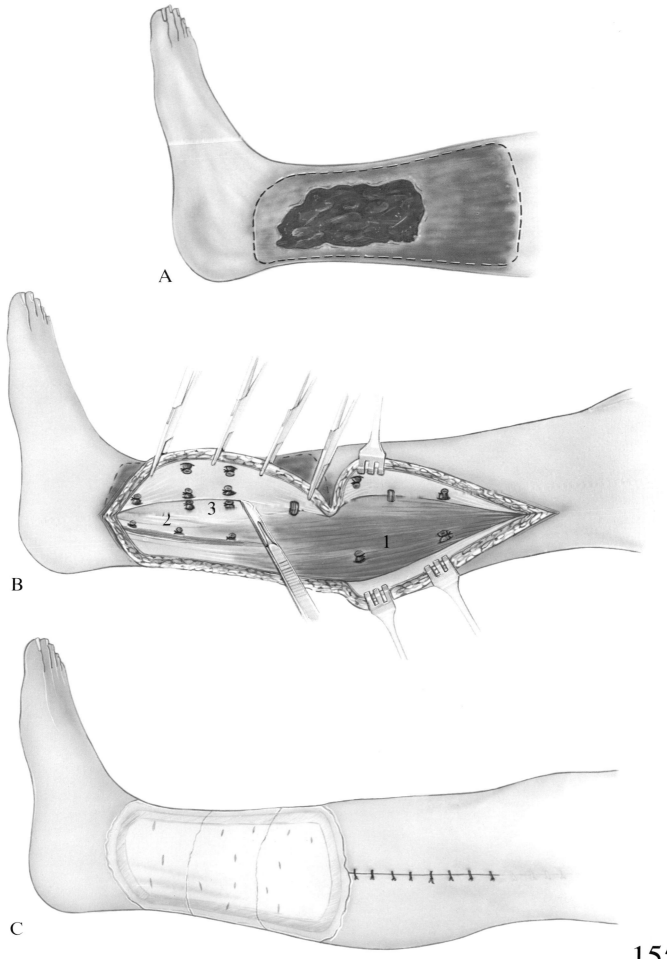

A

B

1

2

3

C

155

Plate 70

TWO-STAGE OPERATIVE PROCEDURE FOR CHRONIC ULCER

Another method of treating large chronic postthrombotic ulcerations is a two-stage procedure, demonstrated here by the color photographs. The first stage requires hospitalization to clean up the ulceration and to apply a skin graft. After complete healing the patient is discharged home until readmission for definitive surgery on the superficial, deep and communicating systems of veins.

I. PRIMARY SPLIT-THICKNESS SKIN GRAFT
II. INTERRUPTION OF THE SUPERFICIAL FEMORAL VEIN, LIGATION AND STRIPPING OF THE LONG AND SHORT SAPHENOUS VEINS, AND INTERRUPTION OF THE COMMUNICATING VEINS OF THE LOWER LEG

A and B. Color photographs showing a large chronic postthrombotic ulceration that almost encircles the left ankle. It first developed 10 years after a postpartum iliofemoral thrombosis and healed off and on for short periods over a term of seven years; it had slowly increased to its present size during the last three years. The photographs were taken after the ulceration had been cleaned up with the patient at bed rest and the legs elevated above the heart level (Plate 59 *A*), and moist dressings of 2 per cent boric acid solution changed once each morning and moistened with the same solution at 12:00 noon, 6:00 P.M. and 10:00 P.M. Split-thickness skin grafts were placed on the clean granulating ulcer and the ankle immobilized with a lower leg plaster cast.

C and D. Color photographs show a complete take of the skin graft. An Elastoplast boot was applied, as shown in Plates 59 and 61, and changed in two weeks. The patient was discharged completely ambulatory to be readmitted to the hospital in one month for the second stage of the procedure.

E. A color photograph taken on readmission to the hospital seven weeks after skin grafting. Note the stasis dermatitis, the skin discoloration and the large varicose veins—all evidence of incompetent superficial, deep and communicating veins and ambulatory venous hypertension. These early signs of skin graft breakdown despite good support to the leg demonstrate the cardinal principle that skin grafts to the granulating ulcer never survive in the postthrombotic extremity unless definitive surgery is performed on the diseased veins.

F. A color photograph taken three weeks after the definitive surgery, as described in Plates 64 to 68. Note the long incision extending behind and distal to the internal malleolus that was carried through the skin graft and ulcer area. The subcutaneous tissues had been replaced with scar tissue 1 cm. thick, which explains the slower healing in this area. Note the normal color of the skin, which is in great contrast to its appearance in *E*. Complete healing was obtained with the use of Elastoplast boots for a few weeks. Since then the patient has continued to wear a heavyweight elastic stocking and applies 0.25 per cent hydrocortisone cream to the skin of the ankle area daily. There has been no recurrence of the ulceration.

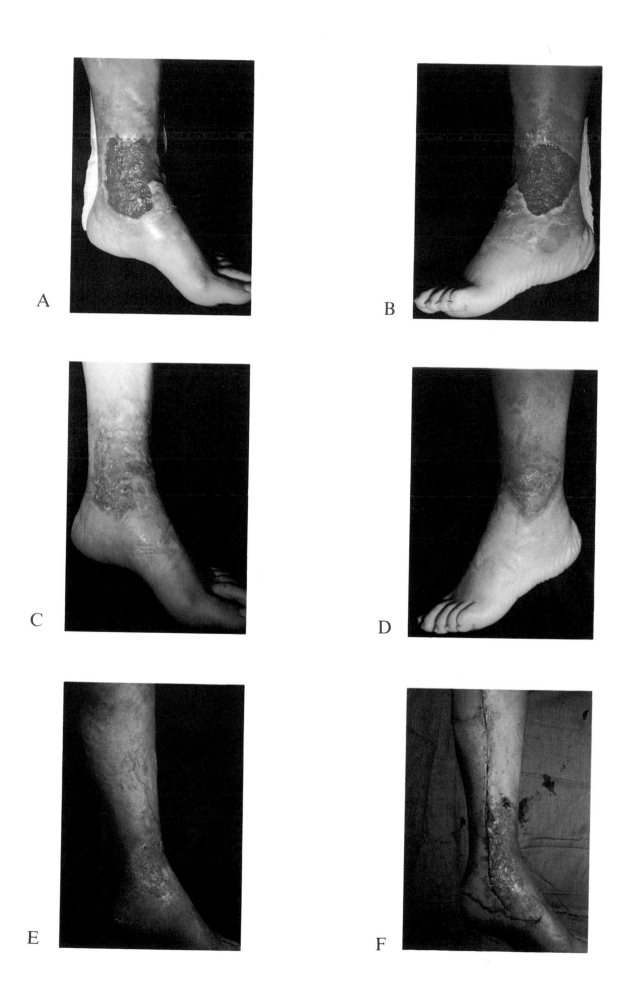

A

B

C

D

E

F

157

BLEEDING ESOPHAGEAL VARICES

Introduction

Esophageal varices develop because of a state of portal venous hypertension, the result of an obstruction to the outflow of the portal venous blood from the portal vein. Portal cirrhosis of the liver is the most common cause of this obstruction and produces an intrahepatic portal venous block. The extrahepatic block is much less common; it is the result of a thrombophlebitis involving the portal vein, probably secondary to omphalitis and thrombophlebitis of the umbilical vein following childbirth. The splenic vein is usually not involved. In some patients with cirrhosis of the liver, secondary thrombosis of the portal vein occurs, resulting in a combined intra- and extrahepatic type of portal bed block. The esophageal varices are large venous channels through which some of the portal blood is being shunted into the systemic venous system by way of the azygos and hemi-azygos system of veins. Unfortunately these communications are not sufficiently large to shunt enough portal venous blood so that a state of portal venous hypertension develops. Many of the tributaries of the portal vein, including the submucous veins of the cardia of the stomach, become greatly dilated. These connect directly with the submucous plexus of veins in the esophagus at the cardioesophageal junction. Esophageal varices, when present, are a constant and serious threat to a patient's life, since many individuals succumb to exsanguinating hemorrhage from their rupture. The point of rupture is invariably within a few centimeters of the cardioesophageal junction, and it is believed to occur as a result of trauma to the distal end of the esophagus where it passes through the diaphragm.

Severe hemorrhage frequently develops without warning, and if some emergency means is not taken to control the hemorrhage the patient succumbs as a result of exsanguination and liver failure. Bleeding from esophageal varices in many patients is not the exsanguinating type, and it is these who do well on medical treatment preparatory to definitive portal systemic venous shunt surgery. An emergency direct anastomosis between the portal vein and the inferior vena cava by the end-to-side technique does control the bleeding in some patients, but it carries a relatively high operative mortality rate of 40 to 50 per cent. In addition, unfortunately, the patients who survive develop a high incidence of postshunt encephalopathy and late death from liver failure because of the total diversion of the portal venous blood by this procedure.

When performed correctly, cardioesophageal tamponage with an intragastric balloon type of tube is a safe method for temporary control of the severe esophageal bleeding that will not stop spontaneously. A number of different types of balloon tubes has been developed. The most effective has proved to be a tube with a large intragastric balloon that holds 700 to

800 cc. of air. Traction on the tube compresses the submucosal veins of the cardia of the stomach, with immediate control of the bleeding varix. As soon as the bleeding is controlled, the patient's blood loss is replaced and his or her condition evaluated; if satisfactory, a more definitive control of the bleeding varix should be obtained within 12 hours by transthoraco-esophageal suture of the distal esophageal varices, to be followed five to six weeks later, preferably, by a splenectomy and an end-to-side splenorenal shunt.

Plate 71

THE EMERGENT TREATMENT OF BLEEDING ESOPHAGEAL VARICES

CARDIOESOPHAGEAL BALLOON TAMPONAGE

A. This shows a triple lumen tube with a single, large, gastric balloon containing 700 cc. of air, known as the "Linton" tube. Use of this has been found to be the most effective method of obtaining immediate temporary control of massive bleeding from esophageal varices. One of the lumens (a) connects with the balloon for inflation and deflation of it; the second (b) connects with the distal end of the tube to permit lavage and aspiration of the stomach; and the third one (c) stops above the balloon and permits aspiration of the esophagus.

B. This depicts a sagittal section of the distal esophagus and the cardia of the stomach to show the varices of the esophagus and the stomach, and that the former are a direct continuation of the latter. Comprehension of this is of fundamental importance when one attempts to obtain immediate control of massive bleeding from rupture of the esophageal varices, because blood that escapes from the esophageal varices all comes from the submucosal veins and varices of the cardia of the stomach.

C. This demonstrates tamponage of the gastric cardal varices with a single intragastric balloon tube that will immediately control bleeding from a ruptured esophageal varix. The tube is inserted through one of the nares and passed down the esophagus into the stomach. Its position in the stomach should be checked by fluoroscopy to avoid rupture of the esophagus if the balloon should be inadvertently inflated in it. After it has been determined that the balloon is within the stomach it is inflated with 700 cc. of air. The proximal end of the tube is pulled back, causing the balloon to impinge against the cardia of the stomach and the undersurface of the diaphragm and permitting slight herniation of the balloon into the distal end of the esophagus. Constant tension is maintained on the tube by attaching a 1-kg. weight to the reinforced tab with a thin cotton line that passes over a pulley at the foot of the bed. It should be noted that the balloon tamponage is resorted to only when the bleeding is so massive that the patient's life is endangered from exsanguination. Bleeding will stop almost instantaneously with this wide type of tamponage if the bleeding is from a ruptured esophageal varix. It is to be emphasized that this tube should be used only for the emergency control of hemorrhage, and tension on it must be maintained for no longer than 24 hours because of the danger of necrosis of the cardioesophageal junction. This balloon tube may be helpful also in the differential diagnosis of upper gastrointestinal hemorrhage since it will not control bleeding from a gastric or duodenal ulcer or that caused by gastritis.

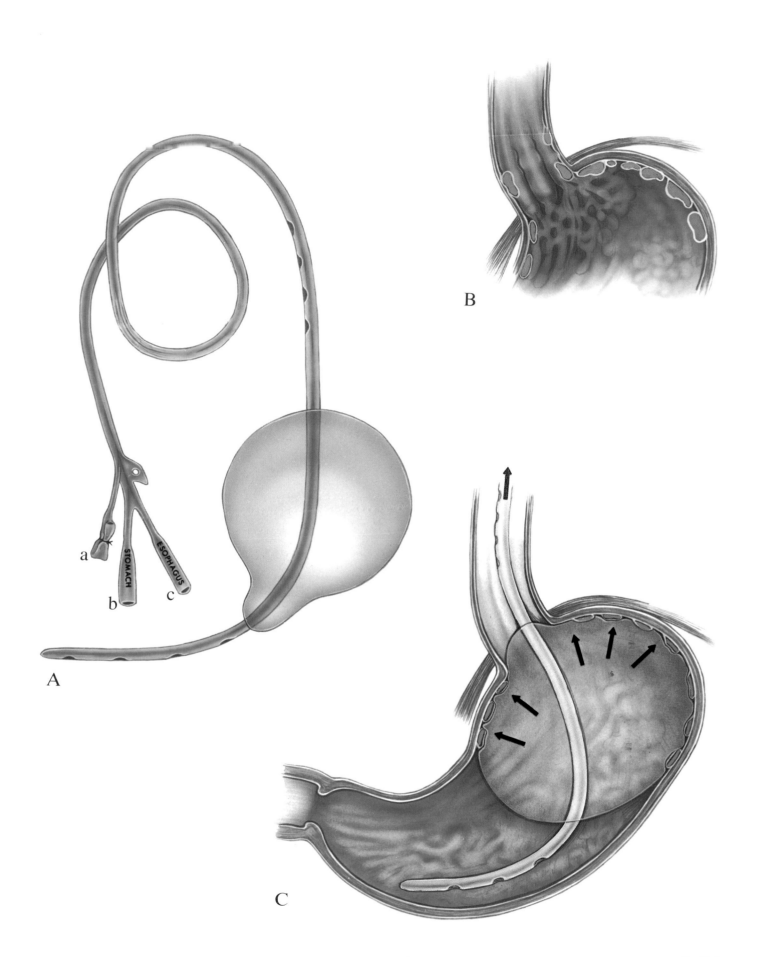

A

B

C

Plate 72

THE EMERGENT TREATMENT OF
BLEEDING ESOPHAGEAL VARICES
(Continued)

TRANSTHORACOESOPHAGEAL SUTURE OF BLEEDING
ESOPHAGEAL VARICES

If balloon tamponage has been necessary to stop the bleeding from esophageal varices, a more definitive control should be obtained. It is a well accepted surgical principle that the best method of controlling a bleeding blood vessel is to either ligate or suture it. The rule I have followed is that if balloon cardioesophageal tamponage has been necessary to save a patient's life from hemorrhage, it is mandatory that as soon as the patient's blood loss has been replaced, and providing he is not in coma or severely jaundiced, more definitive control of the bleeding esophageal varices should be obtained immediately by transthoracoesophageal suture of them. If one relies only on the balloon tube to control the bleeding, too frequently after removal of it in one or two days, the bleeding recurs. If suture of the varices is performed after this delay, the patient will be in a worse nutritional state than when he was first seen and so will be a poorer risk for the operative procedure. The method as described here not only saves lives, but allows a period of six weeks during which the patient can be brought into better condition to withstand the definitive procedure of portal systemic venous shunt.

A. This demonstrates the right lateral decubitus position and the location of the thoracic incision. The left diaphragm of many of the patients rides high because of an enlarged spleen and frequently also as a result of ascites. For this reason the incision should be placed over the sixth or seventh rib. The anesthetic of choice is cyclopropane administered through an endotracheal cuffed tube which is inserted after local cocainization of the pharynx and larynx to prevent aspiration of regurgitated blood and gastric secretions.

B. This demonstrates the operative field and the exposure of the distal esophagus through the left thoracotomy incision after removal of the sixth or seventh rib. The inferior pulmonary ligament has been divided to permit retraction of the left lower lobe of the lung. The esophageal hiatus has been incised to expose a portion of the cardia of the stomach. The balloon tube has been left in place to control the bleeding varices. It also aids in ready location of the esophagus lying medial to the aorta by palpation of the balloon tube within it. The location of the esophagogastric incision is demonstrated by the interrupted line. Note that it is longitudinal and placed equally in the stomach and the esophagus and is about 3 to 4 cm. long.

C. Sometimes the esophagus is surrounded by large veins which must be controlled with ligatures. The pleura is dissected away to expose it (1). The diaphragm (2) is incised to enlarge the esophageal hiatus and to bring a small portion of the fundus of the stomach (3) into view. This is because it is essential to open the stomach to obtain control of submucosal gastric varices. If the patient has ascites, every effort should be made to avoid opening the peritoneum to prevent ascitic fluid from leaking into the pleural space after the operation. Silk guy sutures are placed on each side of the esophagus for control of it. The incision is made with a small knife then enlarged with scissors. Bleeding vessels encountered in the gastroesophageal incision are controlled best by simple sutures of fine silk. Hemostats or curved clamps should not be used because the esophageal wall and the venous channels are so weak they may be severely damaged before the bleeding is controlled. It is better to control them with Allis clamps than suture them.

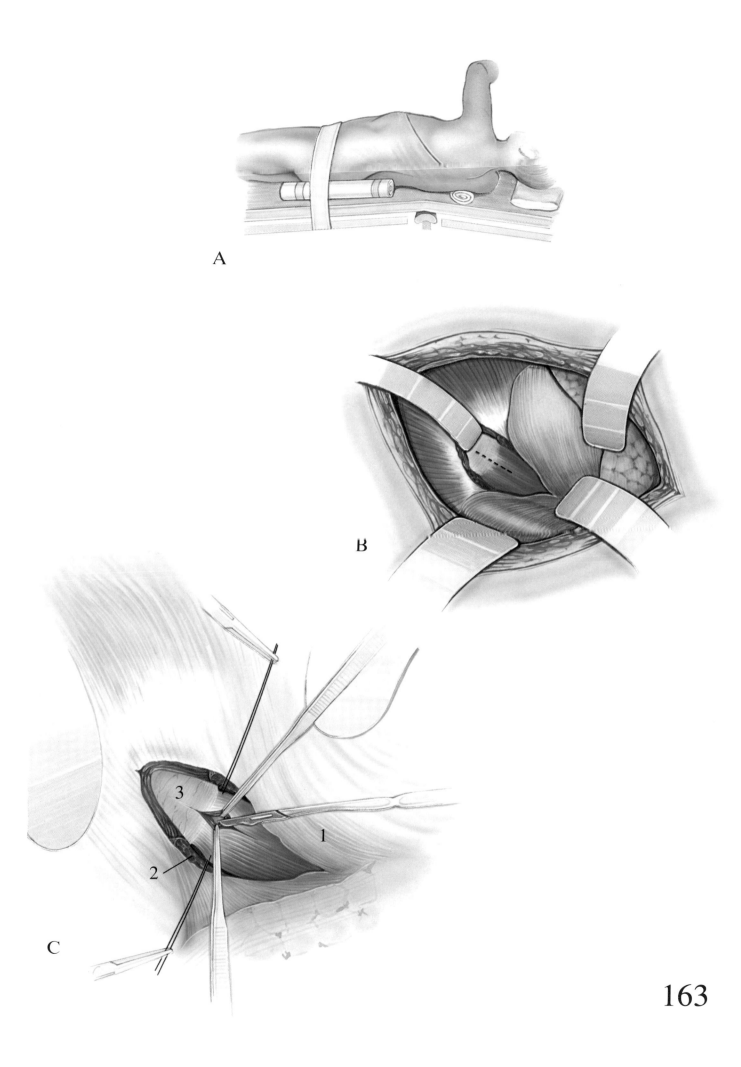

A

B

C

1

2

3

Plate 73

THE EMERGENT TREATMENT OF BLEEDING ESOPHAGEAL VARICES
(Continued)

TRANSTHORACOESOPHAGEAL SUTURE OF BLEEDING
ESOPHAGEAL VARICES *(Continued)*

A. A retractor is in the gastric portion of the incision. Additional guy sutures of silk have been placed through the esophageal wall to give better exposure and control of the varices. The balloon tube is still in place with the balloon deflated to see if the source of bleeding can be found, which occasionally has been possible, as shown. Reinflation and traction on the tube will demonstrate how quickly this type of balloon tamponage controls bleeding. It is then removed. The point of bleeding has never appeared to be ulcerated or due to esophagitis; instead it appears as if a small hole had been punched in one of the varices, the edges are so sharply outlined. It has always been found in the very distal portion of one of the esophageal varices. These large bluish vessels are visible as columns and are similar in appearance to internal hemorrhoids of the anal canal. They have a different appearance from the gastric vessels, as they are very thin-walled, smooth in outline and bluish in color, whereas the gastric vessels are not so distended and the mucosa over them is pink. There is a sharp line of demarcation between the esophageal and gastric mucosa.

B. Each column of varices is sutured by picking it up in its mid portion with the mucosa, using 2-0 chromic catgut on a curved atraumatic needle as a running suture. As a rule, three columns of veins are sutured, commencing in the mid portion of the varix and carrying it down to include some of the gastric varices. The suture is then brought back up to a short distance above where it was started and then back down to the point of origin and ligated. This results in a double hemostatic suture line. Each variceal column is treated in a similar manner. Presuture venous pressures demonstrate the presence of portal hypertension. When these are repeated in the same varix above the point of suturing there is always a marked drop, indicating the blood in the varices was coming from the submucosal gastric vein. As a result of the suturing, immediate control is obtained and usually prevents further bleeding for a period of six to eight weeks.

C. After completion of suturing of the varices, the longitudinal incision in the stomach and esophagus is closed in a transverse manner. This is accomplished with greater ease and security of the suture line if some of the stomach has been exposed as demonstrated by incising the diaphragm, because the stomach is much more readily mobilized in its longitudinal axis than the esophagus, thus permitting it to be pulled upward, with less tension resulting on the suture line. The transverse closure is favored because it does not produce the degree of stenosis that a longitudinal closure does and because it also helps to prevent disruption of the incisions in my experience. Fine interrupted silk sutures are always used. The inner row passes through all layers and they are so placed that the knots lie within the esophageal lumen, as shown. This method of suturing has the advantage that it inverts the edges of the gastroesophageal incision.

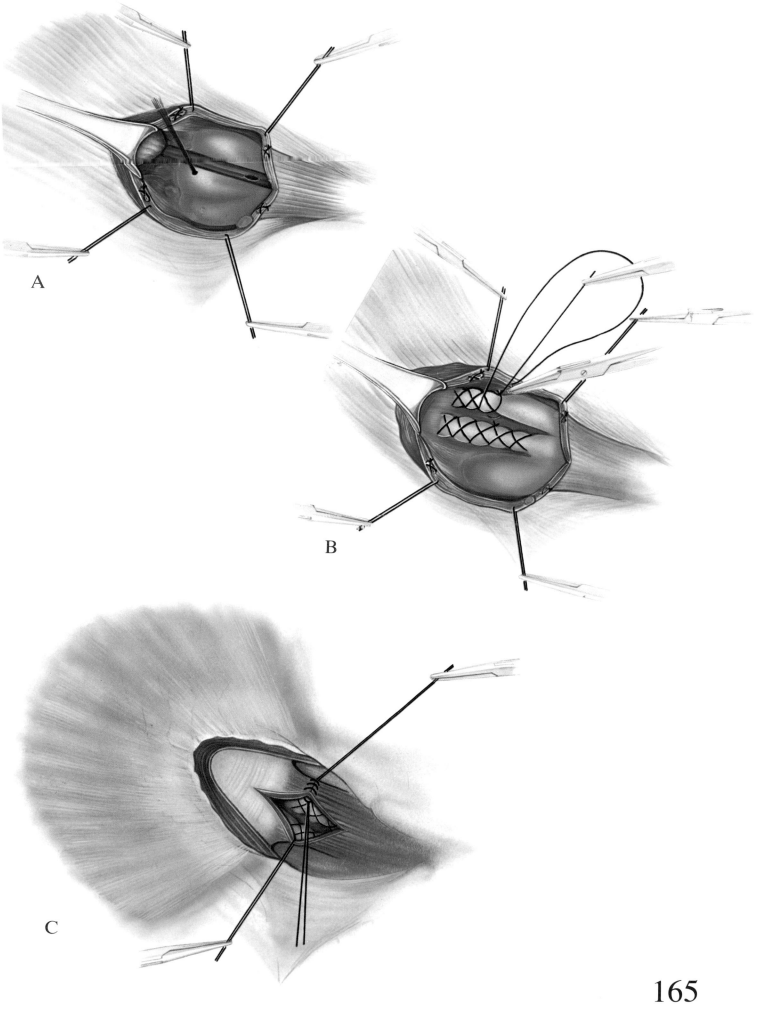

A

B

C

165

Plate 74

THE EMERGENT TREATMENT OF
BLEEDING ESOPHAGEAL VARICES
(Continued)

TRANSTHORACOESOPHAGEAL SUTURE OF BLEEDING
ESOPHAGEAL VARICES *(Continued)*

A. This demonstrates the second row of interrupted infolding mattress sutures of fine silk that are placed next. Again the mobility of the stomach makes it possible to place these sutures without undue tension. Occasionally another layer is placed between the pleura and the stomach to take tension off the gastroesophageal suture line, but as a rule this is not necessary.

B. The incision in the diaphragm is next closed, using interrupted sutures of strong linen or cotton. The esophageal hiatus is reconstructed in this manner, and as a result reflux esophagitis has never been a problem. If the patient has ascites and there has been an ascitic leak as a result of the incision in the diaphragm, every effort should be made to close the point of leakage with sutures at the time the diaphragm is closed to prevent an ascitic fluid leak into the pleural space postoperatively. The lungs are reinflated. A No. 24 Foley catheter with a 30 cc. bag is placed in the pleural space and brought out through a stab incision in the eighth intercostal space. The thoracic incision is closed with interrupted cotton or linen sutures to the intercostal muscles and the muscles of the chest wall and interrupted silk sutures to the skin.

C. This demonstrates the closed incision with the Foley catheter attached to a closed three-bottle suction apparatus with 10 cm. of negative water pressure. This tube is removed 48 hours postoperatively.

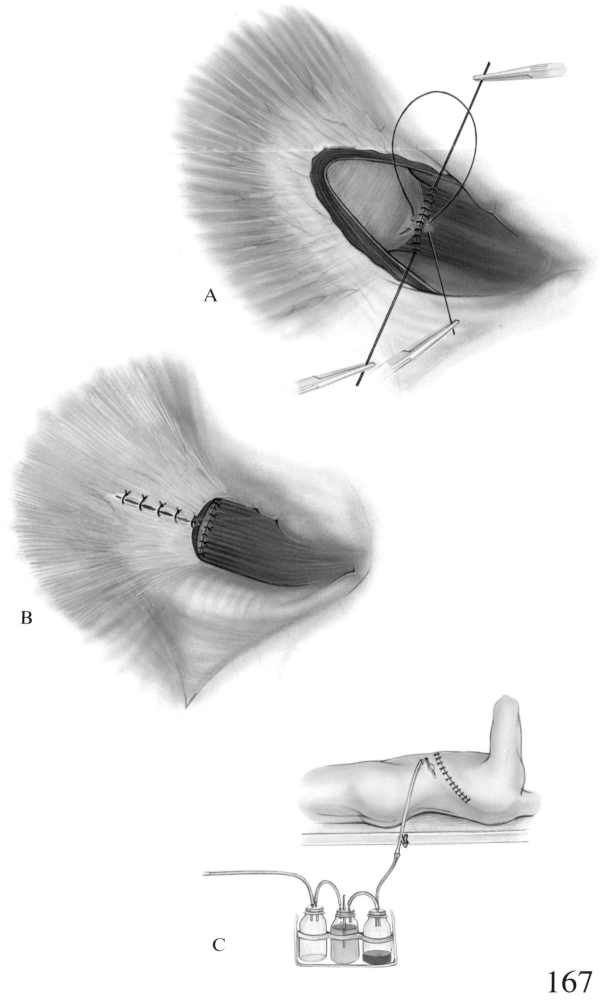

THE DEFINITIVE TREATMENT OF BLEEDING ESOPHAGEAL VARICES

Introduction

End-to-Side Splenorenal Shunt with Splenectomy

Emergent measures to control massive exsanguinating hemorrhage from esophageal varices are important in order to save lives. Unfortunately none of these except one corrects the state of portal hypertension, the primary cause of the esophageal varices. This one is an emergency direct portacaval shunt, which unfortunately is not the best type of shunt because of the high early and late mortality rates from liver failure and the high percentage of postshunt encephalopathy in the survivals. There have been a great many operative procedures devised and reported for reduction of portal hypertension, but one of the earliest was reported by Whipple and Blakemore, an end-to-end anastomosis between the splenic vein and the left renal vein after splenectomy and left nephrectomy. My modification of it has seemed to stand the test of time better than most of the others. This consists of making an end-to-side splenorenal shunt by constructing an anastomosis between the proximal end of the splenic vein and the side of the left renal vein, which results in a much more efficient type of shunt and avoids the necessity of the removal of a normal left kidney. It is too difficult an operative procedure to carry out as an emergency operation, but may be accomplished four to six weeks after the bleeding esophageal varices have been sutured, or as an elective procedure after bleeding has stopped spontaneously.

The reduction of the portal venous hypertension with this type of shunt is not so pronounced as by a direct anastomosis between the portal vein and the inferior vena cava. Experience, however, has shown that with a well constructed end-to-side splenorenal shunt the reduction in pressure is sufficient to prevent further esophageal bleeding in the majority of the patients. It has been observed that a satisfactory shunt can be constructed if the splenic vein is 8 mm. in diameter or larger. When physical examination reveals the presence of a large spleen in a patient with bleeding esophageal varices, this is usually sufficient evidence that the splenic vein will be large enough for the construction of a shunt. If further evidence is desirable or if the spleen cannot be palpated, the size of the splenic vein may be determined by splenoportography or by selective celiac angiography.

Our experience has taught us that this type of shunt can be constructed in the majority of patients with an intrahepatic portal bed block and also in patients with an extrahepatic block if the spleen has not been previously removed. Most patients with this type of shunt live longer and healthier lives than those with direct portacaval shunts because postshunt encephalopathy and liver failure are much less common. It is believed the main reason the splenorenal shunt has fewer postshunt complications is that it is constructed with a smaller anastomosis so that it does not shunt all the portal venous blood as does a direct portacaval anastomosis, yet at the same time a sufficient amount is released to decompress the portal bed. It also effectively clears ascites. For these reasons it is believed this type of shunt should be performed in the majority of patients.

Plate 75

THE DEFINITIVE TREATMENT OF BLEEDING ESOPHAGEAL VARICES

END-TO-SIDE SPLENORENAL SHUNT WITH SPLENECTOMY

A. An artist's drawing demonstrating the venous pathways after a splenectomy and an end-to-side splenorenal shunt for portal cirrhosis with a high degree of postsinusoidal block. The veins of the portal system do not contain valves, so that blood can flow through them in reverse direction from the normal; e.g., some of the hepatic arterial blood can flow in the reverse direction from the hilum of the liver, the result of an abnormal arteriovenous shunting of hepatic arterial blood into the portal venous system. The blood from the stomach, in part, runs into the portal vein through the coronary vein (1), thereby helping to decompress the esophageal varices. Some of the blood from the superior mesenteric vein (2) escapes through the splenic vein (3) and the splenorenal shunt (4) to decompress the entire portal bed.

B. The construction of a splenorenal shunt can be greatly facilitated by the utilization of hypotensive spinal anesthesia administered by the Gillies technique, because this reduces the operative bleeding by lowering the portal venous pressure, thereby facilitating the dissection of the splenic vein and also reducing operative blood loss. This is a color photograph of the sponge rack used during an end-to-side splenorenal shunt and splenectomy. There are 16 small Hibbs sponges, $\frac{1}{2} \times 6$ inches, and 27 regular-sized sponges, 3×12 inches. Note the small amount of blood on these sponges, indicating how little blood loss has occurred. This photograph clearly demonstrates how hypotensive spinal anesthesia can greatly reduce the blood loss during this operative procedure, which otherwise is usually a bloody operation. The patient was a male age 52 years who had a transthoracoesophageal suture of his esophageal varices as an emergent procedure for severe esophageal bleeding on November 28, 1954. Two months later, on January 25, 1955, the splenorenal shunt and splenectomy were performed. He made an uneventful recovery following the operation and was able to return to his work for approximately seven years. Biopsy of the liver revealed portal cirrhosis of the postnecrotic type. Preoperative liver function tests revealed 22 per cent Bromsulphalein dye retention, a serum bilirubin level of 1.7 mg. per cent and serum albumin of 3.6 gm. per cent. Five years postoperative, repeat determinations of these tests revealed 14 per cent Bromsulphalein dye retention, a serum bilirubin of 1.2 mg. per cent and a serum albumin of 3.7 gm. per cent. All were slightly improved, indicating he had suffered no liver injury as a result of either the hypotensive spinal anesthesia or the splenorenal shunt.

C. This is the anesthesia chart for a splenectomy and an end-to-end splenorenal shunt in a woman aged 57 years with portal hypertension and bleeding esophageal varices; the operation was performed under hypotensive catheter spinal anesthesia, supplemented with intravenous pentothal and nitrous oxide and oxygen administered through an endotracheal tube. This was performed by Dr. George E. Battit of the Department of Anesthesia of the Massachusetts General Hospital. Note the lowering of the pulse rate and the reduction in the arterial blood pressure. These are restored to normal by repositioning the patient in slight Trendelenburg position and by the utilization of one to three blood transfusions, depending on the amount of blood loss. This method of producing arterial hypotension has not resulted in injury to the kidneys, liver, heart or brain.

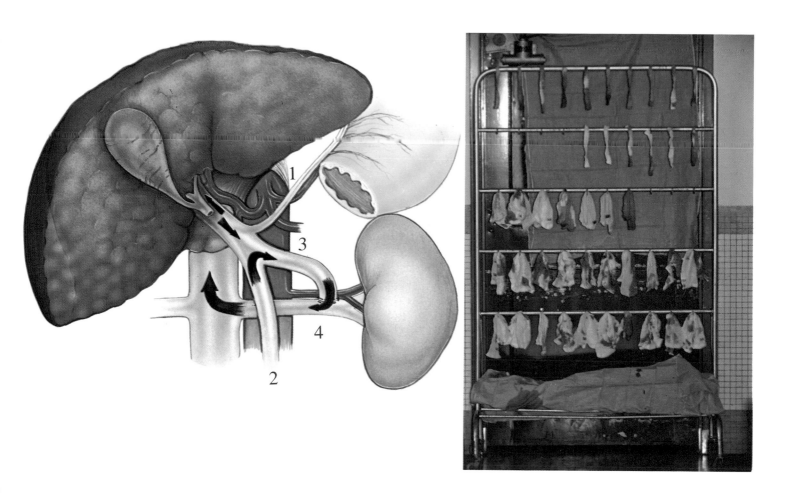

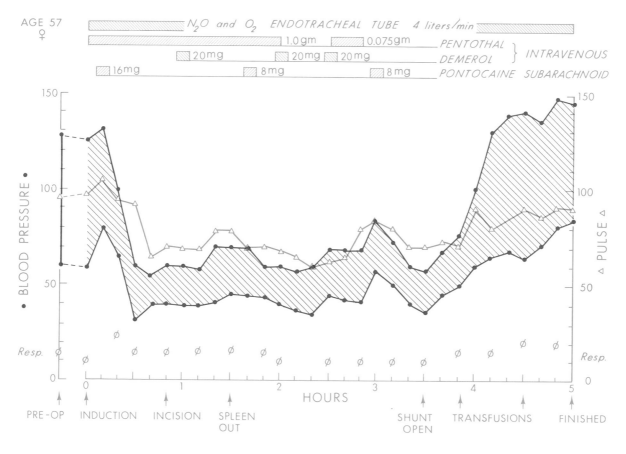

Plate 76

THE DEFINITIVE TREATMENT OF
BLEEDING ESOPHAGEAL VARICES
(Continued)

END-TO-SIDE SPLENORENAL SHUNT WITH SPLENECTOMY
(Continued)

A. This demonstrates the right decubitus position of the patient on the operating table, rotated back at a 45-degree angle with two blanket rolls and one wide strip of adhesive tape to maintain the position. The table is jackknifed and the kidney bar elevated directly underneath the location of the thoraco-abdominal incision, which is shown. It extends obliquely back from above the umbilicus and over the tenth rib. The anesthesia of choice is hypotensive spinal anesthesia and this is supplemented with intravenous pentothal and light gas oxygen anesthesia administered through an endotracheal tube to maintain a systemic blood pressure close to 60 mm. of mercury. This state of hypotension along with positioning the patient so that the operative field is the highest part of the body greatly reduces blood loss and facilitates the operative dissection, especially of the splenic and renal veins, and the construction of as perfect an anastomosis as possible. Before closure of the incision the blood pressure is brought back to normal by leveling the table into slight Trendelenburg position so that any unligated blood vessels may be detected and ligated.

B. The major portion of the tenth rib is removed subperiosteally after division of the external oblique muscle and the anterior portion of the latissimus dorsi muscle and separation of the fibers of the serratus anterior muscle. Anteriorly the internal oblique and rectus muscles are partially divided. The costal cartilage (1) of this rib is divided as shown, leaving both sections to permit an accurate approximation of the costal arch when closing the incision.

C. The peritoneal cavity is opened, separating the fibers of the transversalis muscle and incising the peritoneum and the posterior rectus sheath. The pleural cavity is opened by incising through the periosteal bed of the tenth rib. The diaphragm is partially divided, and guy sutures are placed in each edge to facilitate retraction of them. The inferior edge of the left lower lobe of the lung (1) is seen at the lower portion of the incision. A huge spleen (2) is partially exposed by division of the diaphragm. Above this a grossly nodular left lobe of the cirrhotic liver (3) is seen. The blue ribbonlike structure is a large collateral venous channel (4) in the falciform ligament, an attempt by nature to create a portasystemic venous shunt.

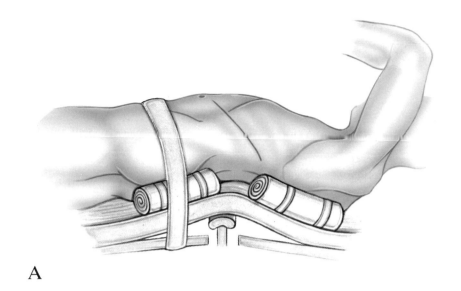

A

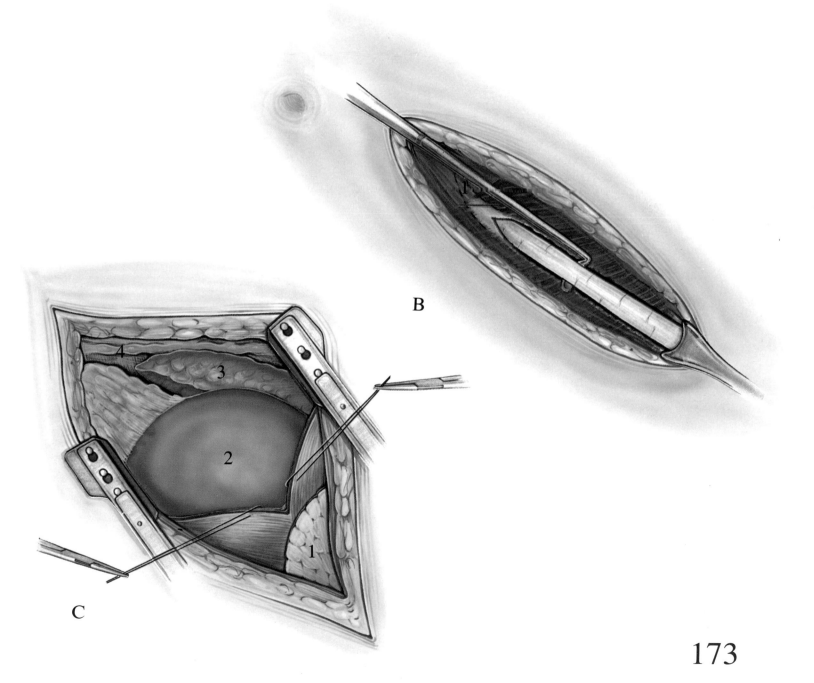

B

C

173

Plate 77

THE DEFINITIVE TREATMENT OF
BLEEDING ESOPHAGEAL VARICES
(Continued)

END-TO-SIDE SPLENORENAL SHUNT WITH SPLENECTOMY
(Continued)

A. The first assistant brings the spleen downward and forward by traction on the superior and lateral borders with his left hand. This brings into view the lienorenal ligament with innumerable small blood vessels in it (1). These are some of the natural shunts that have been developed as a result of the portal bed block. Despite the enormous numbers of them, it is obvious they are very inefficient portasystemic shunts since patients continue to bleed from their esophageal varices.

B. The splenectomy is commenced by dividing this vascular lienorenal ligament between curved clamps. The dissection is carried up to the region of the vasa breva. The blood vessels in the clamps next to the spleen need not be ligated, but those held by the other clamps are best controlled by a running over-and-over suture of 3-0 chromic catgut. Complete hemostasis of these vessels is essential. The advantage of hypotensive spinal anesthesia is especially helpful at this stage as it aids greatly in the control of blood loss in this vascular area.

C. After the lateral attachments of the spleen have been freed up it is turned downward to expose the vasa breva blood vessels (1) between it and the stomach (2) and also some of the left gastroepiploic vessels (3). These are all doubly clamped and divided between small hemostats as they are ligated. Great care is taken not to include the gastric wall in the ligatures because if this is done it could result in necrosis of the stomach wall with a resulting leak of gastric fluid.

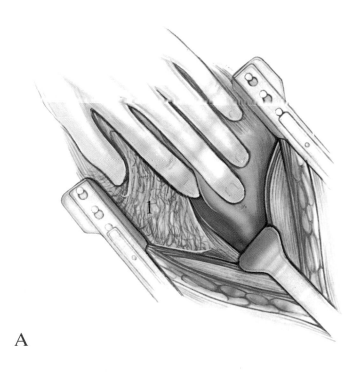

A

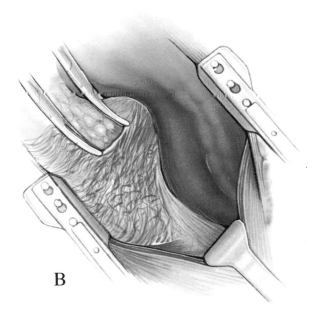

B

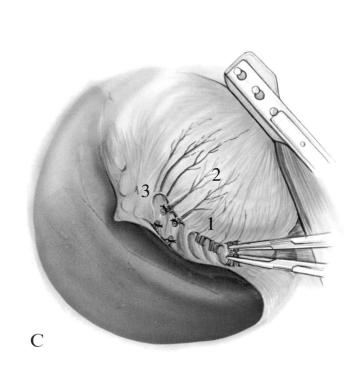

C

175

Plate 78

THE DEFINITIVE TREATMENT OF BLEEDING ESOPHAGEAL VARICES
(Continued)

END-TO-SIDE SPLENORENAL SHUNT WITH SPLENECTOMY
(Continued)

A. The spleen has been completely mobilized and is attached only by its pedicle. It has been lifted up and drawn toward the right side of the patient, demonstrating the splenic vein (1) with a curved clamp beneath it, and next to that the splenic artery (2). They both lie on the posterior superior portion of the pancreas (3). When a surgeon sees a splenic vein of this size and length he knows he can construct a satisfactory and effective shunt.

B. The splenic artery is isolated at this stage since it can be done with less danger of injuring the splenic vein; injury to the vein could prevent a shunt from being constructed. The artery is doubly ligated with linen or cotton ligatures and divided between them. This maneuver prevents engorgement of the spleen which occurs if the splenic vein is ligated first. It also permits the giving of an autotransfusion by squeezing the spleen.

C. The splenic vein is next divided near the hilum of the spleen, between a hemostat and a ligature, to complete the splenectomy. A second ligature with long ends is placed on the proximal end of the vein distal to the hemostatic ligature to mark it and to aid in avoiding injury to it. This ligature is also used as a means of controlling and retracting the vein.

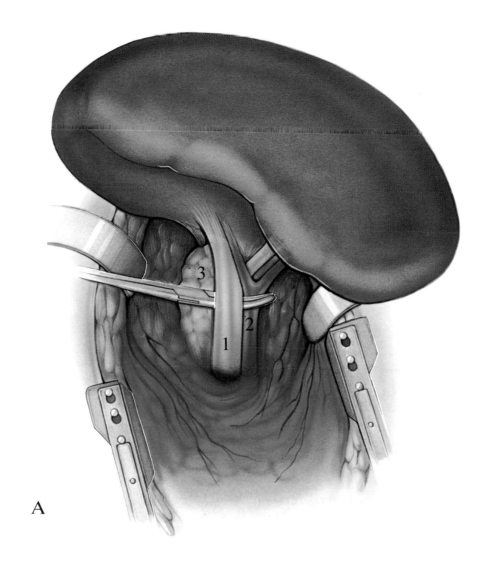

A

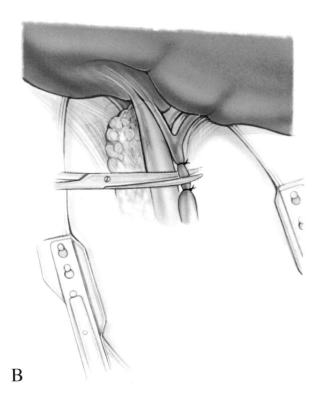

B

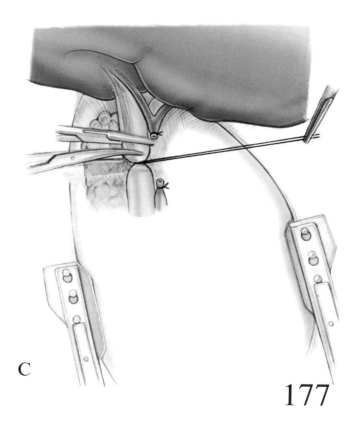

C

177

Plate 79

THE DEFINITIVE TREATMENT OF BLEEDING ESOPHAGEAL VARICES
(Continued)

END-TO-SIDE SPLENORENAL SHUNT WITH SPLENECTOMY
(Continued)

A. After the splenectomy has been completed it is recommended that further dissection of the splenic vein (1) wait until the renal vein has been isolated. This is done by first locating the upper and lower poles of the left kidney (2) between the fingers of the surgeon's two hands. The general location of the renal vein is found by palpating the hilum of the kidney. The fatty tissues and the perirenal fascia medial to it are incised with scissors to expose the renal vein (3) and the renal artery. Sometimes these tissues are quite thick, and vascular, so hemostasis is obtained carefully. Sufficient length of the vein is dissected out in order to determine where in its course the splenic vein will be closest to it, as it is important to use as short a segment of the latter as possible to obtain the best shunt.

B. The dissection of the renal vein has been carried out toward the midline, demonstrating the large suprarenal vein (1) with the curved clamp under it and the spermatic or ovarian vein (2) arising opposite to it on the inferior side of the renal vein. Sometimes the suprarenal vein lies at the site where it is best to make the shunt. If it does, there should be no hesitancy in ligating and dividing it, as this has never resulted in serious damage to the suprarenal gland. The stump of the vein is excised with an ellipse of the renal vein, because it is never large enough to make the shunt directly to it.

C. Attention is next directed to the splenic vein. First the shortest length necessary for constructing the splenorenal anastomosis should be determined. In order to obtain the best permanent shunt it is important to use as short a segment of the splenic vein as possible, so it is important in most patients to free it up proximally to make this possible. In many cases the splenic vein is found to be too long and if used full length probably would result in its kinking and the failure of the shunt. For this reason, the distal part of the vein is not dissected free, thereby saving considerable operative time since sometimes 2 to 3 cm. may be left undisturbed except for ligatures at each end. In order to accomplish this, the splenic vein is carefully separated from the pancreas between its pancreatic branches, doubly ligated and divided. The small round circles on the splenic vein indicate the location of the paired pancreatic branches on its opposite side.

D. One of the most difficult technical procedures in the operation is the ligation and the division of the small very tender pancreatic branches of the splenic vein. If they are torn in freeing up the splenic vein from its bed in the pancreas, serious damage may be done to the splenic vein in obtaining control of them. The bleeding is always profuse because of the high pressure in the vein. If this accident occurs, the small opening in the splenic vein is best controlled by a mattress suture of 5-0 silk on a taper point needle. If care is taken in freeing up the splenic vein from the divided end, and isolating the pancreatic branches, they can be neatly doubly ligated with 5-0 silk ligatures, using a fine, curved, right-angle clamp to pull the ligature through beneath it as shown. These small vessels always come off in pairs about 1 cm. apart. It is usually necessary to interrupt two or three pairs of them.

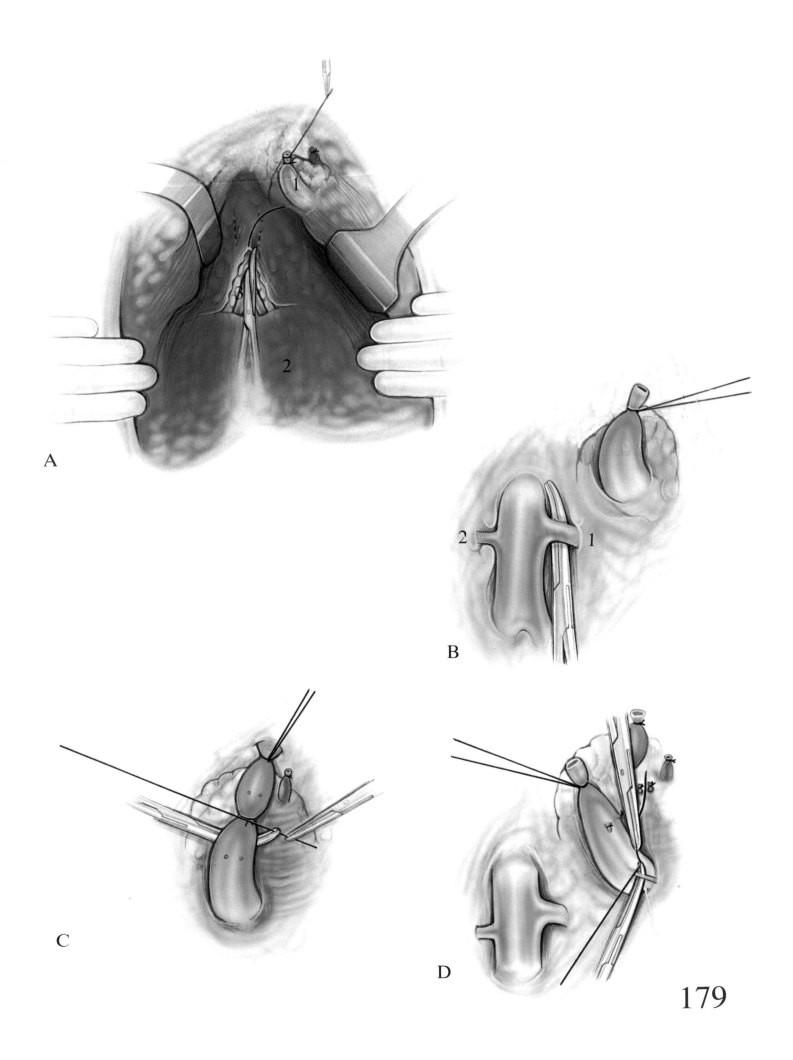

A

B

C

D

179

Plate 80

THE DEFINITIVE TREATMENT OF
BLEEDING ESOPHAGEAL VARICES
(Continued)

END-TO-SIDE SPLENORENAL SHUNT WITH SPLENECTOMY
(Continued)

A. As a result of the dissection and manipulation of the splenic vein, it always becomes reduced in caliber because of vasospasm (1). This natural response to even the slightest trauma that blood vessels, including veins, demonstrate, has caused some surgeons to conclude that the splenic vein is too small to permit the construction of a satisfactory splenorenal venovenous anastomosis.

B. Reversal of this state of vasoconstriction of the splenic vein and restoration of the vessel to its normal size can be accomplished with hydrostatic pressure. This is accomplished by placing a bulldog clamp with cloth-covered blades as far proximal as possible on the vein to occlude it. The constricted vein is dilated by injecting normal saline into it with a small syringe, using a 22-gauge needle. Fortunately, after this hydrostatic pressure method of dilation of the vein, it does not go back into vasospasm but remains dilated, permitting the construction of a satisfactory anastomosis.

C. The length of the splenic vein (1) is checked with the renal vein (2) to make sure a sufficient length has been freed up to permit construction of a satisfactory anastomosis. Note the tail of the pancreas (3), showing the splenic vein bed and the ligated distal ends of the pancreatic branches of the splenic vein.

D. A curved, cloth-covered or fine-toothed nontraumatic clamp is placed on the superior border of the renal vein to partially occlude it. In this case it includes the stump of the suprarenal vein that has been ligated and divided. This site is chosen because the splenic vein lies optimally at this point. There should be no hesitancy in sacrificing the suprarenal vein if necessary, as it is of utmost importance to have a streamlined anastomosis. With the aid of an Allis clamp an ellipse of the renal vein is excised with right-angled, curved scissors. A bulldog clamp covered with cloth to prevent its slipping is placed on the splenic vein, taking extreme care not to twist it during its application, because if this occurs, it will cause the anastomosis to thrombose. The ligature on the end of the splenic vein is next put on gentle traction to determine the proper length at which to divide the vein with fine straight scissors.

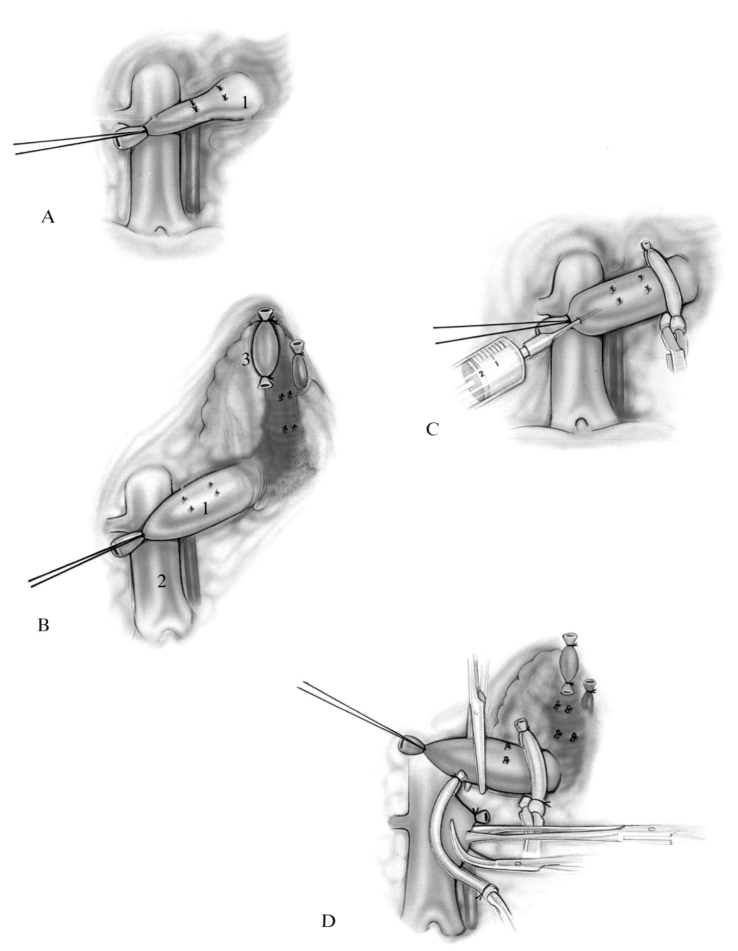

A

B

C

D

181

Plate 81

THE DEFINITIVE TREATMENT OF
BLEEDING ESOPHAGEAL VARICES
(Continued)

END-TO-SIDE SPLENORENAL SHUNT WITH SPLENECTOMY
(Continued)

A.   An ellipse has been cut out of the renal vein and one guy suture (1) has been placed in the cut edge to help to keep the vein from slipping out of the curved clamp. Two guy sutures (2) and (3) have been placed in the edges of the splenic vein for orientation during the construction of the anastomosis and to keep the lumen of the vein open, which greatly facilitates the technique of placing the sutures. The sutures of choice are an atraumatic 5-0, braided Dacron coated with Teflon and waxed thoroughly with bone wax to allow it to slide without picking up the adventitia, since if this occurs, it spoils the streamlining of the anastomosis, or a monofilament synthetic one that accomplishes this without waxing. A fine straight needle such as shown has been found to be the most satisfactory type. The suture (a) commences at the far end of the anastomosis, opposite guy suture (3) in the splenic vein. It goes from outside in, then crosses over and goes from inside out on the renal vein cuff, then outside in and crosses over to the splenic vein, continuing on as seen in *B*.

B.   The posterior suture line continues as a running everting mattress type in order to approximate the intima of the splenic vein with that of the renal vein. The posterior row is always placed first because it is the most difficult to put in and would be almost impossible to do satisfactorily if it were done after the anterior row. After completion of one half, a stay suture (4) is placed and tied. The running mattress suture is pulled taut by grasping each end of it, then tied to the stay suture (4), taking care that the knot does not slip to cause a purse string effect with narrowing of the anastomosis.

C.   One half of the posterior suture line has been completed. A new suture (b) has been placed and tied to itself and the loose end of the running mattress suture (a), again with care not to let the knot slip but keeping it secure enough so the mattress suture is not too loose. As the drawing shows, there is excellent intima-to-intima approximation, so that no suture material, knots or rough edges of the veins are visible within the anastomotic lumen. The next step is to complete the remaining half of the posterior row in the same manner as the first half.

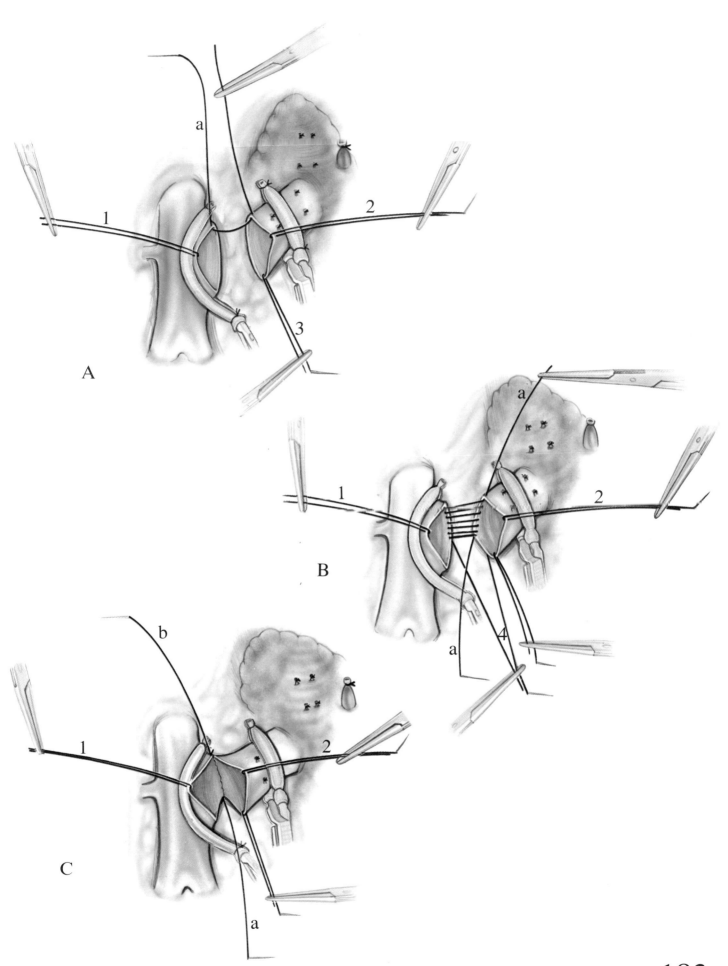

A

B

C

183

Plate 82

THE DEFINITIVE TREATMENT OF BLEEDING ESOPHAGEAL VARICES
(Continued)

END-TO-SIDE SPLENORENAL SHUNT WITH SPLENECTOMY
(Continued)

A. The posterior suture line has been completed and anchored at each end so that it will not loosen. Note how accurately the edges of the veins have been brought together, with excellent intima-to-intima approximation and no suture material, knots or rough vein edges visible since they all lie extravascular. Careful attention to these technical details of venovenous anastomosis that have a relatively slow flow of blood through them is of extreme importance in maintaining patency. Under no conditions should the veins be sutured together with a running over-and-over suture placed from inside the venous lumen, as this leaves the suture, the knots and the raw edges within the lumen. This is especially bad if silk sutures are used, because this is much more thrombogenic than synthetic suture materials. It is well worth the extra time and effort it takes to put in the running everting mattress suture.

B. This demonstrates the beginning of the anterior running everting mattress suture line with suture (b). It is much easier to place since the needle is passed through both vein cuffs at the same time, as shown. It is carried to the mid point, where guy suture (2) is used as a stay suture to secure the two vessels together, then the running suture (b) is tied to it to anchor it.

C. The first half of the anterior suture line has been completed. The bulldog clamp is released temporarily to flush out any thrombi that might have formed in the splenic vein since it was occluded. Note the marked gush of blood from the splenic vein, indicative of a high portal venous pressure, which gives the surgeon assurance that the shunt, if well constructed, should function satisfactorily to decompress the portal venous bed. After reclosure of the bulldog clamp, the venous channels are flushed out with normal saline solution to remove any remaining blood. The suture line is then completed with suture (a), making certain that the posterior wall of the anastomosis is not caught with the suture since this, if not detected and corrected, will result in failure of the shunt.

D. This demonstrates a well constructed end-to-side splenorenal anastomosis with excellent eversion of the edges of the splenic and renal vein cuffs and without any stenosis at the suture line or twisting of the splenic vein. The tail of the pancreas appears normal, indicating that it has a good blood supply. The distal section of the splenic vein that was not needed is shown, as well as the ligated proximal end of the splenic artery. Note that there is a relatively short segment of splenic vein exposed from where it comes out of the pancreas to the anastomosis. This is essential for a permanent, long-functioning shunt, since it prevents kinking of the splenic vein and decreases the danger of thrombosis.

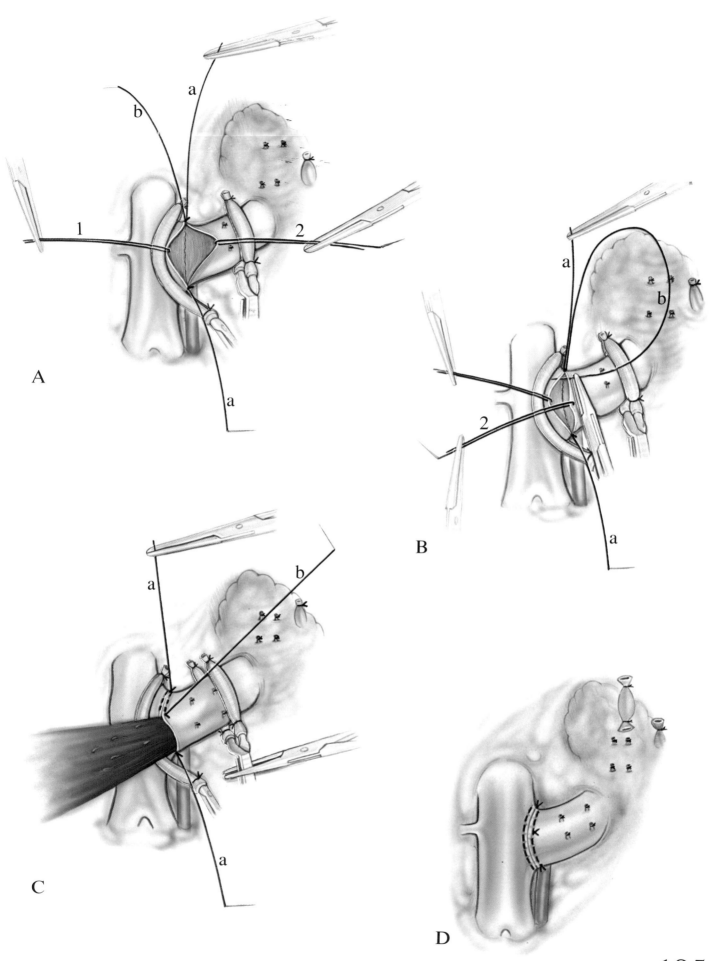

A

B

C

D

185

Plate 83

THE DEFINITIVE TREATMENT OF· BLEEDING ESOPHAGEAL VARICES
(Continued)

END-TO-SIDE SPLENORENAL SHUNT WITH SPLENECTOMY
(Continued)

A. This shows a well constructed end-to-side splenorenal shunt. However, in order to obtain sufficient length of the splenic vein it was necessary to dissect more of it from the pancreas than is usually necessary. As a result, the distal end of the pancreas, because of its length and size, tends to impinge on the anastomosis when it returns to its normal position, so that from its weight alone it may tend to obliterate the shunt since the venous pressure when open may be only about 20 cm. of water. For this reason it is best to resect the distal end of the pancreas with a knife just proximal to the shunt. A "V" type of incision is made to facilitate closure.

B. The resection has been completed and the blood vessels ligated. The pancreatic duct is carefully isolated and ligated. The pancreas is closed with a few mattress sutures of fine silk and simple sutures of the same. Drainage of the pancreatic stump is not necessary. It should be noted that resection of the tail of the pancreas should also be performed if it loses its pink color and develops a bluish purple discoloration. This sometimes occurs if the splenic artery is interrupted too far medially and also if much of the splenic vein has been freed up. In some patients beginning fat necrosis may also be noticed. If the tail is not excised when these conditions exist, it usually goes on to necrosis, with sepsis and thrombosis of the shunt and even death of the patient. As yet, I have never been sorry I resected the pancreas, whereas in some patients, in retrospect, I wish I had.

C. This drawing demonstrates a frequent anatomical variation in which the splenic vein lies directly anterior and parallel to the renal vein. The construction of the end-to-side anastomosis under these conditions is much more difficult to perform. It helps to completely occlude the renal vein between two bulldog clamps and make the anastomosis between them. The renal artery should also be occluded with a bulldog clamp. Renal artery occlusion for periods of 45 minutes has not caused renal damage and provides ample time for the performance of a carefully constructed anastomosis. The splenic vein is divided at an angle so that it will join the renal vein at an acute angle. The method of suturing is the same except that it is commenced with a double needle suture placed as a mattress suture at the acute angle of the anastomosis. Each side is completed as a running everting mattress suture. It is important under these conditions to use a short segment of splenic vein to prevent its kinking.

D. This shows the completed shunt with a satisfactory anastomosis. Note that the distal end of pancreas was resected because it tended to occlude the anastomosis when it was placed back in its normal position.

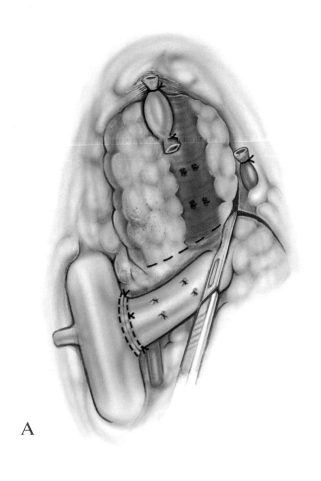

A

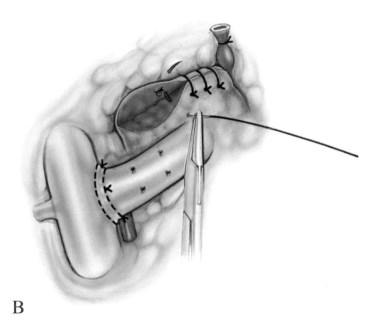

B

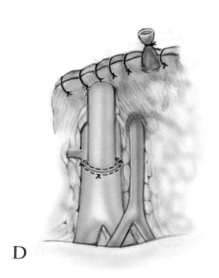

C

D

187

Plate 84

THE DEFINITIVE TREATMENT OF
BLEEDING ESOPHAGEAL VARICES
(Continued)

END-TO-SIDE SPLENORENAL SHUNT WITH SPLENECTOMY
(Continued)

A. Postshunt venous pressures are taken before closing the abdominal incision to help to determine whether the shunt is functioning by comparing the readings taken before and after the shunt was performed. They are obtained by direct measurements in the manometer with normal saline solution tinged with blood. An 18-gauge needle that has been bent and attached to the manometer with fine rubber tubing is inserted through the inferior surface of the renal vein, then through the anastomosis into the splenic vein (1). Note that the portal pressure has dropped from a preshunt level of 35 cm. to a postshunt level of 18 cm., which is good evidence of a well functioning shunt. The needle is partially withdrawn so that the point is in the renal vein lumen and then is advanced medially, keeping the tip of it in the renal vein. The manometer level falls again to give the systemic venous pressure, which is 3 cm. higher than the preshunt level and further evidence of a functioning shunt. The needle is withdrawn after obtaining the pressure readings. Sometimes a single stitch of fine silk may be needed to control the bleeding from the needle puncture site.

B.   The entire operative field is shown after completion of the shunt. The following structures are shown: the splenorenal shunt (1), the left kidney (2), the sutured proximal end of the pancreas (3), the splenic flexure and transverse colon (4), the stomach (5), the cirrhotic liver (6), the left lower lobe of the lung (7) and the upper and lower portions of the diaphragm (8). The operating table is straightened and placed in moderate Trendelenburg position to allow the blood stored in the large venous channels of the body to recirculate and to restore the patient's blood pressure to normal. This sometimes causes some bleeding that had not occurred during the hypotension, so the field is carefully examined and any bleeding points ligated or cauterized with the diathermy. The diaphragm is closed securely with closely spaced interrupted sutures of linen or cotton, making sure it is water tight, especially if the patient had ascites at the time of operation. A needle biopsy site in the liver may require a catgut suture to stop the bleeding from it.

C.   A No. 26 Foley catheter with a 30 cc. bag is placed in the left pleural space and brought out through a stab incision in the eighth interspace (1). Another similar tube should be placed in the left subphrenic area if oozing from the operative site continues, and brought out through a stab incision in the left upper quadrant (2). Each of these catheters is connected to 10 cm. of negative water pressure with a three-bottle suction apparatus, then removed in 48 hours. The abdominal wall portion of the incision is closed with a running suture of 0 chromic catgut to the peritoneum, posterior rectus sheath and transversalis muscle and fascia. The same is used to suture the internal and external oblique muscles and the anterior rectus sheath with a few interrupted mattress sutures. Nylon stay sutures are placed through all layers of the abdominal portion of the incision, except the peritoneum. The costal arch is reconstituted with interrupted mattress sutures of heavy linen or cotton to approximate the two sections of the tenth costal cartilage which were preserved when the incision was made. The muscles of the chest wall are sutured with interrupted sutures of 0 chromic catgut. The skin is closed with interrupted silk sutures.

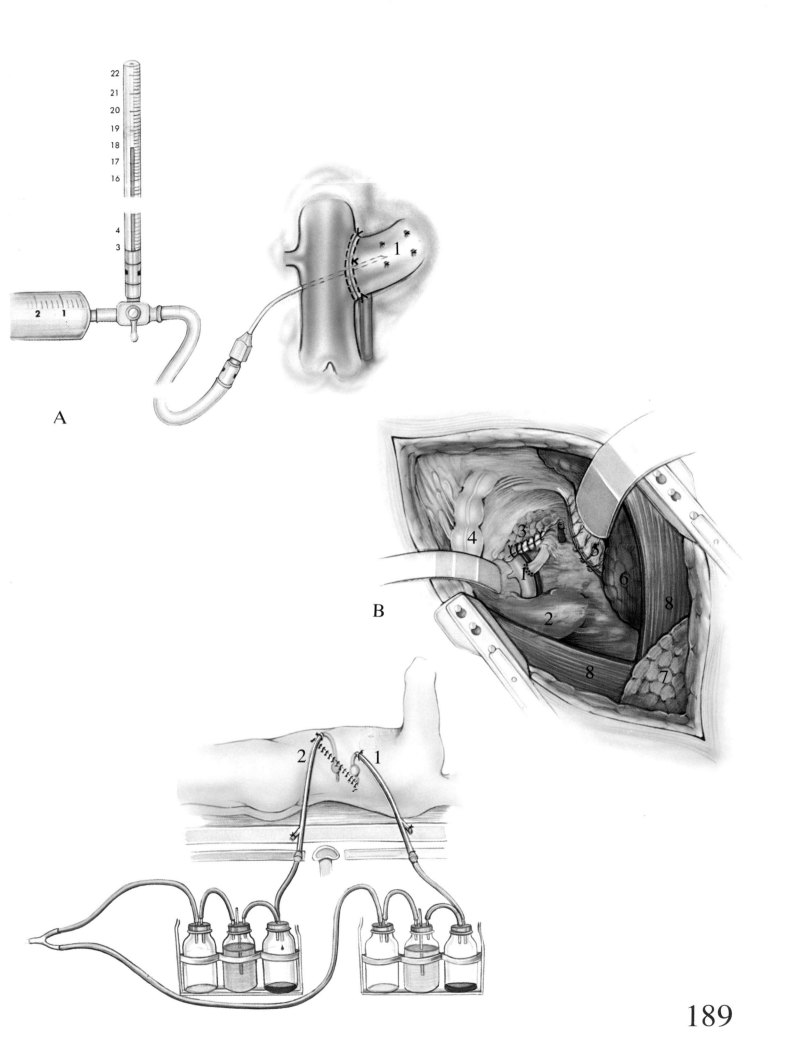

A

B

189

Plate 85

THE DEFINITIVE TREATMENT OF
BLEEDING ESOPHAGEAL VARICES
(Continued)

END-TO-SIDE SPLENORENAL SHUNT WITH SPLENECTOMY WITH
OTHER ANATOMICAL VARIANTS

The preceding illustrations of the construction of an end-to-side splenorenal shunt represent the anatomical relationships of the splenic and renal veins and the renal artery in the great majority of patients. It seems worthwhile to show a few of the variations in these relationships and to demonstrate that they do not preclude the construction of a satisfactory shunt.

A. This demonstrates an anomalous course of the renal artery that is important to recognize in order to prevent injury to the blood supply of the kidney and still complete a satisfactory shunt. In this and similar cases encountered, the renal artery bifurcates earlier than usual so that a portion of it and the branch supplying the lower half of the kidney are found lying over the renal vein. The artery and vein must be carefully separated to avoid injury to them and to permit retraction of the artery upward. This will then allow the curved clamp to be applied to the renal vein for the construction of the shunt without interference with the blood supply to the lower half of the kidney.

B. This demonstrates a rare and unusual anatomical variant in that the pancreas, splenic vein and artery lie caudad to the renal vein. The anomalous position of the vessels is usually detected after the splenectomy when the search is being made for the renal vein. Detection of the position of the kidney and its hilum by palpation is the first thing that draws one's attention to the possibility that this reversed position of the renal and splenic vein is present. Once they are dissected out, the anastomosis is constructed in the routine manner but placed at the inferior margin of the renal vein.

C. A more difficult problem is encountered when the renal and splenic veins lie so far apart it is impossible to anastomose them. Under these conditions a portion of the long saphenous vein is removed from the left groin for a graft. Unfortunately it is usually too small in caliber to use, so a paneled graft is made. A section three times longer than the defect between the splenic and renal veins is removed. It is incised lengthwise then cut in equal lengths. The graft is constructed over a large-sized polyvinyl catheter, using a running, over-and-over, 6-0 Teflon-coated Dacron suture. It is important to sew the two suture lines in opposite directions to prevent the graft from twisting. A successful triple panel graft has been performed in one patient.

D. The anastomosis of the paneled graft (1) to the end of the splenic vein (2) should be made first, using a polyethylene catheter stent. The location of this anastomosis should be carefully selected on the splenic vein to make certain the other end of the graft will be the correct length to permit a satisfactory anastomosis without tension or too much redundancy. The end-to-end anastomosis of the graft and the splenic vein is best done over a stent, utilizing the end-to-side technique with 6-0 Teflon-coated Dacron sutures. The anastomosis of the graft to the renal vein is performed in the routine manner. The completed shunt is shown in the drawing. In this patient it was necessary to make the anastomosis to the larger of two branches of the renal vein.

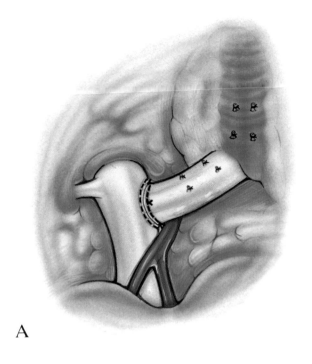

A

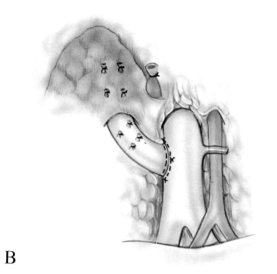

B

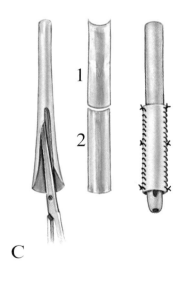

C

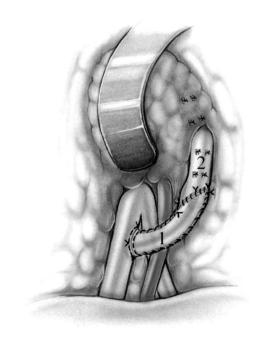

D

Plate 86

THE DEFINITIVE TREATMENT OF BLEEDING ESOPHAGEAL VARICES
(Continued)

DIRECT PORTACAVAL SHUNTS

Hemodynamics of Direct Portacaval Shunts

A direct portacaval shunt performed by constructing an anastomosis between the portal vein and the inferior vena cava was performed on animals by a physiologist, Professor N. V. Eck, a Russian of German descent, in 1877. This type of shunt has been used by many surgeons during the last 25 years in the treatment of bleeding esophageal varices and ascites secondary to portal cirrhosis of the liver because it decompresses the portal venous system more effectively and completely than any other type of shunt. In addition, it has been favored by surgeons because in most patients it is the easiest to construct from the technical viewpoint. Unfortunately it does not give the best long-term results because of a much higher incidence of postshunt encephalopathy and a higher early and late mortality rate from liver failure. If the patient has had a previous splenectomy or the splenic vein is too small to construct a satisfactory splenorenal shunt, a direct portacaval shunt may be the most satisfactory procedure to perform.

A. This artist's drawing demonstrates the blood flow of the hepatic artery through a liver with portal cirrhosis and the bypassing of the entire portal venous blood from the liver into the inferior vena cava through an end-to-side type of direct portacaval anastomosis after division of the portal vein, with ligation of the hepatic end and the construction of the shunt with the distal end. It is to be noted with this type of direct portacaval shunt none of the portal venous blood passes through the liver, which probably explains the high incidence of postshunt encephalopathy. On the other hand, however, all the hepatic arterial blood must pass through the liver and out the hepatic veins, so that this organ, although deprived of portal venous blood, does have its arterial blood supply maintained. The gallbladder is shown, but for clarity the bile ducts are not depicted.

B. This artist's drawing demonstrates the hepatic arterial and portal venous blood flow, as indicated by the arrows, after the construction of a side-to-side anastomosis between the portal vein and the inferior vena cava. In the presence of a high degree of postsinusoidal intrahepatic block this will deprive the liver not only of its portal venous blood, but also of the arterial blood because of the reflux of the blood into the intrahepatic portal venous system and thence through the portacaval shunt because of a reversal of blood flow in this portion of the system. A small amount of the arterial blood may make its way out through the hepatic veins, but in some patients the liver will be so deprived of arterial blood that it develops massive necrosis, causing the death of the patient. It is recommended, because of these pressure relationships of the hepatic arterial and portal venous blood flow, that a side-to-side direct portacaval anastomosis should not be done in the presence of a high degree of postsinusoidal intrahepatic portal bed block.

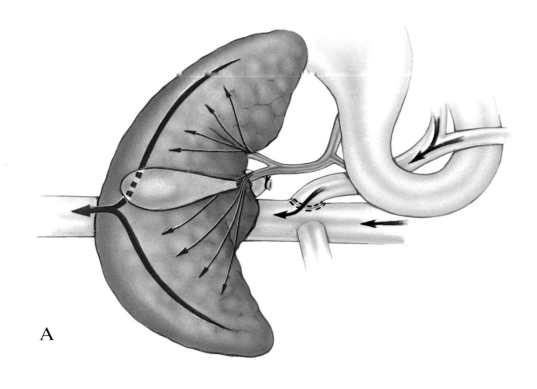

A

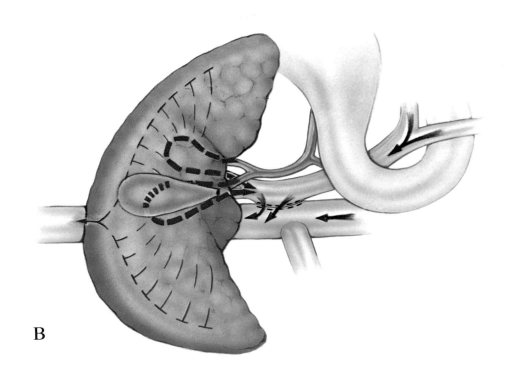

B

193

Plate 87

THE DEFINITIVE TREATMENT OF BLEEDING ESOPHAGEAL VARICES
(Continued)

DIRECT PORTACAVAL SHUNTS *(Continued)*

Hemodynamics of Direct Portacaval Shunts (Continued)

A. This demonstrates the hepatic artery and the portal vein in the gastrohepatic ligament, and the inferior vena cava with the right renal vein lying posterior in a patient with portal cirrhosis of the liver. A portion of the gallbladder is shown, but the bile ducts have been omitted for the sake of clarity. A venous pressure is being obtained in the portal vein with a manometer filled with normal saline solution colored with a small amount of blood; it registers 35 cm. of water. The patient had a systolic blood pressure of 80 mm. of mercury, as hypotensive spinal anesthesia had been used. The portal venous pressure has been found to be directly proportional to the systolic blood pressure, so that under normotensive conditions the portal venous pressure would have been between 50 and 60 cm. of water.

B. Differential pressures following temporary occlusion of the portal vein are recorded in the same patient shown in *A* in the distal extrahepatic portal venous bed (1), and in the proximal intrahepatic portal bed (2). Note that the extrahepatic pressure has dropped from 35 to 25 cm., whereas the intrahepatic pressure has risen from 35 to 38 cm. These observations demonstrate that in this patient there is a high degree of postsinusoidal intrahepatic block that causes reflux of hepatic arterial blood into the portal venous system, resulting in a reversal of blood flow in the portal vein, which is a contributing factor to the state of portal hypertension.

C. Additional evidence of the reflux of hepatic artery blood into the portal venous system may be readily demonstrated by recording the intrahepatic portal venous pressure after occlusion of the hepatic artery in the gastrohepatic ligament with a bulldog clamp while still maintaining occlusion of the portal vein. In this patient, the same as in *A* and *B*, it dropped abruptly to 10 cm., whereas the distal extrahepatic pressure remained the same. It is recommended, therefore, that these pressure readings be taken before performing a side-to-side portacaval anastomosis. Under such conditions the patient's liver will be deprived not only of portal venous blood but also, more vital to its survival, the hepatic arterial blood, since both will take the path of least resistance, which is the side-to-side direct portacaval shunt. This definitely indicates that this type of shunt should not be performed and instead an end-to-side portacaval anastomosis should be constructed even in the presence of ascites.

D. The degree of postsinusoidal intrahepatic block may be less than demonstrated in *B* and *C*. In this patient the preocclusion portal venous pressure was 32 cm., as shown in the manometer (a). After occlusion of the portal vein the intrahepatic pressure fell to 23 cm. (b), and the distal extrahepatic pressure rose to 38 cm. (c). These findings demonstrate a lesser degree of intrahepatic portal bed block, so that under these conditions a side-to-side portacaval anastomosis could be performed with less danger of depriving the liver of its hepatic arterial blood supply and probably also less shunting of the portal venous blood from it.

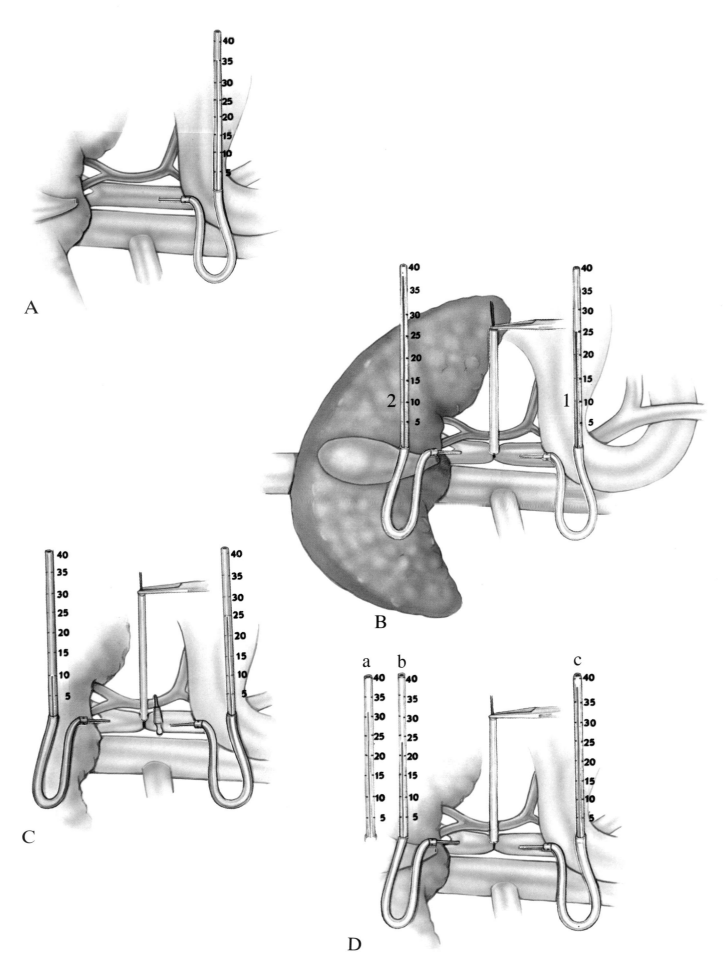

A

B

C

D

a b c

1

2

195

Plate 88

THE DEFINITIVE TREATMENT OF BLEEDING ESOPHAGEAL VARICES
(Continued)

TECHNIQUE OF CONSTRUCTION OF DIRECT PORTACAVAL SHUNTS

A.   This demonstrates the position of the patient for the construction of a direct portacaval shunt using a thoraco-abdominal incision. This is recommended because it gives the best exposure of the portal vein and the inferior vena cava for the performance of an anastomosis and also for avoiding injury to the common bile duct and the hepatic artery. The patient is placed in the left decubitus position at approximately a 90-degree angle after hypotensive spinal anesthesia has been instituted. To reduce bleeding the table is jackknifed and the kidney bar elevated so that the operative field is the highest portion of the body. The incision is made over the tenth rib and carried anteriorly to partially divide the external oblique, the internal oblique and the rectus abdominalis muscles slightly above the umbilicus. The transversalis muscle is divided in the line of its fibers and the peritoneum incised to open the peritoneal cavity. A subperiosteal resection of the anterior two thirds of the tenth rib is performed. This opens the right pleural space.

B.   The exposure of the operative field has been completed in the following order: The right diaphragm (1) has been partially divided. A small portion of the left lower lobe of the lung (2) is visible above the diaphragm. The right lobe of the liver (3) and the gallbladder (4) are displaced upward and into the right pleural space, and the first portion of the duodenum (5) and the head of the pancreas (6) are retracted downward. The portal vein (7) is next isolated, sometimes with the coronary vein showing, preserving it if possible for drainage through the shunt. The common bile duct (8) is carefully retracted forward, if it lies in the way, as well as the hepatic artery (9), which is usually not exposed but may sometimes have an anomalous course, coming from behind the portal vein to pass lateral to it up to the liver hilum. Under these conditions this method of exposure is a great help in preserving this artery and at the same time constructing a satisfactory portacaval anastomosis. The inferior vena cava (10) is readily exposed in the retroperitoneal area. Not infrequently it is necessary to divide and ligate a few small hepatic veins that go from the caudate lobe of the liver (11) to the inferior vena cava, in order to have sufficient length of vein to construct a satisfactory anastomosis. In some patients it may even be necessary to resect a portion of the caudate lobe to be able to perform the shunt.

C.   After freeing up the portal vein in the gastrohepatic ligament and the inferior vena cava retroperitoneally, venous pressures in them are recorded. A long, angled, tourniquet clamp (1) is placed around the distal end of the portal vein (2). In addition to controlling bleeding from the vein after its division, the clamp enables the assistant to control the end of the vein to facilitate performing the anastomosis; it also acts as a retractor. The hepatic end of the portal vein (3) is secured as close as possible to the hilum of the liver with a transfixion suture of linen or cotton. This permits use of the entire length of the portal vein if it is separated a considerable distance from the inferior vena cava by the caudate lobe of the liver.

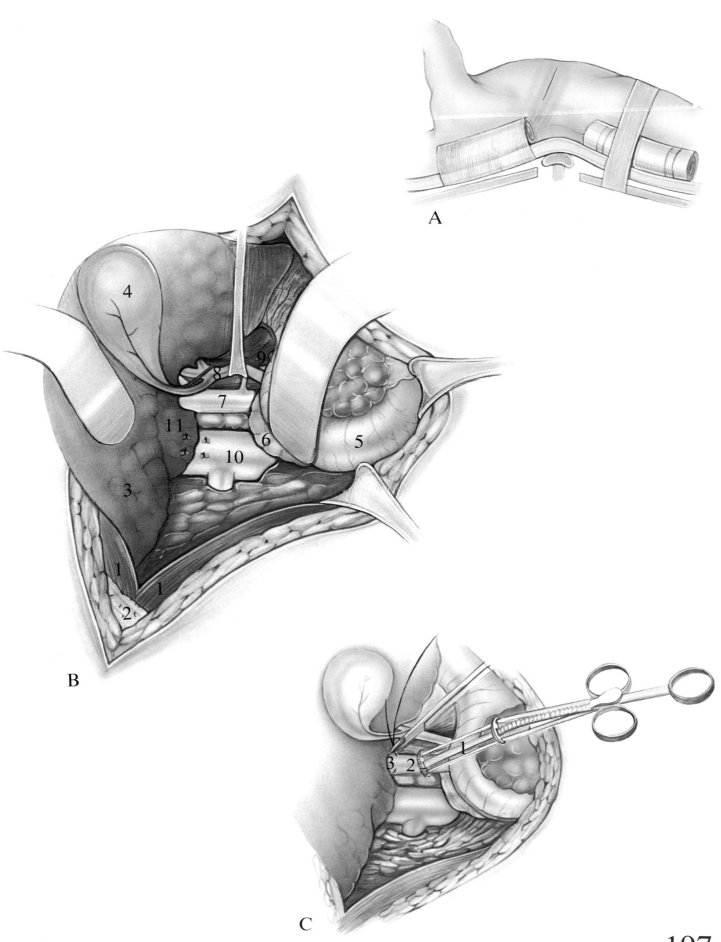

A

B

C

Plate 89

THE DEFINITIVE TREATMENT OF
BLEEDING ESOPHAGEAL VARICES
(Continued)

TECHNIQUE OF CONSTRUCTION OF DIRECT PORTACAVAL
SHUNTS *(Continued)*

A. The portal vein has been divided as close to the transfixion suture as is safe. Guy sutures are placed in the distal end (1). Then the optimum site for the anastomosis is determined so that the portal vein will join the vena cava at an acute angle for better streamlining of the blood flow. At the same time it should be made certain that the tourniquet clamp (2) has not twisted the portal vein as it was applied; if it has, it should be released and reapplied. A large curved clamp (3) with the blades covered with shoelace is placed on the inferior vena cava (4), isolating a portion of the anteromedial wall, so that the portal vein will not be angulated at the anastomosis; this may occur, with early thrombosis of the shunt, if the anastomosis is made to the anterior surface of the vena cava, because the portal vein lies to the left. A small ellipse of the isolated segment of the vena cava is pulled upward with an Allis clamp and excised with curved scissors. This venotomy should not be larger than the diameter of the portal vein. In order to reduce the possibility of postshunt encephalopathy, a serious complication of direct portacaval shunts (especially when they are of large caliber), the anastomosis should be made small, but not with so much narrowing that it will interfere with its streamlined characteristics. A good rule is to not make it greater than 1 cm. in diameter.

B. The long angulated tourniquet clamp on the portal vein gives excellent control. The first assistant can be most helpful in the construction of this anastomosis. The posterior suture line, a 5-0 Teflon-coated Dacron suture (a), preferably with a straight needle, is placed first as a running everting mattress type suture in order to obtain an intima to intima approximation. It is begun at the left and continued to the middle of the posterior row where it is tied to a stay suture after pulling it taut. The other end of suture (a) is tied to the end of the suture for the anterior row at the left end of the anastomosis. Suture (a) is continued to complete the posterior suture line and tied to a stay suture at the end after pulling it taut. Care must be taken when tying these knots that they do not slip, because this will purse string the suture line, producing too much narrowing of the anastomosis.

C. The posterior suture line has been completed, and by use of the running everting type of mattress suture, excellent intima to intima approximation of the portal vein and inferior vena cava has been obtained without the sutures or any rough edges of the vessels showing in the anastomotic lumen. The same type of closure of the anterior suture line is carried out using suture (b) and interrupting it at the halfway point to pull it taut and tie it to a stay suture. The portal vein is released to flush out any thrombi that may have formed beyond the tourniquet clamp. The suture line is then completed from the other end with suture (a). Great care must be taken in placing the anterior suture line that the opposite wall of the anastomosis is not caught with the suture, since if this occurs and it is not detected, early thrombosis of the shunt will develop.

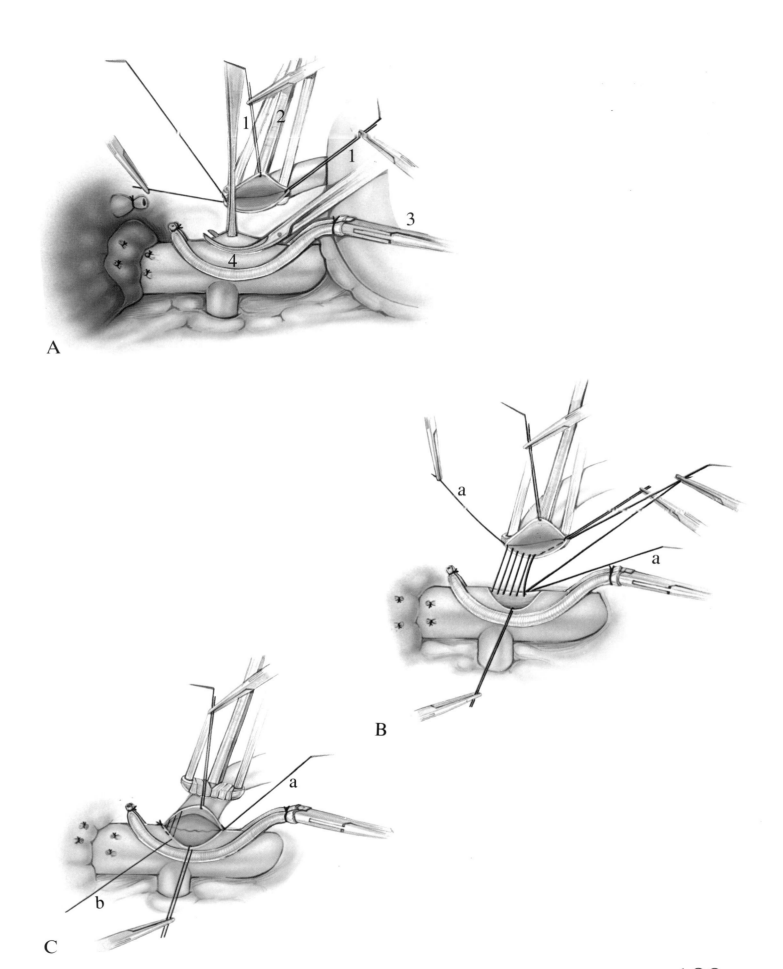

A

B

C

199

Plate 90

THE DEFINITIVE TREATMENT OF
BLEEDING ESOPHAGEAL VARICES
(Continued)

COMPLETED END-TO-SIDE AND SIDE-TO-SIDE DIRECT
PORTACAVAL SHUNTS

A. This demonstrates a completed streamlined end-to-side direct portacaval shunt. Note the acute angle at which the portal vein has been anastomosed to the inferior vena cava with the running everting mattress suture method. In this case it was necessary to interrupt the coronary vein in order to free up the portal vein to permit it to lie without angulation or kinking of it which would have occurred if it had been left intact. Before replacing the structures held back by the retractors to their normal position, hemostasis is checked. In addition, every effort should be made to control by ligatures any lymph vessels that were not controlled during the dissection of the structures in the gastrohepatic ligament. This is because if they are not ligated, the lymph from both the splanchnic and the hepatic ends of these vessels may cause postshunt ascites. Venous pressures are taken in the portal vein and the inferior vena cava. A well functioning shunt shows a decrease in the former and usually a slight increase in the latter. No attempt is made to reperitonealize the operative field. The diaphragm is closed with interrupted linen or cotton sutures, making it fluid tight so that ascitic fluid will not escape into the pleural space, which is drained with a No. 24 Foley catheter in the routine manner. It is placed on 10 cm. negative pressure with three-bottle suction for 48 hours postoperatively and then the catheter is removed. The peritoneal cavity is not drained. The peritoneum is closed tightly with a running suture of 0 chromic catgut. The thoracic and abdominal portions of the incision are closed in individual muscle layers with interrupted nonabsorbable sutures. Nylon stay sutures are placed in the abdominal portion of the incision through all layers of the abdominal wall except the peritoneum. The skin is closed with interrupted sutures of silk.

B. This shows a completed side-to-side direct portacaval shunt performed by anastomosing the adjacent sides of the portal vein and the inferior vena cava; this leaves the portal vein in continuity. In the presence of a high degree of intrahepatic postsinusoidal block, this type of shunt should not be performed because all the portal venous blood and most of the arterial blood supply to the liver will pass through the shunt, thereby depriving it not only of its portal venous blood supply but also of its life-supporting arterial blood. If the procedure has any place in the treatment of bleeding esophageal varices, it should be performed only when there is a relatively low degree of intrahepatic postsinusoidal portal bed block that permits the arterial blood to pass through the liver instead of bypassing it through the shunt. It is also worth pointing out that the portal vein and the vena cava are so often separated by a large caudate lobe of the liver that it is not possible to bring them together without resecting the caudate lobe or utilizing some type of prosthetic graft. It is believed, since direct portacaval shunts result in such a high incidence of postshunt encephalopathy and early and late deaths from liver failure, that they should be used only when a splenorenal or some other type of shunt cannot possibly be performed.

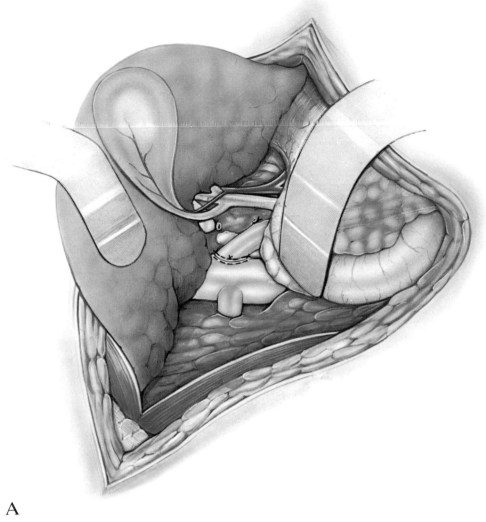

A

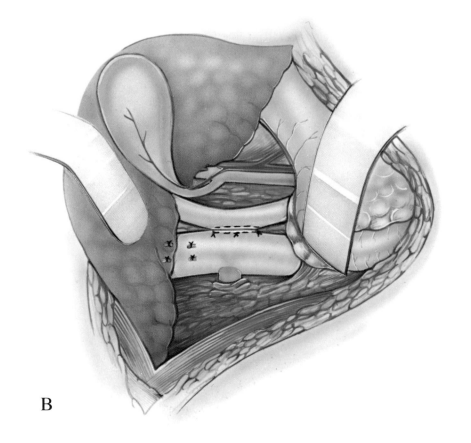

B

201

Plate 91

THE DEFINITIVE TREATMENT OF
BLEEDING ESOPHAGEAL VARICES
(Continued)

CORONACAVAL SHUNTS

During the past decade a tremendous number of different types of portasystemic venous shunts have been reported in the literature, each an attempt to prevent the postshunt complications of the direct portacaval type and to find one that can be more easily accomplished than the end-to-side splenorenal type. Additional time and experience are needed to determine which of them are going to give the best long-term results, with control of the esophageal varices, the prevention of postshunt encephalopathy, and low operative and the late mortality rates from liver failure. The procedures described here and in Plate 92 have been found by the author to give excellent results so are included here.

A. This shows a coronacaval shunt between the left gastric or coronary vein and the inferior vena cava. The exposure is obtained through a right thoraco-abdominal incision, the same as for a direct portacaval anastomosis. The left gastric vein (1), which may be 7 to 8 mm. in diameter, is isolated along the lesser curvature of the stomach (2) and followed distally, then ligated and divided at its termination in the portal vein. The inferior vena cava (3) is readily exposed by opening the posterior peritoneum. An end-to-side anastomosis is then performed between the coronary vein and the inferior vena cava by the technique that has already been described for other end-to-side types of anastomoses. This type of shunt, performed in one patient with cirrhosis of the liver, is still functioning after 17 years, and in another with an extrahepatic portal bed block after 14 years, with the disappearance of the esophageal varices in both, with no further esophageal bleeding or any signs of postshunt encephalopathy.

B. This is a schematic drawing demonstrating the connections of the esophageal varices, the veins of the lesser curvatures of the stomach and the submucosal veins of the cardia of the stomach with the coronary vein and its branches, indicating the direction of the flow of blood through them after a coronacaval shunt in a postsplenectomy bleeding patient with an extrahepatic portal bed block. The direction of the flow of the venous blood in these vessels, which is reversed so that it flows toward the esophageal varices in patients with a high degree of both intrahepatic and extrahepatic portal bed block, is changed after construction of the coronacaval shunt so that again the flow is in a normal direction, with the one exception that it now empties into the low pressure venous system of the inferior vena cava instead of the higher pressure system of the portal vein. As can be seen by the drawing, it is the most direct method of decompressing the veins of the lower esophagus and the proximal portion of the cardia of the stomach. It is believed that it is also a more selective type of decompression because of its location and the fact that the coronary vein is a relatively small one and does not decompress the entire portal bed to the same extent that a direct portacaval shunt of necessity does. As a result, it prevents postshunt encephalopathy and liver degeneration, but at the same time it decompresses the esophageal varices sufficiently to prevent further bleeding. Extreme care must be taken in constructing the anastomosis because of the relatively small size of the coronary vein and the necessity to make sure there is not too much tension on it. In some patients a venous graft of the saphenous vein may need to be inserted.

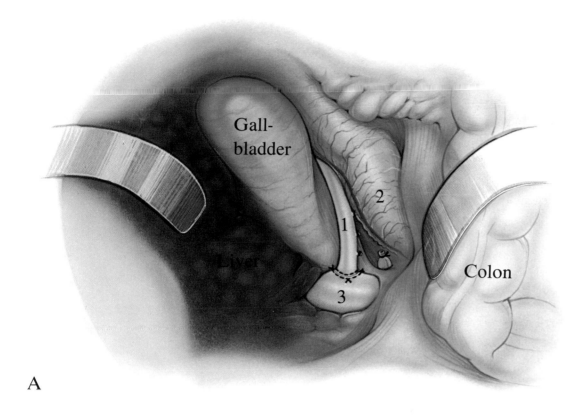

A

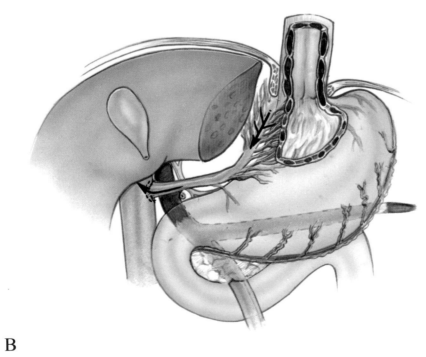

B

Plate 92

THE DEFINITIVE TREATMENT OF
BLEEDING ESOPHAGEAL VARICES
(Continued)

MESOCAVAL SHUNT WITH AUTOGENOUS SAPHENOUS VEIN
GRAFT

A. This is the venous phase of a celiac angiogram made in an attempt to demonstrate the superior mesenteric and portal veins in a man aged 20 years with an extrahepatic portal bed block and bleeding esophageal varices in whom a splenorenal shunt and later a transesophageal suture of the esophageal varices had both failed to control esophageal bleeding. Both had been followed by numerous severe esophageal hemorrhages. Note the segmental nature of the venous pattern in the mesentery of the small intestine without any large vein or the superior mesenteric vein being visualized.

B. The abdomen was opened through a right paramedian incision. The superior mesenteric and portal veins were both fibrous scarred channels unsuitable for shunts. One short segment of a dilated vein (1) was found at operation at the base of the small bowel mesentery above the third portion of the duodenum (2) and the inferior vena cava (3). It would have been impossible to anastomose the inferior vena cava to this vein as had been originally planned, because it was so thin-walled and too difficult to free up any farther than is shown without injury.

C. A mesocaval shunt was constructed, however, using a segment of the proximal part of the long saphenous vein that was 8 mm. in diameter. It is seen crossing over the third portion of the duodenum. Both anastomoses were performed by the end-to-side technique. The result has been most gratifying, with disappearance of the esophageal varices and no further bleeding episodes or signs of postshunt encephalopathy after eight years. This type of shunt is of small caliber like the splenorenal and coronacaval shunts; it functions better than the large ones since it does not shunt too much of the portal venous blood but does carry enough to decompress the esophageal varices and prevent them from bleeding.

END-TO-SIDE MESOCAVAL SHUNT

D. This demonstrates another type of mesocaval shunt by an end-to-side anastomosis between the proximal end of the divided inferior vena cava and the side of the superior mesenteric vein. The superior mesenteric vein is first isolated at the base of the transverse mesocolon just distal to the right colic vein and the third portion of the duodenum to determine if it is satisfactory for the construction of a shunt. If it is, the inferior vena cava is isolated through the posterior peritoneum or by elevation of the right colon. For ease of manipulation the common iliac veins are divided. The distal ends are secured by suturing them with arterial silk. The lumbar veins are isolated, doubly ligated and divided as the vena cava is elevated until a sufficient length has been freed up, usually just distal to the renal veins. The end is then brought through an opening made in the mesentery of the jejunum just distal to the duodenum and anastomosed end-to-side to the superior mesenteric vein. A variant of this method has recently been reported in which a Teflon prosthesis 18 mm. in diameter was used to make the mesocaval shunt and implanted by the end-to-side technique to both vessels so that it was unnecessary to interrupt the interior vena cava. Further experience with these two methods is necessary to determine their long-term results.

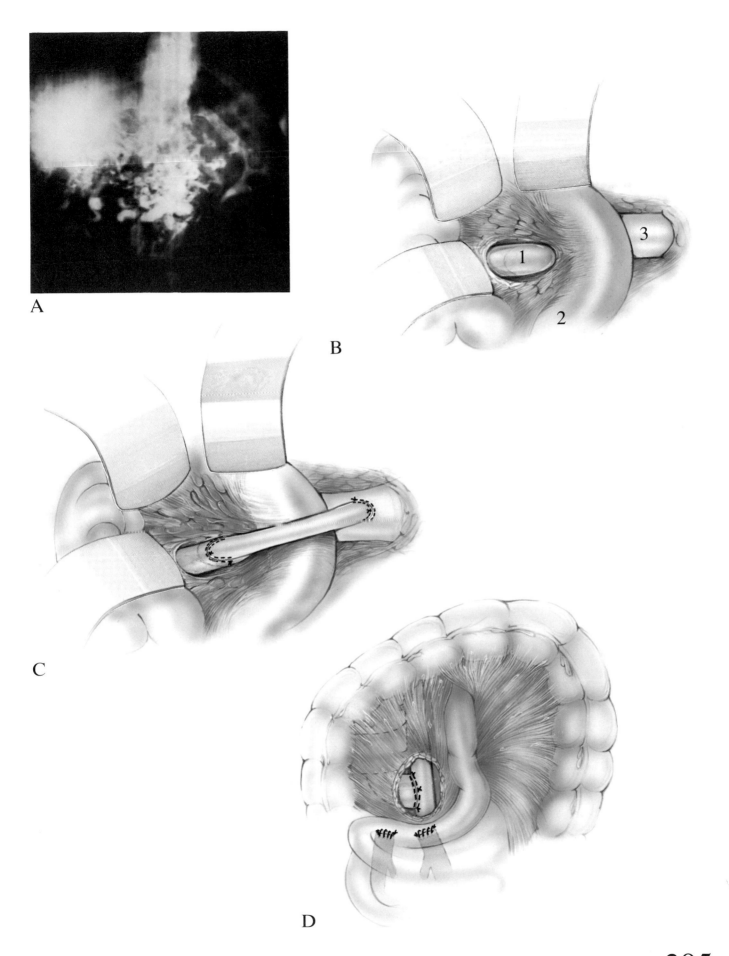

A

B

C

D

205

Part II

Diseases of the Arteries

ABDOMINAL ARTERIOSCLEROTIC AORTIC ANEURYSMS

Introduction

The diagnosis of an abdominal arteriosclerotic aortic aneurysm should be made on physical examination in the majority of patients. In some individuals who are very obese, large abdominal arteriosclerotic aortic aneurysms may not be palpable because of marked obesity of the abdominal wall and also of the intraperitoneal structures, such as the mesentery of the small bowel, overlying the aneurysm. The diagnosis in many cases, however, is missed on physical examination because the examining doctor fails to palpate the abdomen carefully for this condition; because the majority of them are asymptomatic for many years, the physician is not examining for an aortic aneurysm. As a result, it is not surprising that the diagnosis is frequently made from study of a roentgenogram of the abdomen made as part of a gastrointestinal examination or, more often, from a urological work-up that includes an intravenous pyelogram. Many arteriosclerotic aortic aneurysms have some calcification in their walls that may not be visible on an anteroposterior roentgenogram of the abdomen unless the aneurysms are larger in diameter than the bodies of the lumbar vertebrae, because the latter hide them. For this reason, if the diagnosis is suspected on physical examination because of an increased pulsation over the abdominal aorta opposite and a little above the umbilicus, it is important to obtain a lateral roentgenogram of the lumbar spine that includes the abdominal area. In some cases additional information may be obtained also by oblique views of the lumbar spine. Utilizing this technique it is possible to visualize most abdominal aortic arteriosclerotic aneurysms because there are no bony structures to hide the calcified plaques in the walls. In the majority of abdominal aortic aneurysms aortography is unnecessary and may even result in failure to make the diagnosis, because many of them contain a large amount of intravascular thrombus through which a channel has formed the size of the normal aortic lumen, so that the angiogram does not show the true size of these large aneurysms. When an aneurysm extends high in the epigastrium it is useful to determine preoperatively by aortography whether or not the renal and superior mesenteric arteries arise from it, because if this occurs, a much more extensive operative procedure is necessary than if the aneurysm arises distal to the renal arteries. Fortunately the great majority are limited to the infrarenal portion of the aorta, so that they can be removed safely and aortic continuity restored with a knitted Dacron prosthesis without great difficulty.

A preoperative intravenous pyelogram should always be obtained to determine if the patient has two functioning kidneys. In some cases it may help to determine the course of the ureters in relation to the aneurysmal

208

walls. In the great majority of resections of abdominal aortic aneurysms the ureters are readily visualized and so can be protected from injury.

There is still not complete agreement among surgeons with reference to how large an aneurysm should be before one advises a patient to have an elective operation to remove it. My. rule has been to recommend the operation if the aneurysm is 5 cm. or more in its greatest diameter and providing the patient's age and general condition from a cerebrovascular, cardiac, pulmonary and renal status are satisfactory. An increase in the size of the aneurysm over months or a few years to the 5-cm. size is a strong indication for removal in the near future. The operative mortality rate is so low for the resection of moderate-sized abdominal aortic aneurysms and the replacement of them with a knitted Dacron bifurcation prosthesis, and the results so uniformly excellent, that it is inexcusable for the surgeon or physician not to recommend the operation to patients who otherwise are in a good state of health. The final decision, of course, must rest with the patient.

There is no comparison between the morbidity and the mortality of the elective procedure and those of the emergency one done because of massive rupture of a large aneurysm in patients who are ten years older than when the diagnosis should have been made and the operation performed. Such patients are poorer operative risks because of their increased age and especially because of the condition of their hearts, lungs and kidneys. However, the operation must be performed even under these conditions, because a fair percentage of patients survive, but not nearly so many as those done at a younger age when the aneurysms are smaller in size and the patients are better operative risks. Elective resections of large abdominal aortic aneurysms or even small ones in patients beyond 80 years of age should not be performed unless the heart, lungs and kidneys are in good condition so that the operative risk, especially from the cardiac aspect, is not too great.

Plate 93

THE TECHNIQUE FOR THE ELECTIVE RESECTION OF ABDOMINAL ARTERIOSCLEROTIC AORTIC ANEURYSMS WITH THE INSERTION OF KNITTED DACRON PROSTHESES

THE POSITION OF THE PATIENT AND THE DRAPING ON THE OPERATING TABLE

A. This demonstrates the patient lying supine on the operating table. He is a thin individual with a large abdominal aortic aneurysm which can be seen pushing the anterior abdominal wall forward. Prophylactic intramuscular antibiotic therapy of 500,000 units of penicillin and 250 mg. of streptomycin is given on call to the operating room. In addition, a slow drip of 5 per cent dextrose in distilled water with 1 gram of erythromycin is also given during the operation. This prophylactic antibiotic therapy is continued postoperatively for five days. It not only results in clean surgery but also reduces pulmonary and urinary complications. The principles of aseptic surgery must also be scrupulously carried out. The skin of the patient's abdomen is prepared with an aseptic solution and dried thoroughly with ether; then a self-adhering thin plastic sheet is applied as shown so that the hands of the surgeon and his assistants and the instruments never come in contact with the skin throughout the operation. In order to provide more room for the surgeon and his assistants, the arms are suspended on a frame over the head of the patient.

The anesthesia is administered, using intravenous pentothal supplemented with a muscle relaxant and gas oxygen administered through a cuffed endotracheal tube. For aid in closure of the abdominal incision a little ether may be helpful. A central venous pressure cannula, an intra-arterial cannula in the radial artery to monitor the blood pressure, and a third cannula for intravenous fluids and transfusions are placed. A Foley catheter is inserted into the bladder. Spinal or epidural anesthesia administered through a catheter is an excellent method in good risk patients and in some with pulmonary problems.

B. This demonstrates the operative view of the patient's abdomen after application of the sterile drapes. A special method is shown of applying them at the foot of the table to prevent the instruments from falling on the floor. The space between the legs is filled with folded sheets or gowns. A half sheet is fastened with Kelly clamps to the Mayo stand that holds the instruments. The other corners of the end of the half sheet are fastened to the towel on the sides of the patient at the groin levels in a similar manner.

A long right paramedian muscle retracting incision is preferred, extending from the ensiform process down to the symphysis pubis, as shown by the line on the abdomen. The closure of this incision gives such excellent results, without dehiscence or postoperative incisional hernias, that the extra time required to make it is worthwhile, unless the situation requires a rapid exposure of the great vessels of the abdomen. A long transverse incision across the abdomen just above or below the umbilicus in patients with very wide abdominal girths and costal arches gives excellent exposure if the aortic aneurysm does not extend too far proximally and if there are not large common iliac aneurysms distally. A midline incision the full length of the abdomen is recommended in emergency procedures for ruptured abdominal aortic aneurysms when speed can be of such great importance.

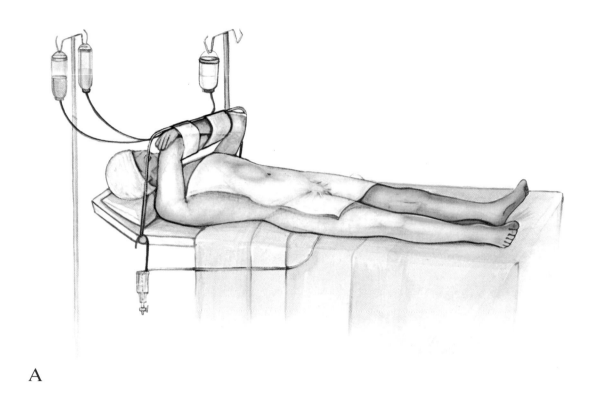

A

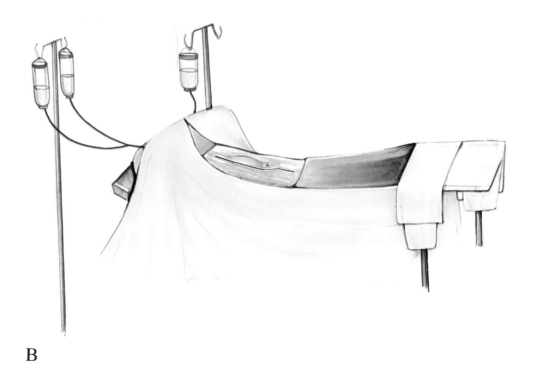

B

Plate 94

EXPLORATION FOLLOWED BY EXPOSURE OF THE ANEURYSM AND THE USE OF LINTON INTESTINAL BAG

A. After the abdomen has been opened through a long right paramedian muscle retracting incision, an abdominal exploration is carried out. This shows the hand inserted cephalad to palpate the liver, the gallbladder, the stomach and the esophageal hiatus to determine if there is any pathology associated with these organs and structures. The position of the Levin tube that has been passed into the stomach is also determined, as it is important to keep the stomach on suction during the operation to prevent distention of it and of the intestines. The small and large intestines are examined carefully and, in the female, the uterus and its adnexa. This thorough exploration paid off in one patient especially, because a carcinoma of the third portion of the duodenum was found. This was removed after completion of the aneurysmectomy and the grafting procedure. The patient is alive and well without evidence of recurrence of the malignant disease 15 years after the operation. This type of case demonstrates that the transperitoneal approach, in addition to making the procedure easier and safer, permits discovery and safe removal of other serious intraperitoneal lesions, which of course is not possible by the extraperitoneal method.

B. The transverse colon and the greater curvature are retracted upward to expose the small intestines. The surgeon draws these into a large rubber bag which has been constructed with a sleeve through which his hand can be inserted to pull the intestines into the bag. His assistant holds the large end of the bag open and firmly against the right side of the incision to facilitate this procedure. Draw strings at the large end are pulled to narrow this opening, but it is important not to close it too tightly because of the danger of strangulating the bowel. A moist towel is placed over the bag and against the opening, which helps to keep the intestines within it.

C. The hand is withdrawn and the sleeve is tied very tightly with a strong piece of cotton tape. This method keeps the small intestines out of the way, and also in excellent condition throughout the operative procedure. During the time they are in the bag sometimes as much as 200 cc.'s of plasma will exude; this is replaced into the abdomen at the end of the operation. Were the bag not used, this would be lost in the gauze packs. It is essential that the bag be washed out thoroughly before use with normal saline to remove all traces of the surgical starch powder which is used in making the bags and also is sometimes dusted into the bag before sterilization. This material is very irritating to the bowel and the starch particles can cause serious granulomatous lesions.

D. Note there are two Deaver retractors on the left side of the incision and a large six-inch one against the right side. They are covered with very fine meshed cotton stockinet so that it is unnecessary to insert large gauze packs. Towels have been fastened to the skin edges of the abdominal incision with towel clips. The one on the right side is now used as a hammock-like support for the rubber bag containing the small intestines, because otherwise it will slip off the intestines. The towels are fastened at the upper and lower ends of the incision to the drapes by means of Kelly clamps. A large abdominal aortic aneurysm is shown with a portion of the duodenum (1) adherent to the right of it. Crossing above it is the transverse colon (2), and at the lower end of the incision the sigmoid colon (3) is visible.

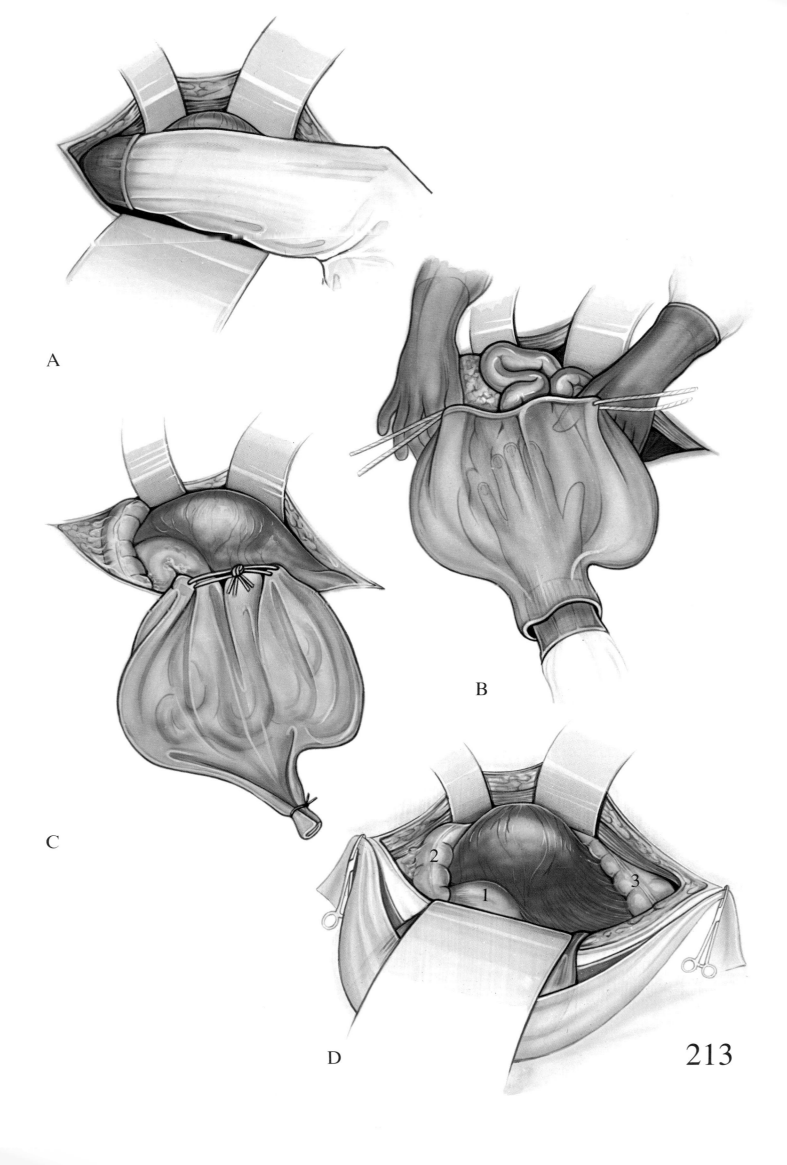

A

B

C

D

1

2

3

213

Plate 95

DISSECTION OF THE NECK OF THE ANEURYSM WITH PLACEMENT OF THE PROXIMAL TOURNIQUET CLAMP

A. The dissection is commenced on the anterior wall, cutting through the posterior peritoneum that overlies the aneurysm. There are a few blood vessels in it that require ligation. It is important to preserve these peritoneal flaps both on the right and the left sides in order to use them as one layer of a two-layer closure over the aortic graft after it has been implanted. On the right side it is always left attached to the third portion of the duodenum and the proximal jejunum. In most cases this portion of the intestinal tract will free up very readily from the aneurysm along with its peritoneal flap, but in some instances it may be so adherent to a scarred and sclerotic type of aneurysmal sac that it is necessary to dissect away a thin layer of the aneurysmal wall to prevent injury and opening of the duodenal lumen (Plate 127*A*). This complication is a serious one when it occurs because of the resultant bacterial contamination in the operative field where a Dacron prosthesis is to be implanted.

B. This demonstrates the exposure of the proximal aorta, or what is often called the "neck" of the aneurysm. It is the aorta just distal to the left renal vein, as shown. The inferior vena cava is separated from the aneurysmal wall and the neck of the aneurysm by careful dissection, ligating a few small vessels arising from the proximal portion of the aneurysm that are encountered. The dissection is carried out on the left side in a similar manner. The left renal vein is shown at its termination in the inferior vena cava, and the left spermatic vein can be seen arising from it toward the left kidney. Sometimes this vessel is so adherent to the aneurysmal wall that it must be ligated and divided. After carrying out this dissection it is usually possible with the thumb and forefinger of the right hand to almost completely encircle the proximal aorta, although in some cases it may be quite adherent posteriorly; this requires careful separation of it from the anterior longitudinal ligament. When this is accomplished it is very easy to gently pass a large right-angled clamp around the proximal aorta, as shown, without tearing a lumbar artery or a vein. The end of a shoestring is placed in the jaws of the clamp and pulled through behind the aorta to be used in the tourniquet clamp later to occlude the aorta. The inferior mesenteric artery is ligated and divided. Before ligating the distal end, the retrograde blood flow from it should be checked. This is known as the Henle-Coenen sign. The surgeon does not need to worry about ischemia of the sigmoid colon if the back flow is brisk, and especially if it is pulsatile—a positive Henle-Coenen sign. If the inferior mesenteric artery is widely patent and obviously a main source of blood supply to the sigmoid, it may be necessary in a rare instance to anastomose it to the graft to preserve the blood supply of the colon.

C. This shows the tourniquet clamp in place, with a shoestring threaded through the clamp and then tied. The distal end has been wrapped with a cotton tape to cushion the metal crossbar and to give it a rough surface so that it does not slip after it is closed.

D. This shows that the shoestring has been tied with a square knot on the back side of the clamp so that it is ready to be closed when the resection of the aneurysm is commenced. The common iliac arteries are shown coming off the aneurysm but have not been completely freed from the vena cava and the iliac veins; this will be shown in the next plate.

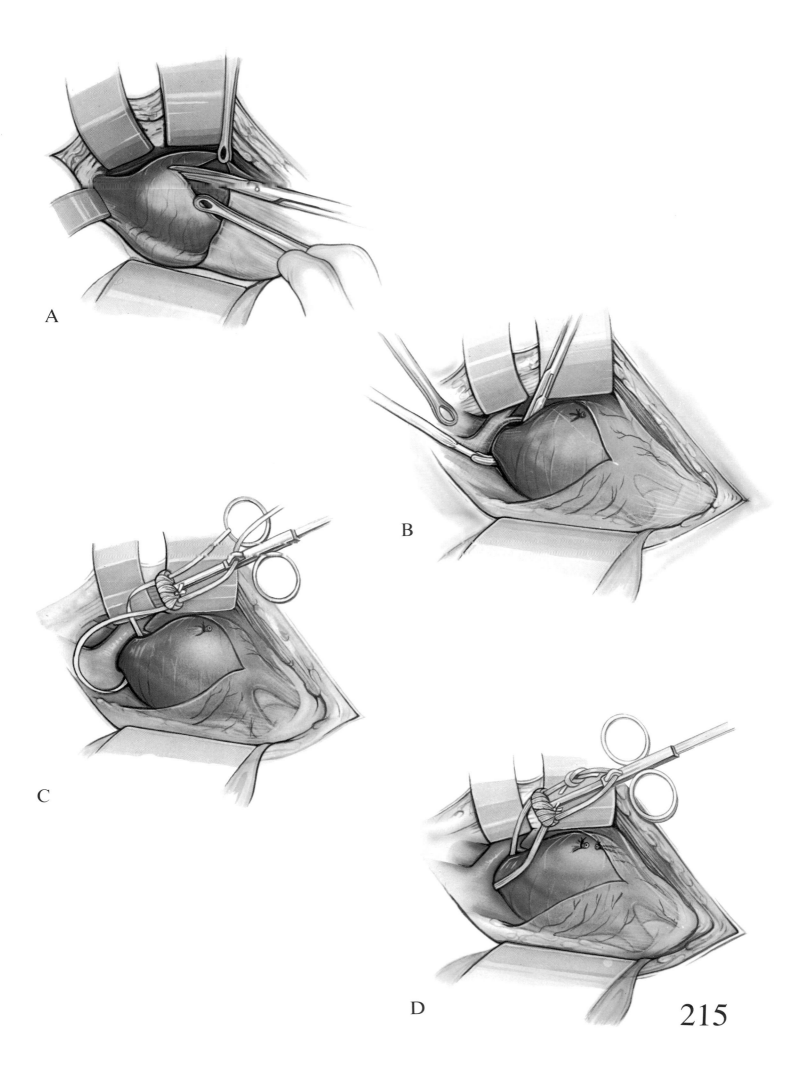

A

B

C

D

215

Plate 96

TOTAL HEPARINIZATION OF THE PATIENT; DISSECTION OF COMMON ILIAC ARTERIES

A. Total heparinization of the patient prevents blood clots from forming in the aorta and arteries of the lower extremities between the time of occlusion of the abdominal aorta and the restoration of the circulation after implanting of the aortic bifurcation graft. Without heparinization, thrombi may form proximal to the aortic clamp, resulting in embolization of the kidneys since the renal arteries are part of the outflow tract of the aorta; this can prove fatal. Thrombosis distal to the common iliac arteries in the external iliac and femoral arteries may also develop, with resulting ischemic problems in the lower limbs; this unnecessary complication requires thrombectomy. It has been demonstrated that the injection of 4000 units, or 40 mg., of heparin into the inferior vena cava 15 minutes before occluding the aorta, with an additional injection of 20 cc. of dilute heparin solution, containing 400 units or 4 mg., in each distal common iliac artery prevents these complications from developing. In order to make sure that the heparin is effectively injected intravenously, the surgeon should aspirate 4 cc. of the concentrated solution containing 4000 units of heparin from an ampule which has been gas sterilized and then inject it himself into the inferior vena cava. In this manner he can be absolutely certain that the heparin is injected intravenously without having to rely on other personnel who may not realize the importance of its use, and so may fail to give it.

B. This demonstrates the injection of the heparin into the inferior vena cava, which has always been exposed by this stage of the operative procedure. This vessel is chosen because it is the largest one available and one can be certain that the heparin is injected intravenously. It will also be circulated very rapidly from this vessel, so it is an ideal site for the injection. The dissection and isolation of the common iliac arteries have purposely been delayed until the heparin has been injected. The time taken to do the dissection gives sufficient time to make sure that the heparin has been well distributed throughout the blood stream. My rule has been to permit at least 15 minutes to elapse between the time of injection and the occlusion of the proximal aorta.

C. The right common iliac artery is first isolated by separating it very carefully with sharp, curved, slightly dull pointed scissors from the right common iliac vein and the bifurcation of the inferior vena cava. The use of ring forceps greatly facilitates the traction on the artery and the vein, which is so important to facilitate the separation of them.

D. After the right common iliac artery has been freed up over a distance of 2 to 3 cm., a similar procedure is carried out on the left common iliac artery. This drawing demonstrates the utilization of a right-angled clamp to perform the final separation and to pull a thin-walled Penrose tube beneath it for additional traction.

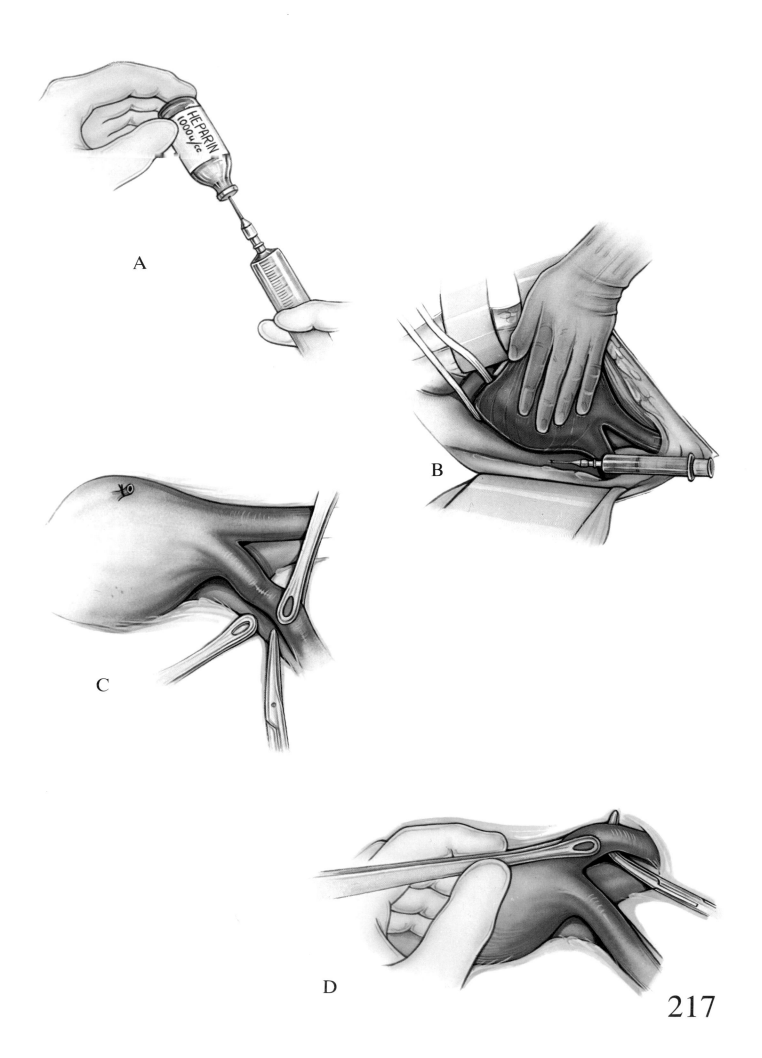

A

B

C

D

217

Plate 97

REPAIR OF A LACERATION OF THE LEFT COMMON ILIAC VEIN; CLOSURE OF PROXIMAL AORTIC TOURNIQUET CLAMP AND METHODS OF CONTROL OF COMMON ILIAC ARTERIES

A. This demonstrates the most satisfactory method of controlling a laceration of the left common iliac vein. This occurs more frequently than injury to the right common iliac vein because a small branch of it is more often torn in the dissection. The point of laceration is grasped with a fine-tipped Allis clamp which, if placed properly (this can be done very readily), will control the bleeding instantaneously. It is recommended that the laceration be sutured with interrupted mattress sutures of 4–0 arterial silk on curved needles rather than using a running over-and-over suture. This method has been found most satisfactory because the mattress sutures will not tear through even the thinnest walled vein.

B. By this time at least 15 minutes has elapsed since the heparin was injected, so the closure of the tourniquet clamp proximal to the aortic aneurysm is performed as demonstrated. This clamp has the great advantage that it occludes the aorta with the least trauma of any instrument, and it may be loosened and reapplied with utmost ease and without injury to the aortic wall. It is held out of the way of the operative field by a long ligature placed through the upper ring and passed around a Kelly clamp attached to the drapes, with another one fastened to the end of the ligature. This is allowed to hang at the side of the patient so that the weight of it maintains gentle traction on the tourniquet clamp handle. It is inadvisable for a member of the operating team to hold it by hand because this tends to produce a lever-like action which always makes it slip.

C. The distal control of the common iliac arteries is usually performed with cloth covers on the jaws of the bulldog clamps. The cloth covering prevents the clamps from slipping, so that a crushing type of occluding clamp is unnecessary in most cases. The covering is a short section of a white shoestring, a hollow tube, slipped over the jaws and tied at each end.

D. In some instances the distal common iliac arteries may be very short and sclerotic, so that the bulldog clamps will not control the retrograde flow from them; in this case it is very helpful to apply separate tourniquet clamps to control them as shown. They are not yet closed in the drawing, but this may be accomplished very quickly after placing them.

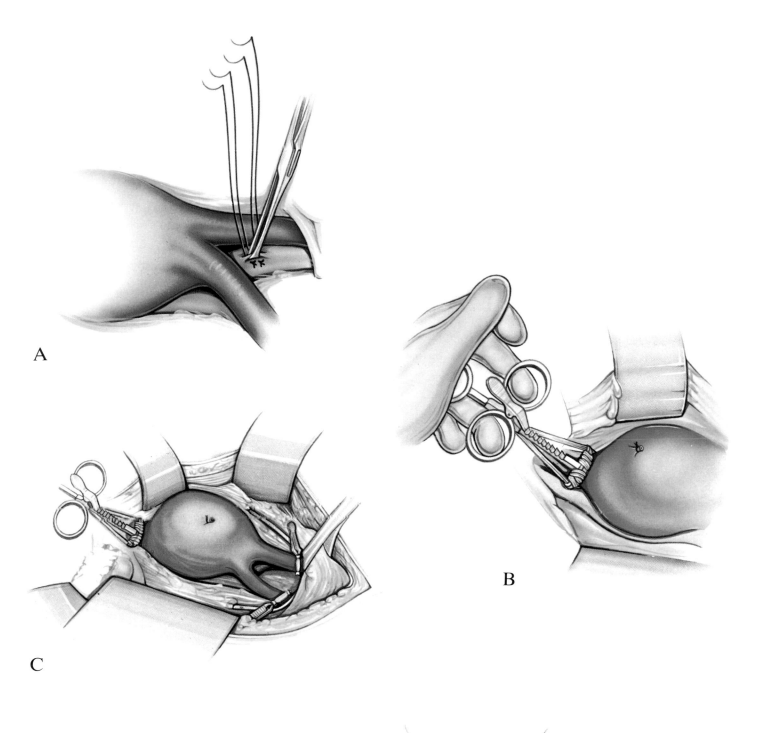

A

B

C

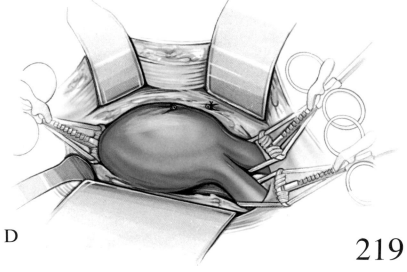

D

219

Plate 98

FLUSHING OF THE PROXIMAL AORTA THROUGH AN INCISION IN THE ANEURYSM; DIVISION OF THE RIGHT COMMON ILIAC ARTERY

A. In addition to general heparinization of the patient, it is also advisable to perform an immediate flush of the proximal aorta after occluding it and the common iliac arteries. This is especially true when by palpation of the neck of the aneurysm one feels the presence of intraluminal material, usually an amorphous partially organized thrombus. The reason for this is that when the aortic clamp is closed it often crushes this material and fragments it. If it is not flushed out immediately it may embolize the renal arteries and sometimes the superior mesenteric artery, since these are the most distal outflow vessels of the aorta when it is occluded just distal to the renal arteries. The illustration demonstrates the making of the incision through the aneurysmal wall with a knife.

B. This demonstrates the opening of the tourniquet clamp and the consequent gush of blood and numerous small pieces of thrombi that are potential emboli if not flushed out in this manner. The aorta is then readily and quickly occluded again with closure of the tourniquet clamp, which is another great advantage of this method of aortic control, since it can be performed without the necessity of visualizing the aorta; the tourniquet clamp always remains in place and so can be closed easily and quickly.

C. Kocher clamps have been placed on both common iliac arteries proximal to the bulldog clamps. These arteries are divided with scissors, after making sure that the right one has been separated from the inferior vena cava to prevent laceration of the vena cava while applying the clamp and dividing the artery.

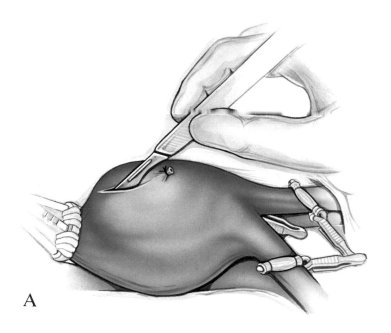

A

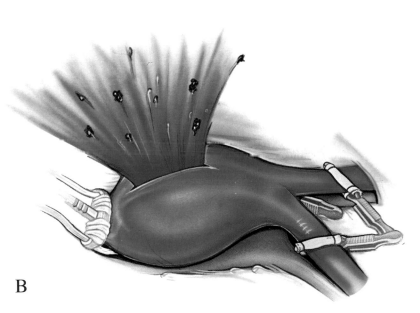

B

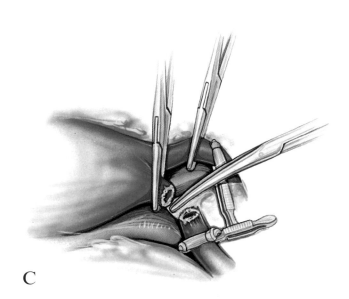

C

Plate 99

FLUSHING OF THE PROXIMAL AORTA THROUGH RIGHT COMMON ILIAC ARTERY; DISSECTION OF THE POSTERIOR WALL OF THE ANEURYSM; METHOD OF CONTROL OF LACERATION OF INFERIOR VENA CAVA

A. This demonstrates another method of an aorta flush which is satisfactory if the lumen of the iliac artery is of large size. It is easily accomplished by release of the tourniquet clamp. After the flush it is reset and the common iliac artery is again secured with a Kocher clamp. This method makes the total removal of the aneurysmal sac less bloody, especially if there is a large retrograde flow of blood from the lumbar arteries.

B. This demonstrates the separation of the aneurysmal sac from the inferior vena cava with curved blunt pointed scissors, while maintaining traction on the iliac arteries. The separation of the inferior vena cava from the lateral edge of the origin of the right common iliac artery is the place laceration is most apt to occur because the inferior vena cava is tented up at this point. It is important, therefore, to visualize the edge of it in order to separate the aneurysm from it or, if necessary, to leave a small portion of the outer layer of the aneurysmal sac to avoid lacerating it.

C. This illustration demonstrates the large pool of blood that forms quickly after a moderate laceration of the inferior vena cava. This may result in the loss of a considerable amount of blood before it is controlled, especially if the usual hemostatic types of clamps are used to grasp the laceration. Under these conditions the surgeon will usually end up with a larger laceration than the original one, because the venous wall is so fragile and tears so easily.

D. It is recommended that a wide-tipped Allis clamp be used to grasp the wall of the vena cava as near as possible to the laceration. It is not necessary to place the clamp directly on it because, with gentle twisting, immediate temporary control of the bleeding will be obtained, since the venous blood is at a low pressure. This step in the procedure can be facilitated a great deal by the first assistant's applying pressure proximally over the vena cava by pressing on the aneurysm with the fingers of the right hand, and distally to the common iliac veins with the fingers of the left hand. In this way the bleeding can be temporarily stopped so that the Allis clamp can be placed more accurately. Then, if necessary, additional clamps can be applied. Care must be taken, of course, that the clamps are not pulled on too strongly because they will tear the vena cava, making a much larger laceration. The advantage of the Allis clamp is that it grasps the venous lacerations from each side and does not push the edges away as the ordinary hemostatic type of clamp tends to do; thus, the edges of the laceration can be more accurately secured.

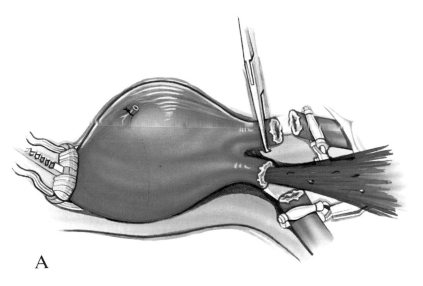

A

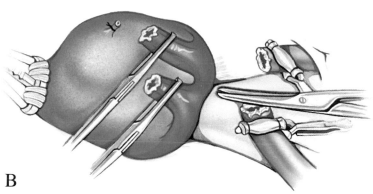

B

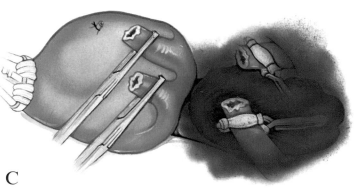

C

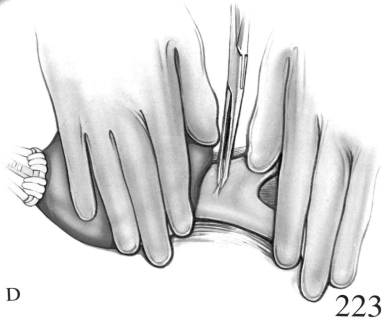

D

223

Plate 100

METHOD OF SUTURE REPAIR OF INFERIOR VENA CAVA LACERATION; INJECTION OF DILUTE HEPARIN SOLUTION IN DISTAL COMMON ILIAC ARTERIES; FURTHER DISSECTION OF THE AORTIC ANEURYSM

A. This demonstrates the method of suture of the inferior vena cava laceration with the Allis clamp in place and with the utilization of interrupted mattress sutures of 5-0 silk on curved needles. With this method, much larger lacerations than shown have been repaired with relatively little loss of blood. Well trained assistants can be of inestimable value, both in preventing and in the repair of these complications.

B. This demonstrates excellent control of a laceration of the inferior vena cava; the interruption of the mid-sacral artery in the curved hemostat; and the injection of 20 cc. of dilute heparin in normal saline solution (100 units, or 1 mg., of heparin per 5 cc. of solution) into the distal ends of the common iliac arteries through a small polyvinyl tube that has been passed beyond the bulldog clamp. As a result, in addition to the 4000 units, or 40 mg., of heparin that were given initially, the patient receives another 800 units, or 8 mg., intra-arterially. The latter is very important, especially in patients with severe atherosclerotic disease of the iliac and femoral arteries, because they are prone to thrombose during the operative procedure unless they are well protected with heparin.

C. In order to facilitate the extirpation of the aneurysmal sac, the contents of it are evacuated by finger dissection through a linear incision, as shown. In this manner, a large amount of solid thrombus and sometimes partially liquefied clot are evacuated.

When the aneurysm is very adherent to the surrounding structures it is safer to leave the posterior wall in place. (See Plates 121, 122 and 125.) This decision is made as one dissects out the anterior and anterolateral sides of the aneurysm after the cleaning out of the aneurysmal sac. If it is decided to remove the aneurysmal sac because it is relatively nonadherent, the emptying out of the aneurysm makes it much easier to separate the aneurysm from the inferior vena cava and to isolate the lumbar arteries.

D. This demonstrates the separation of the aneurysm from the inferior vena cava and a lumbar vein, which permits ready isolation of the lumbar arteries. The distal arteries are secured with curved clamps so that each one can be ligated securely; the proximal ones are first ligated near the aorta and controlled distally with a curved clamp, then divided. The reason for this is that the proximal arteries sometimes lie in the cuff of the proximal aorta that may be used for the proximal aortic anastomosis, so it is important to control the proximal end of these lumbar arteries with ligatures.

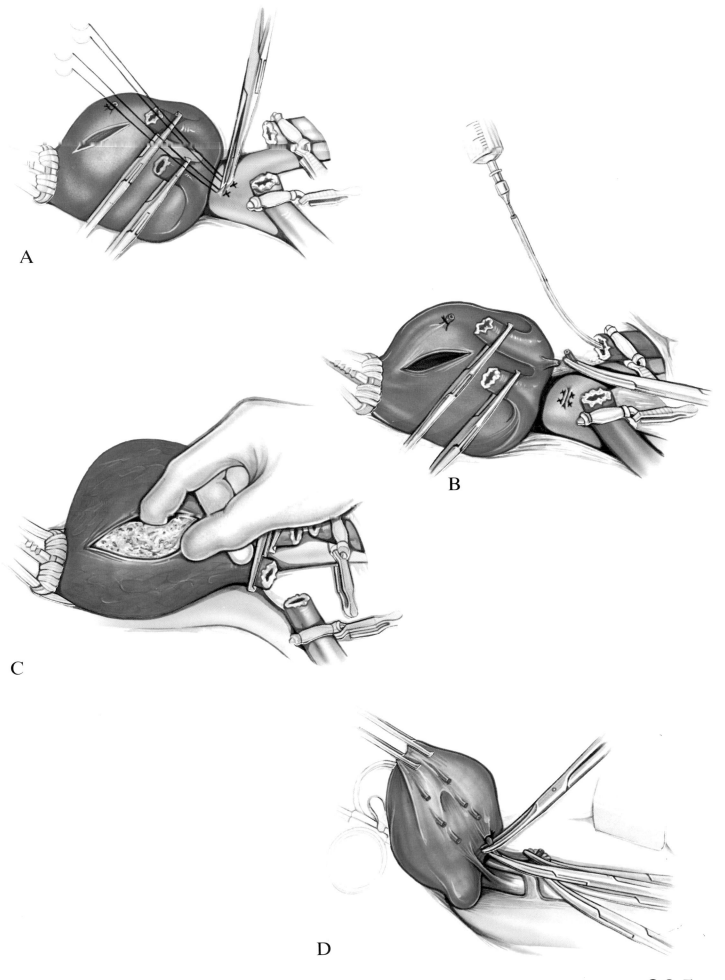

A

B

C

D

Plate 101

METHOD OF INTERRUPTION OF THE LUMBAR ARTERIES; RESECTION OF THE ANEURYSMAL SAC; ENDARTERECTOMY OF THE PROXIMAL AORTIC CUFF

A. This demonstrates the method of ligating the proximal end of the proximal right lumbar artery by use of a right-angled clamp and a ligature that is being placed around the proximal end of it. This is tied before dividing the lumbar artery. The distal ends are controlled, before division, with curved Schnitt clamps.

B. The aneurysmal sac and the aorta proximal to it have been isolated sufficiently so that it now can be excised by dividing the aorta at its junction with the aneurysm and approximately 1.5 cm. distal to the tourniquet clamp, using a right-angled type of scissors.

C. This demonstrates an endarterectomy of the proximal cuff of the abdominal aorta. In many instances there will be considerable calcification of the media and intima, which makes it very difficult to pass a needle through it for suturing the prosthesis to it. For this reason it is better to endarterectomize the aortic cuff by removing the media and the intima up to the level of the tourniquet clamp. This can be done very readily in most instances and will leave a rather thin-walled but tough adventitial cuff. At first this seems unusually thin and as if it would not withstand aortic pressure, but in no instance has it ever been known to give way if the anastomosis is performed properly.

D. This demonstrates the endarterectomized cuff to which the Dacron aortic bifurcation prosthesis will be anastomosed.

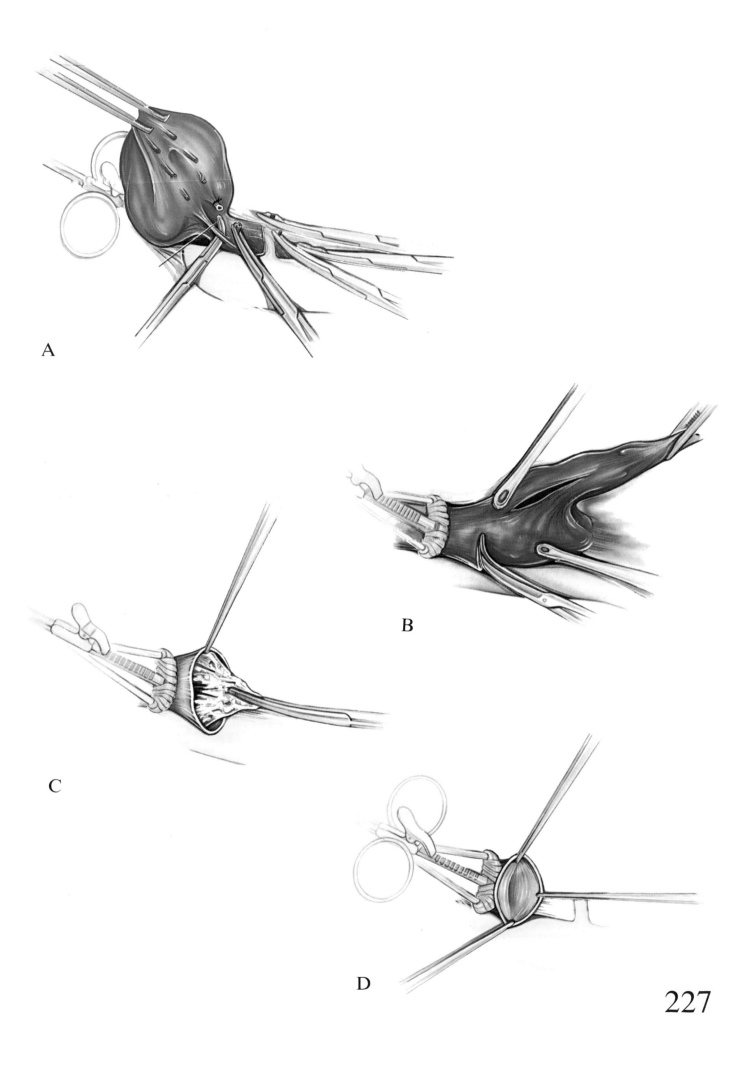

A

B

C

D

227

Plate 102

METHOD OF PERFORMING THE AORTIC PROSTHETIC END-TO-END ANASTOMOSIS UTILIZING A TWO-LAYER SUTURE LINE; INSERTION OF PRIMARY RUNNING POSTERIOR EVERTING MATTRESS SUTURE

A. The aortic bifurcation prostheses are manufactured with much longer aortic portions to the graft than are necessary for infrarenal aortic replacements. In order to maintain a streamlined flow it is best to cut off all except 2 or 3 cm. of the aortic portion of the graft so that the iliac limbs will come off distally almost parallel instead of at a right angle, which will happen if a long aortic cuff is used. The illustration demonstrates the division of the aortic portion of the graft close to its bifurcation.

B. This demonstrates the placing of a running everting mattress suture of 4-0 braided Dacron coated with Teflon; in addition, the suture has been made more slippery by rubbing it with bone wax so that it will slide readily. The suture is started on the left side, beginning from the outside of the aortic cuff well back from the cut edge, and then carried over to the prosthesis, then back and forth as is shown in the illustration to the opposite side halfway around the circumference of the aorta and the graft. This suture is placed loosely, with the ends of the aorta and the graft well separated, as shown.

C. The two ends of the suture are then pulled taut in a straight line as demonstrated, which brings the graft and the aortic cuff in close approximation with the edges everted. It is at this step in the procedure that the suture must slip easily through the aorta and the graft in order to take up all the slack. Note that there is an excess of the aortic cuff; this will be trimmed later.

D. After the initial mattress suture has been pulled taut the inner surface of the aorta and the graft at the site of anastomosis are carefully inspected to make sure that no loose loops of the suture are still lying within the lumen, and also to make certain there has been good approximation of the aortic cuff in the prosthesis as shown. Another 4-0 Dacron suture coated with Teflon (but not coated with wax) is commenced at the same place as the original mattress suture; it is ligated, then the ends of these two sutures are tied together. The stay suture, which is usually placed on the side opposite to where the suturing stopped, is ligated and the initial suture ligated to it. Great care is taken that these knots are made very secure, but in placing the first two or three throws make certain the knot does not slip; otherwise it causes a purse string effect, which should be avoided as it will produce a constriction at the site of the anastomosis. This complication is best prevented by placing a curved Schnitt clamp on the edge of the prosthesis at each side of the anastomosis. The clamps are then stretched apart to make the graft taut while the sutures are tied.

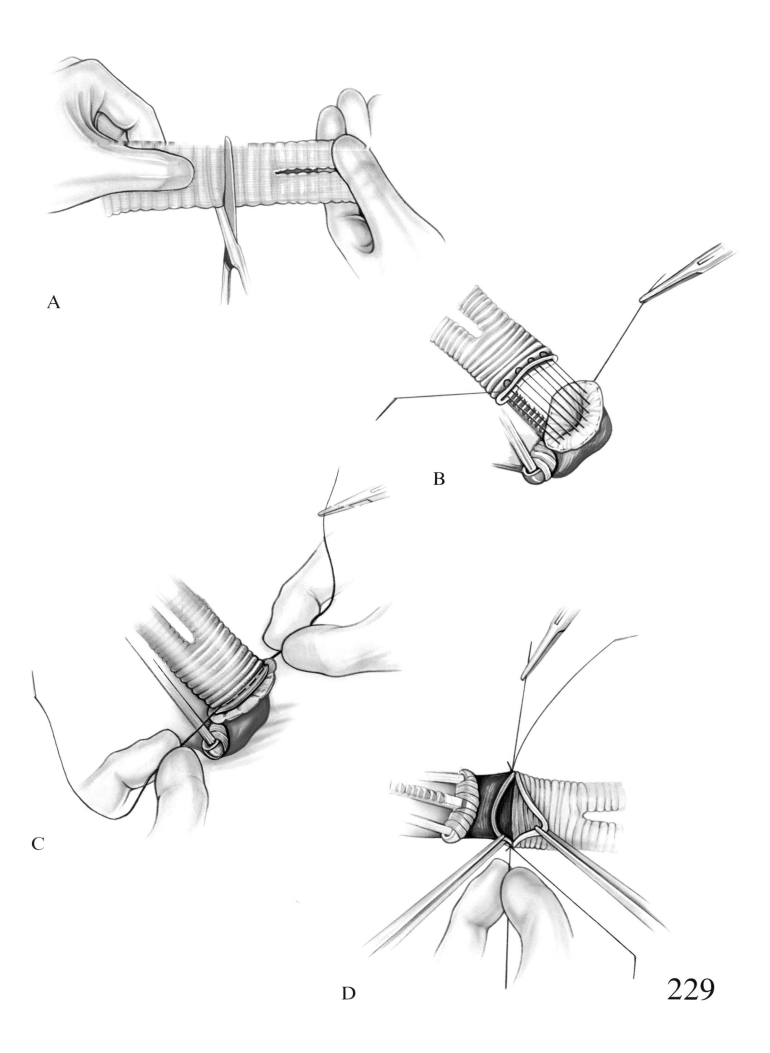

A

B

C

D

229

Plate 103

COMPLETION OF POSTERIOR SUTURE LINE WITH RUNNING OVER-AND-OVER HEMOSTATIC SUTURE; PLACING OF ANTERIOR SUTURE LINE WITH COMPLETION OF END-TO-END PROXIMAL AORTIC ANASTOMOSIS

A. The running everting mattress suture (a) has been ligated on the right to a new suture (c), which is to be used as a running over-and-over stitch for hemostasis since a running everting mattress suture is not hemostatic unless it is pulled so tight that it produces too much constriction at the suture line. The other end of suture (a) on the left has been secured by ligating it with a stay suture (b). Frequently there is additional cuff on the posterior wall of the aorta, which is trimmed away as shown with fine angled or curved scissors.

B. This demonstrates the placing of the over-and-over hemostatic suture on the posterior suture line. Note that the needle is passed through the cuff of the graft and the aorta outside the running everting mattress suture. Note that there should be sufficient cuff of the graft and the aorta so that this can be accomplished without danger of cutting the running mattress suture with the cutting point needle. Again these sutures should be placed close together to prevent constriction of the anastomosis. It is important that each stitch be pulled very taut to make the suture line hemostatic. It is important also not to go proximal to the mattress suture, especially in the aorta, because it is so thin-walled that the thin adventitial wall may tear, with resulting leakage that may be difficult to control after the blood flow is restored.

C. This demonstrates the completed posterior row of the anastomosis, with the ends of the running mattress suture (a) and of the over-and-over suture (b) held as stay sutures while the anterior rows are placed. The end with the needle on it is used in completion of the anastomosis as the running over-and-over suture after the anterior running mattress suture has been placed.

D. This demonstrates the anterior everting mattress suture while traction is maintained on sutures (a) and (b) in order not to constrict this suture line.

E. The aortic anastomosis has been completed, using a two-layer suture line consisting of a primary running everting stitch for strength and a secondary running over-and-over stitch outside the former for hemostasis. Both are interrupted on each side of the anastomosis by ligation to each other at these points. Note the proximal tourniquet clamp still occluded and in place just distal to the left renal vein and that there is good matching in size of the aorta and the graft without stenosis at the suture line. This method of aortic anastomosis gives excellent results and has never leaked, disrupted or resulted in an aortoduodenal fistula.

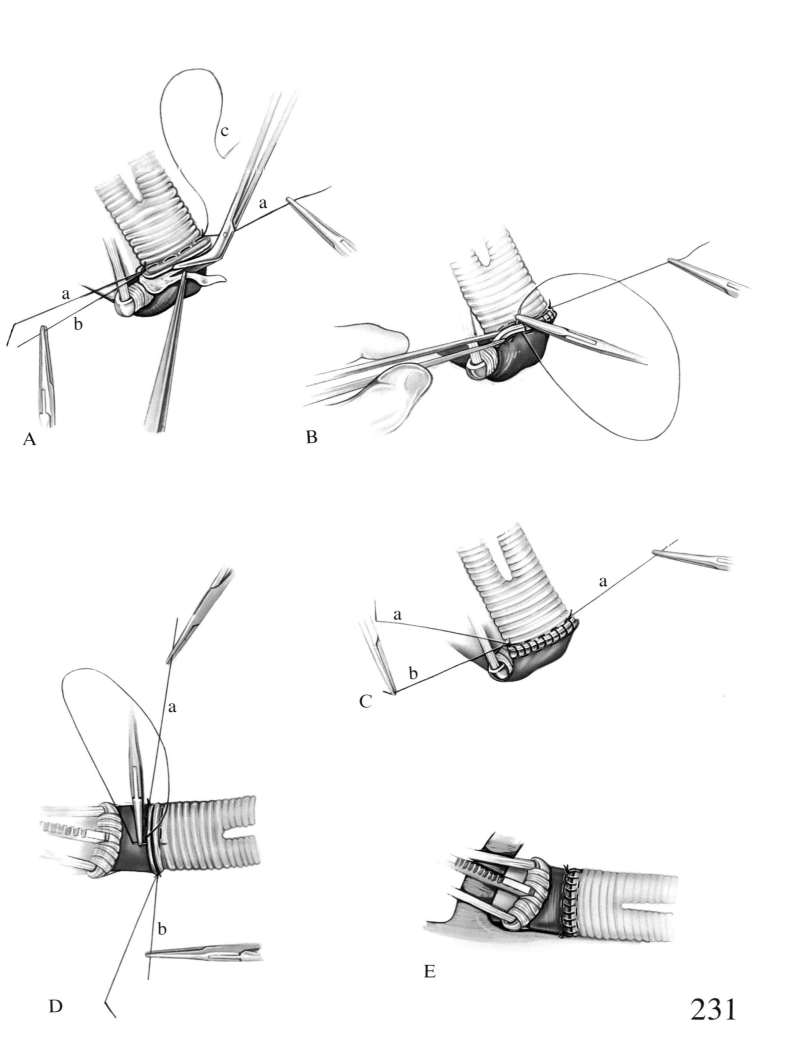

A

B

C

D

E

231

Plate 104

METHOD OF IMPLANTATION OF AN AORTIC GRAFT WITH THE ANEURYSM EXTENDING TO THE LEVEL OF THE LEFT RENAL VEIN

A. The aneurysm has been dissected out as previously described and the main portion of the aneurysm is being removed by cutting across the proximal part of the aneurysmal sac. In this case the aorta at the level of the left renal vein was of satisfactory size so that a graft could be implanted. The method used is similar to that described in Plates 102 and 103. The portion of the cuff that has been left distal to the tourniquet clamp is usually endarterectomized.

B. This demonstrates the method of implanting the running everting mattress suture by reaching well up inside the aortic cuff proximal to the aneurysmal sac at the level that the aorta is relatively normal in diameter and which is just distal to the occluding tourniquet clamp.

C. The everting mattress suture is then pulled taut, which leaves the aneurysmal portion of the cuff distal to the suture line. The ends of the running mattress suture are then anchored by ligating them to other sutures, as demonstrated in Plates 102 and 103.

D. This shows that the primary everting mattress suture (a) has been placed and ligated to the new suture (c) and the stay suture (b) at the left. The excess of the aneurysmal sac beyond the suture line is cut away, but sufficient of it is left so that the running over-and-over suture can be placed as shown.

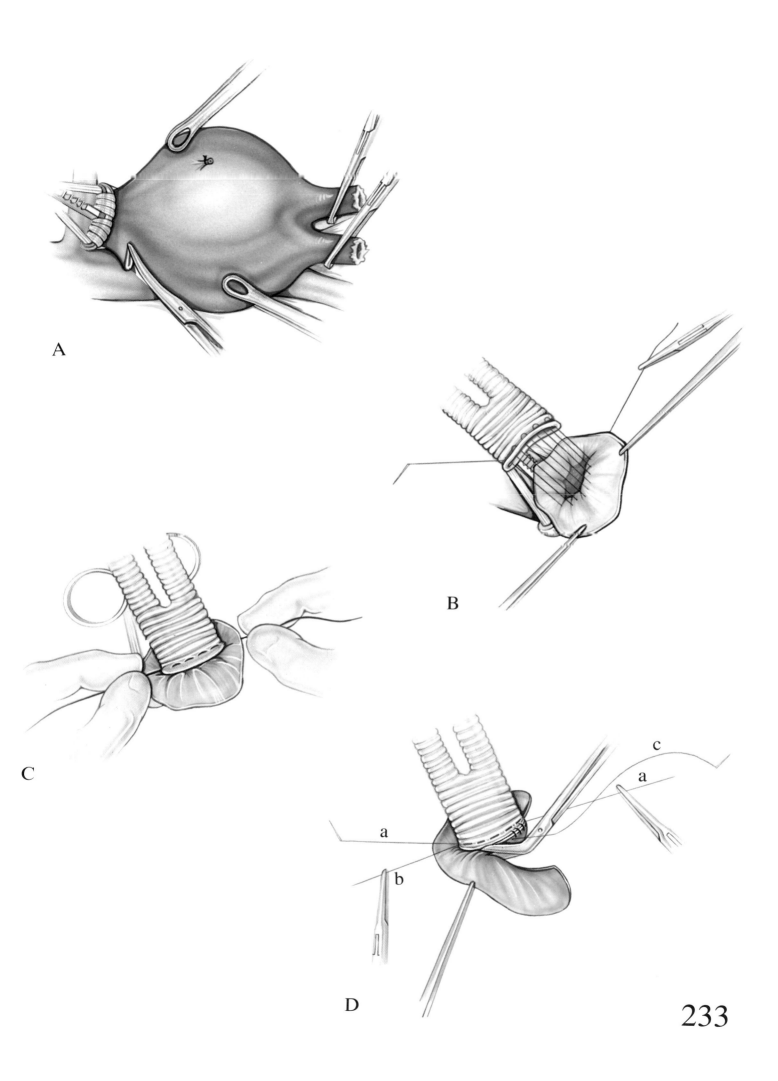

A

B

C

D

233

Plate 105

METHOD OF IMPLANTATION OF AN AORTIC GRAFT WITH THE ANEURYSM EXTENDING TO THE LEVEL OF THE LEFT RENAL VEIN *(Continued)*

A. This demonstrates the completion of the posterior half of the suture line, with the running everting mattress suture and the running over-and-over suture outside it. Note how close the suture line is to the occluding clamp. This is possible if one utilizes the technique of placing the running everting mattress suture well up inside the proximal aortic and aneurysmal cuff. The anterior portion of the aneurysmal cuff, still attached, is seen partially hidden behind the graft. It will be trimmed off after the placement of the anterior running everting mattress suture.

B. This demonstrates the placement of the running everting mattress suture and the beginning of the over-and-over suture commenced on the left side using the needle end of the suture (a), that is, the same one that commenced the anastomosis on the posterior suture line. Note that the large portion of the aneurysmal sac is being resected, leaving sufficient cuff of the aorta to place the running suture distal to the running everting mattress suture. It may be necessary to use a curved suture needle to place these two suture lines because of the close proximity of the occluding aortic clamp.

C. This demonstrates the completed anastomosis. Note the close proximity of the occluding clamp and also that the left renal vein lies against the proximal edge of the clamp. If this method is utilized, it is seldom if ever necessary to interrupt the left renal vein.

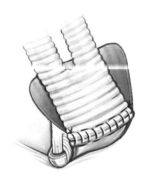

A

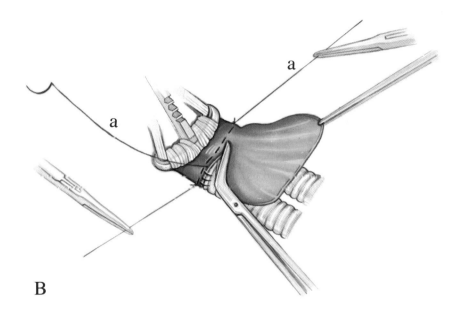

B

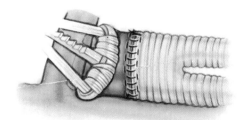

C

235

Plate 106

METHOD OF IMPLANTATION
OF AN AORTIC GRAFT WITH
A VERY SHORT AORTIC CUFF,
USING INTERRUPTED
MATTRESS SUTURES

A. This demonstrates a large abdominal aortic aneurysm that extends up to the level of the renal vein, making it necessary to displace it cephalad to place the tourniquet clamp above the aneurysm. In order to accomplish this at this level, occlusion of the aorta proximal to the renal vessels is obtained by pressure on the aorta against the lumbar vertebrae, using the fingers of the left hand as demonstrated. It is much easier to place the tourniquet clamp slightly higher by retracting the left renal vein while collapsing the aorta by a temporary proximal control and, at the same time, pushing the tourniquet clamp more proximally.

B. This demonstrates the short cuff that results after excising the aneurysmal sac when the technique shown in Plates 104 and 105 cannot be used. It is too short to use the double suture line that has been demonstrated in the previous plates and not safe for a single over-and-over running type suture, so interrupted mattress sutures are used.

C. This demonstrates the placing of the interrupted mattress sutures, requiring curved needles because of the short aortic cuff. Each mattress suture is made by tying two sutures together as demonstrated in Plate 189. The additional knot in the middle of these sutures acts as a buttress against the thin wall of the aorta; small buttons of prostheses do not have to be used. All sutures are placed by passing the needles through the aortic cuff and then the prosthesis, leaving them loose until they are all in place before tying any of them.

D. Each suture is ligated as demonstrated, leaving the two lateral ones for guy sutures. The anterior suture line is constructed in the same manner.

E. This illustration demonstrates the completed anastomosis. This method of constructing an anastomosis with an aortic cuff only a few millimeters in length gives excellent results; none has ever given way or caused trouble at a later date. The sutures are placed about 1 to 2 mm. apart as it is not necessary to interlock them.

F. This demonstrates another technique for control of the proximal abdominal aorta when dealing with a very short aortic cuff. A large Foley catheter (No. 22) with a 30-cc. bag is inserted into the aorta through the proximal aneurysmal sac. It is passed proximal to the superior mesenteric artery, so that after inflation of the bag with saline solution it does not slip out. The renal arteries are exposed and bulldog clamps applied. After resection of the aneurysmal sac the arteries are injected with dilute heparin in normal saline solution to prevent thrombosis. The prosthesis is preclotted before implantation. The Foley catheter is threaded through the aortic prosthesis and its right iliac limb while it is temporarily clamped near the aortic cuff. The aortic anastomosis is constructed with interrupted mattress sutures as shown in the preceding figures. A tourniquet clamp is placed distal to the aortic anastomosis but not closed. The balloon of the Foley catheter is then emptied and the catheter removed. The proximal aorta is flushed out, using finger pressure on the aorta for temporary control. The tourniquet clamp is then closed distal to the anastomosis and the bulldog clamps removed from the renal arteries, thus restoring the blood supply to the kidneys.

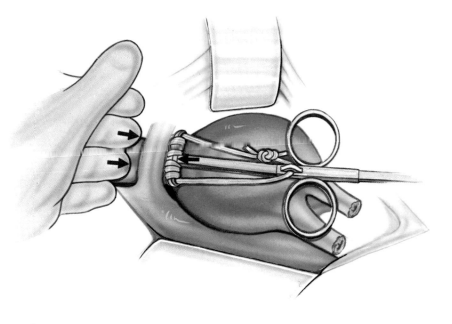

A

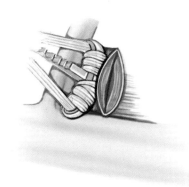

B

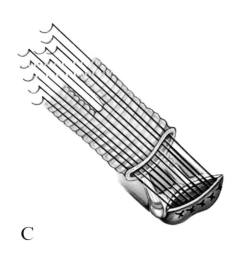

C

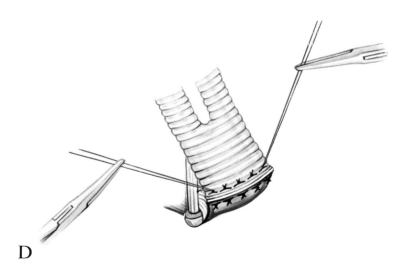

D

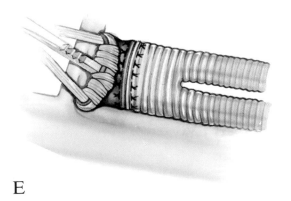

E

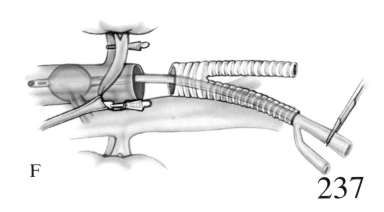

F

237

Plate 107

METHOD OF PRECLOTTING
THE AORTIC BIFURCATION GRAFT

A. Knitted Dacron prostheses are preferred to a woven type because they are porous. Because of the porosity they must be preclotted before allowing blood to flow through them; otherwise, a large amount of blood will be lost as a result of leakage through the interstices of the graft. The advantage of this type of graft, however, far outweighs this disadvantage, because it allows fibroblast of the host to go through the meshes so that it becomes incorporated as part of the body; this does not occur with woven grafts that are made so tight they do not need preclotting. These cellular elements may also play a part in the formation of the pseudo-intima lining the graft. The most satisfactory method of preclotting is to occlude the iliac limbs as shown and then release the aortic tourniquet clamp for a few seconds, allowing approximately 150 to 200 cc. of blood to escape through the interstices of the graft; this forms a pool of blood in the intraperitoneal operative field. A 50-cc. plastic syringe is used to aspirate the blood and inject it into one of the limbs while the other one is occluded. This is repeated 20 to 30 times, injecting each limb the same number of injections. After four to five minutes the graft will be so completely preclotted it does not leak, even in a totally heparinized patient. This is also a good test of the suture line. Preclotting with blood collected in a basin requires much longer than letting the blood pool in the abdominal incision because of tissue thrombokinase in the latter. The preclotting is much more effective if blood is forced out through the interstices of the graft in the manner described.

B. This demonstrates a final injection of blood into one of the iliac limbs without blood leaking out; the aorta is still occluded.

C. A final test is made by occluding both limbs of the graft and then opening the tourniquet clamp to make sure that the suture line of the anastomosis is tight.

D. Light-weight knitted Dacron prostheses are more difficult to preclot than the thicker standard type. Preclotting can be hastened and maintained in this type of graft and in any of the other types that are taking too long to preclot by pulling a large short section of a Penrose rubber tubing over the aortic segment of the prosthesis and smaller long ones over the iliac limbs. The proper size should be selected so that the tubing fits snugly when the prosthesis is distended. Rubber is very thrombogenic, so it hastens preclotting; because it is smooth, it does not pull the clot off when it is removed. The tubing should be left on the graft until it has been implanted; then make sure that it is removed completely.

E. The limbs and the aortic portion of the graft are cleaned out thoroughly with a glass drinking tube connected to the wall suction to remove all blood and blood clots. This should be done as soon as possible after the preclotting; otherwise the clots become very adherent and are impossible to remove, which undoubtedly interferes with the functioning of the graft. This method of preclotting will last for 30 to 40 minutes before it begins to liquefy, so that there is ample time to perform the two distal anastomoses.

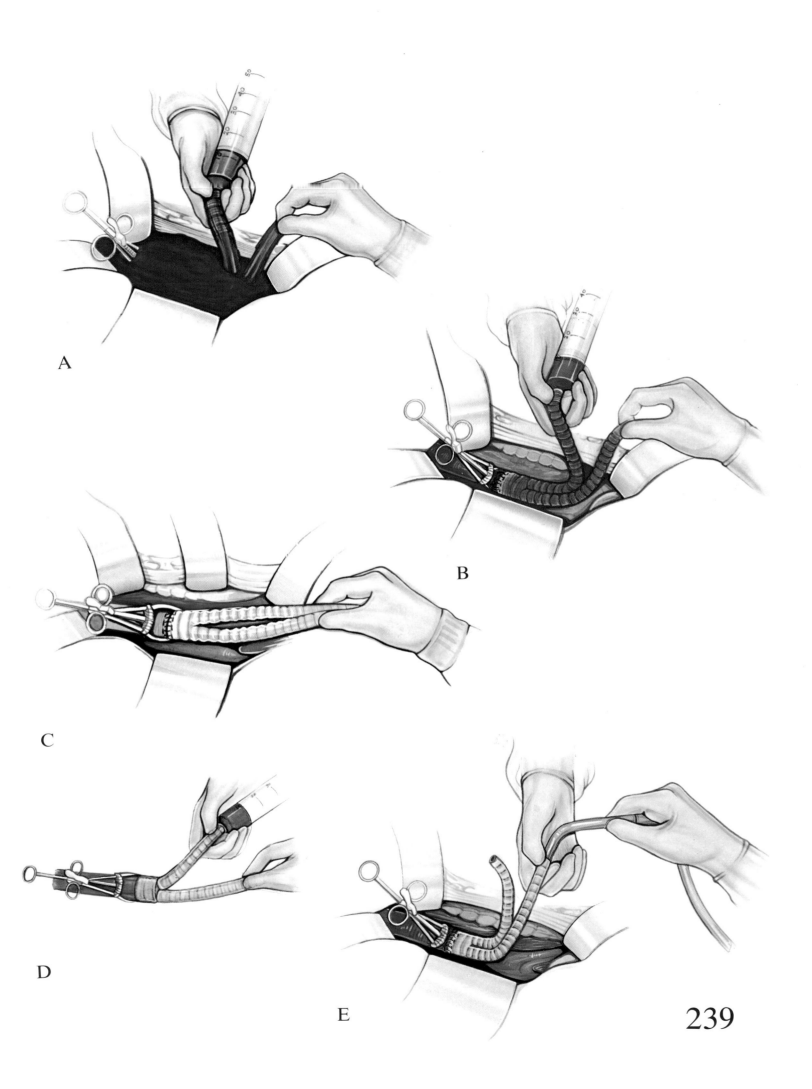

A

B

C

D

E

239

Plate 108

END-TO-END ANASTOMOSIS BY THE END-TO-SIDE TECHNIQUE OF LEFT ILIAC LIMB OF GRAFT TO DISTAL END OF LEFT COMMON ILIAC ARTERY AFTER ENDARTERECTOMY

A.   This demonstrates the aortic graft with the proximal anastomosis completed. The sigmoid colon is retracted distally to show the bifurcation of the common iliac arteries, with bulldog clamps on the left external iliac and hypogastric arteries and one on the right common iliac artery. A large atheromatous plaque was found at the bifurcation of the left common iliac artery, so it was necessary to endarterectomize it in order to perform an end-to-end anastomosis by the end-to-side technique which has been found to be much more satisfactory than a direct end-to-end anastomosis. In order to construct a satisfactory anastomosis of this type under these conditions it is necessary to control the distal blood flow by placing bulldog clamps on the external iliac and hypogastric arteries as shown.

B.   The distal end of the left common iliac artery has been incised with scissors down to and including the origin of the external iliac artery. This arteriotomy should be placed on the anterior wall, staying away from the origin of the hypogastric artery.

C.   The endarterectomy is then readily accomplished by grasping the atheromatous plaque including the media and intima with angled forceps and carefully dividing it cleanly near the origins of the hypogastric and the external iliac arteries. If this is done carefully with fine-pointed scissors, making sure not to leave a loose distal flap of intima and media, it is never necessary to suture the intima and media down to the adventitia. If suturing is done it often results in further fragmentation of the loose flaps that tends to favor thrombus formation at the site of anastomosis. This is a serious error because it may result in an occlusion of the origin of the external iliac artery, which is the main outflow tract beyond the graft. Anything that may cause narrowing of the artery at this point should therefore be avoided if possible.

D.   This shows the distal end of the left common iliac artery with the media and intima still adherent to the adventitia of the distal segment. The arteriotomy can be seen extending a short distance down the external iliac artery to eliminate a narrowing at this point as the graft is implanted. The end of the left iliac limb of the graft is beveled obliquely so that it will match in length the distal end of the common iliac artery and arteriotomy. The prosthesis has been twisted slightly, as shown by the arrows, to demonstrate the method of performing this. It should be pointed out that the section that is removed is on the posterior side of the prosthetic limb, so that the graft and artery will be approximated accurately without a twist after completion of the anastomosis.

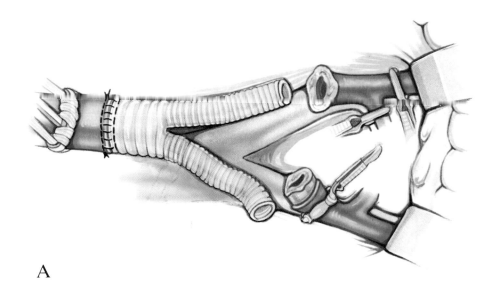

A

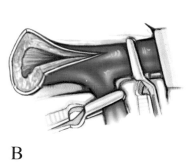

B

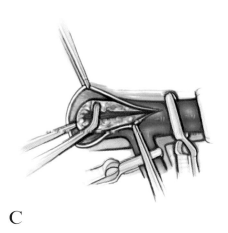

C

D

241

Plate 109

COMPLETION OF THE LEFT COMMON ILIAC ANASTOMOSIS AND THE START OF THE RIGHT ONE BY THE DIRECT END-TO-END TECHNIQUE

A. This shows the proximal mattress 4-0 Teflon-coated Dacron suture being placed first through the iliac prosthesis from the outside in and through the posterior wall of the common iliac artery from the inside out. This suture is then tied as the assistant stretches the prosthesis distalward. It is important that the prosthetic limb should be on a slight degree of tension; otherwise, it will be too long and tend to kink after blood is allowed to flow through it. If the mattress suture is placed in this manner the stitch will not pull through the arterial wall, as may occur if an over-and-over stitch is used.

B. The proximal half of each suture line has been completed and the sutures tied at the midway point of the anastomosis to a stay suture. The distal anterior mattress stitch has been placed and is ready to be tied. The curved needles used here are made by bending straight needles. This facilitates the placing of the mattress stitch, especially if it is a very small artery. The remainder of the anastomosis is then completed, using the distal sutures and sewing back to the original ones at the midpoint of the anastomosis. Further details of the technique for this type of anastomosis will be found in Plates 138 and 139.

C. This demonstrates the completed aortic and left common iliac anastomosis. The bulldog clamps on the external iliac and hypogastric arteries are first removed; then, without any clamp on the right iliac limb and with the aorta still occluded, any backflow from the left side is observed as blood coming from the open end of the right limb of the graft. Once this is tested, the left iliac limb is temporarily occluded with a bulldog and the aorta is flushed out through the right iliac limb. The bulldog is then removed from the left iliac limb and placed on the origin of the right one so that blood can flow down the left side into the lower extremity. Note that there is a short section of a piece of Penrose tubing that has been slipped over the right iliac limb and pulled up to the crotch of the graft. The bulldog clamp goes over this small section of tubing as shown. Because the pressure of the bulldog clamp often destroys the preclot at the point it is placed, it is not uncommon for a large amount of blood to leak through the iliac limb after the clamp is removed if the rubber is not used. Being thrombogenic, the rubber prevents this from occurring. The surgeon must remember, of course, to remove the tubing after all the occluding clamps have been removed and the graft is functioning.

D. Attention is then directed to the right common iliac artery. It will be noted that there is retraction of the adventitia with protrusion of the thick media and intima. It is extremely important to recognize this if it occurs and to make sure in doing the distal anastomosis, if it is done end-to-end as shown, that the sutures include the adventitia because of lack of tensile strength in the media and intima; if only these latter are sutured, a disruption of the anastomosis will result.

E. This demonstrates the method of trimming the thickened media and intimal plaques flush with the adventitia. This safeguards the suture line because, when the suturing is done, the adventitia must be included; it also results in a better streamlined anastomosis.

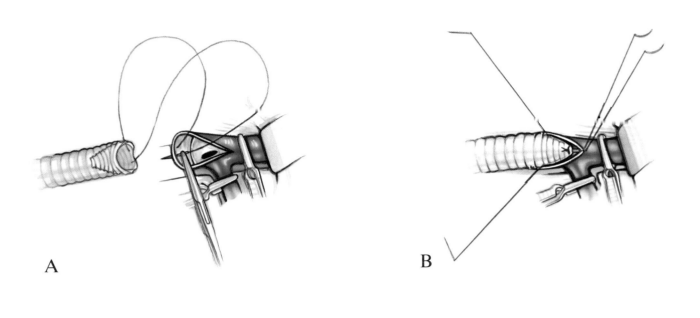

A

B

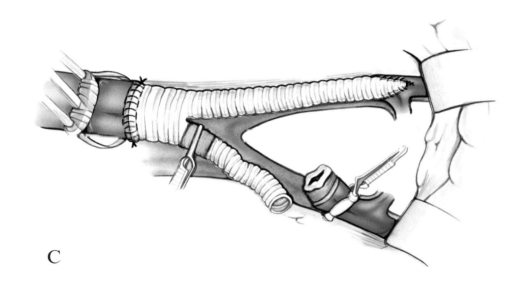

C

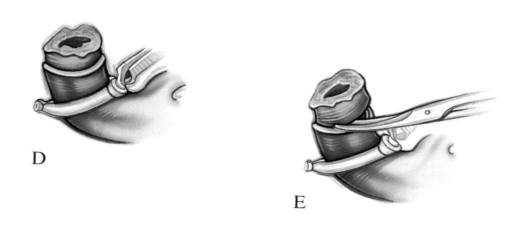

D

E

243

Plate 110

COMPLETION OF THE RIGHT COMMON ILIAC ANASTOMOSIS BY THE DIRECT END-TO-END TECHNIQUE AND THE IMPLANTATION OF THE BIFURCATION AORTIC PROSTHESIS

A. The end of the prosthesis and the common iliac artery are approximated, with the mattress suture in the midline posteriorly. They are then sutured in both directions with each end of this mattress suture. This will be a running suture that is passed from outside in on the prosthesis and inside out on the artery in order not to loosen the intima in the latter. This suturing can also be done from the inside if the artery is large by use of a curved needle. In this case the needle should go from within out on the artery and from without in on the prosthesis. Again, this is done in order not to separate the intima from the adventitia.

B. This demonstrates completion of the posterior half of the suture line with good approximation. Since the sutures are synthetic, made of Dacron, the fact they show within the lumen is not serious since one is suturing a Dacron tube to the iliac artery with a Dacron suture; the small additional amount of Dacron will not cause any complication.

C. This demonstrates that one half of the anterior suture line has been completed. At this stage of the anastomosis the occluding bulldog on the external iliac artery is released to make sure there is backflow from it and that a thrombus has not formed in it; if it has, it can usually be removed by using a Fogarty catheter, but this creates an unnecessary operative complication. Total heparinization and additional dilute heparin injected into the common iliac artery will prevent it. It is not necessary to flush the proximal aorta since the occluding clamp is at the bifurcation on the prosthesis. A small polyvinyl catheter, No. 12 French, has been inserted through the anastomosis to aspirate any blood or blood clots that may have collected in the iliac limb of the graft, a simple safeguard against flushing them down the distal arterial tree when the graft is opened. The small catheter is then removed and the anastomosis completed by continuing the suture on the inner side of the artery and tying it to the one that was carried to this point. The bulldog clamp on the hypogastric artery is removed, which allows blood to reflux up into the iliac limb. A small 5-cc. syringe with a No. 26 needle is then inserted into the limb of the graft to evacuate the air that has been retained in it so that it will not be carried distalward. After completing this, the bulldog clamp on the external iliac artery and then the one on the limb of the graft are removed, in that sequence. The small piece of Penrose tubing is allowed to remain on for a few more minutes and then it is removed by cutting it longitudinally. This simple procedure may save a large amount of blood from being lost at the point where the graft has been occluded.

D. This demonstrates the graft functioning after its implantation and the three types of anastomoses that were used. The tourniquet clamp has been loosened but it has not been removed. It is always the last clamp to be taken off, after making sure that there are no leaking points in the suture lines that may need proximal aortic control while they are secured with interrupted sutures. When complete hemostasis has been obtained, the tourniquet clamp is removed by simply cutting the shoestring where it goes around the aorta.

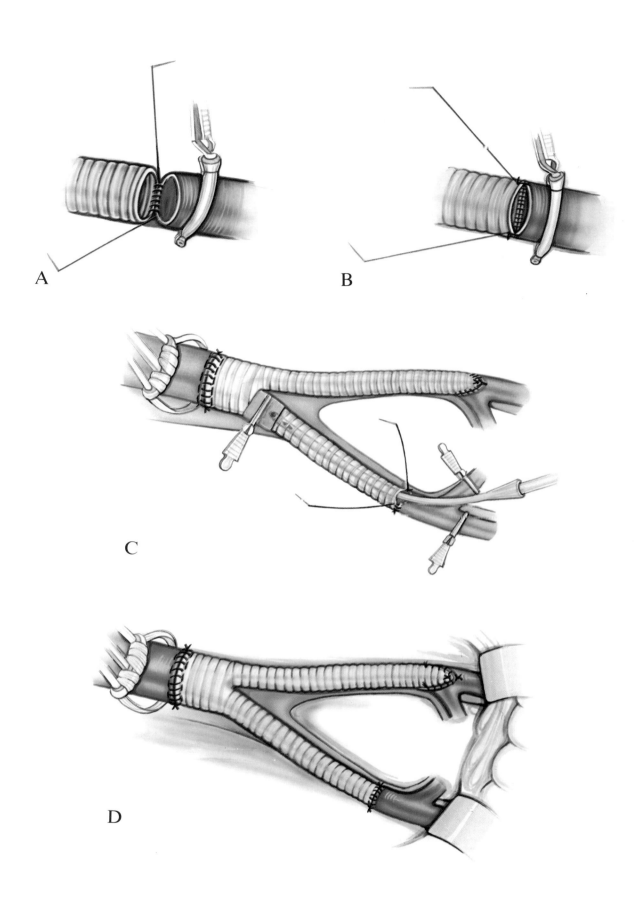

A

B

C

D

Plate 111

END-TO-END ANASTOMOSIS BY THE END-TO-SIDE TECHNIQUE OF LEFT ILIAC LIMB OF GRAFT TO THE DISTAL END OF THE ENDARTERECTOMIZED LEFT COMMON ILIAC ARTERY

A. This demonstrates a more distal exposure of the bifurcation of the left common iliac artery. An incision has been made through the peritoneum in the left iliac fossa to expose the distal end of the common iliac and the proximal ends of the external iliac and hypogastric arteries. A wide Penrose tubing with a small retractor against it has been placed around the sigmoid and the mesosigmoid; included in this is the left ureter to protect it from injury. These are all retracted cephalad. Bulldog clamps have been placed on the external iliac and hypogastric arteries to control the arterial backflow. Note the very thick atheromatous circular plaque and the small lumen of the distal common iliac artery, which would not make a satisfactory direct end-to-end anastomosis.

B. The distal end of the common iliac artery has been opened longitudinally and the arteriotomy continued distally into the external iliac artery where the atheromatous plaques have thinned out and the lumen is of essentially normal caliber, so that a graft implanted to this level will have a good outflow tract.

C. This demonstrates the removal of the large atheromatous plaque, which is readily accomplished by carefully separating it from the adventitia proximally and the media of the arteries distally.

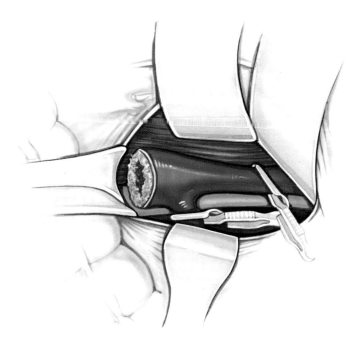

A

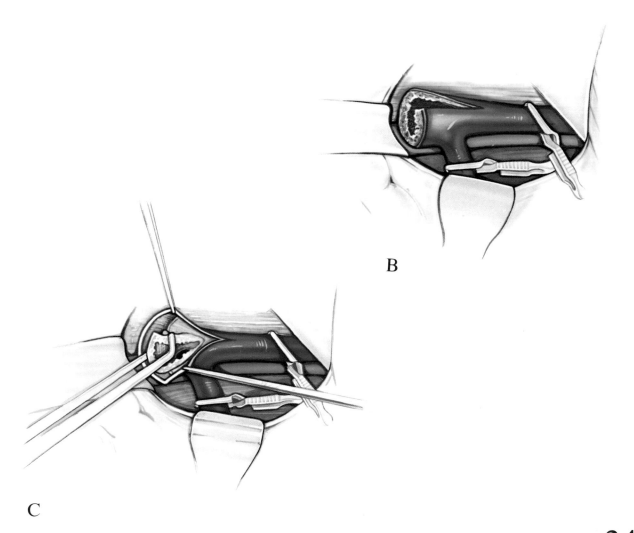

B

C

Plate 112

COMPLETION OF THE END-TO-END ANASTOMOSIS BY THE END-TO-SIDE TECHNIQUE OF LEFT ILIAC LIMB OF GRAFT TO THE DISTAL END OF THE ENDARTERECTOMIZED LEFT COMMON ILIAC ARTERY

A. The left iliac limb of the prosthesis has been brought down under these structures. A further toilet has been made of the intima of the common iliac and external iliac arteries. Sometimes the atheromatous plaque involves the first portion of the hypogastric artery and can be removed readily by careful dissection with a curved hemostat to restore the lumen of this vessel as shown. Again, as noted previously, if this procedure is done carefully and accurately without leaving any distal flaps, it is unnecessary to suture the distal ring of the media and intima.

B. The end of the prosthesis has been brought down, the correct length being determined by cutting away a portion of the posterior portion to bevel the end. It is important to make sure that the right length has been selected; it should not be too long or too short, but under a slight amount of tension. The posterior mattress suture is being placed and the anastomosis will be completed as shown in Plates 138 and 139.

C. This demonstrates the completed anastomosis with a very satisfactory matching of the size of the iliac limb of the graft and the distal arteries. This is one of the advantages of this type of anastomosis; it is possible to accomplish it by taking larger bites of artery and smaller ones of the prosthesis, so that a very excellent streamlined anastomosis can be constructed, which cannot be accomplished by the direct end-to-end technique.

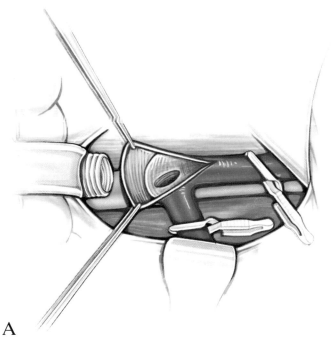

A

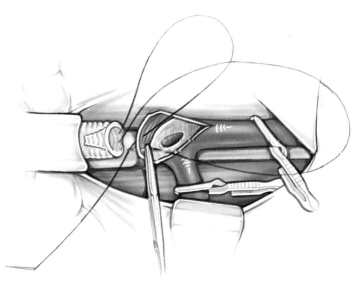

B

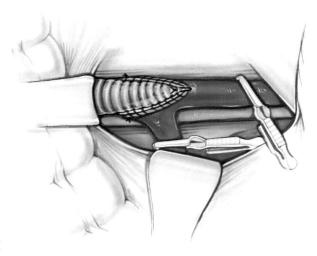

C

249

Plate 113

END-TO-SIDE ANASTOMOSIS
OF LEFT ILIAC LIMB OF GRAFT
TO PROXIMAL LEFT EXTERNAL
ILIAC ARTERY

A. This and Plate 114 demonstrate the anastomosis of the iliac limb of the graft to the left external iliac artery, which in some instances is necessary because of the large amount of atheromatous material in the origin of the left external iliac artery and the poor adventitia in this location; a local endarterectomy and implanting the graft to the distal end of the common iliac artery would be poor judgment. An incision is made through the peritoneum in the left iliac fossa to expose the distal common iliac and proximal external iliac and hypogastric arteries. The arteries are exposed better by proximal retraction of the sigmoid colon, its mesentery and the left ureter.

B. This demonstrates one method of determining the location where one can make a satisfactory end-to-side anastomosis. After the external iliac artery has been freed up, a small right-angled retractor is placed under it and pulled upward. The illustration demonstrates how the artery is flattened out, showing it obviously has a good lumen. This step has been found useful in addition to careful palpation of the artery. With favorable findings it is safe to proceed with an end-to-side anastomosis.

C. The distal end of the common iliac artery is secured with a running over-and-over suture of 4-0 Dacron.

D. The iliac limb of the graft is brought down into the operative field, posterior to the sigmoid colon, its mesentery and the ureter. A longitudinal incision is made in the external iliac artery. If necessary, of course, this arteriotomy can be made more distal, depending on the distribution of the atheromatous plaques.

E. This demonstrates excision of the distal posterior portion of the graft to bevel it for the anastomosis. The length of the piece that is removed should be approximately twice the diameter of the prosthesis because it is then possible to make a more streamlined type of anastomosis with the longer bevel. A more detailed description of this type of anastomosis will be found in Plates 135, 136 and 137.

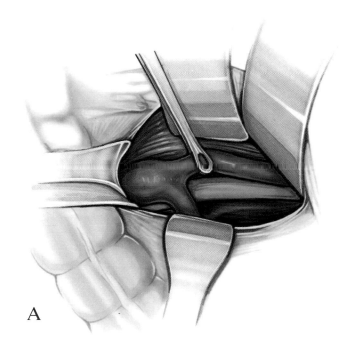

A

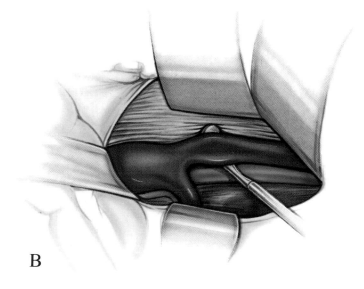

B

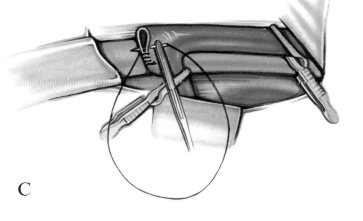

C

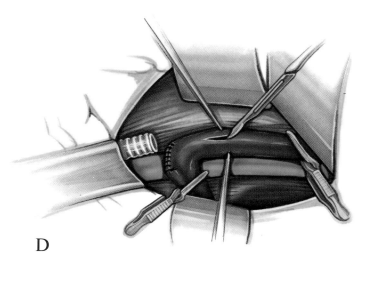

D

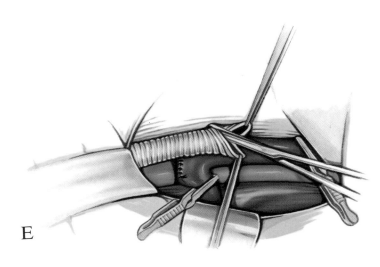

E

251

Plate 114

COMPLETION OF END-TO-SIDE ANASTOMOSIS OF LEFT ILIAC LIMB OF THE GRAFT TO PROXIMAL LEFT EXTERNAL ILIAC ARTERY

A.   The posterior mattress suture is being placed. Note the relatively long arteriotomy and also the beveling of the distal end of the graft.

B.   The suturing is continued on the far side of the anastomosis. Note that the needle goes through from the outside to the inside of the graft and inside out on the artery. This prevents the loosening of the media and the intima during the suturing. It is also important that the first assistant maintain firm tension on the suture after each stitch is taken, as shown; otherwise, the anastomosis will leak because the suturing is not snug and tight. Because of its elasticity, it is also important to maintain firm tension on the prosthesis with the long fine forceps during the suturing; otherwise, there will not be sufficient length of the graft to reach to the distal end of the arteriotomy to complete the anastomosis.

C.   The proximal half of the suture line on each side has been completed. Each suture is ligated to a stay suture that has been placed at this point to prevent it from loosening while the remainder of the anastomosis is completed. A distal mattress suture is then implanted as shown.

D.   The mattress suture has been ligated, and one end of this suture is now being used as a running over-and-over type of suture to complete the suture line on the far side. It will be tied to the end of the other suture, which has been saved. After completing this part of the anastomosis a similar closure of the fourth quadrant of the anastomosis is completed, again always sewing from the graft to the artery.

E.   This demonstrates the completed anastomosis after removal of the bulldog and aortic clamps to allow blood to flow down the arteries to the left lower extremity and pelvis. It is much easier to construct a faultless end-to-side anastomosis with a Dacron graft if this technique is followed, because if both the proximal and distal mattress sutures are tied first, the edges of the graft curl in so much that it is especially difficult to obtain satisfactory suturing at the proximal end of the anastomosis, where a suture line leak after completion of the anastomosis is hard to control.

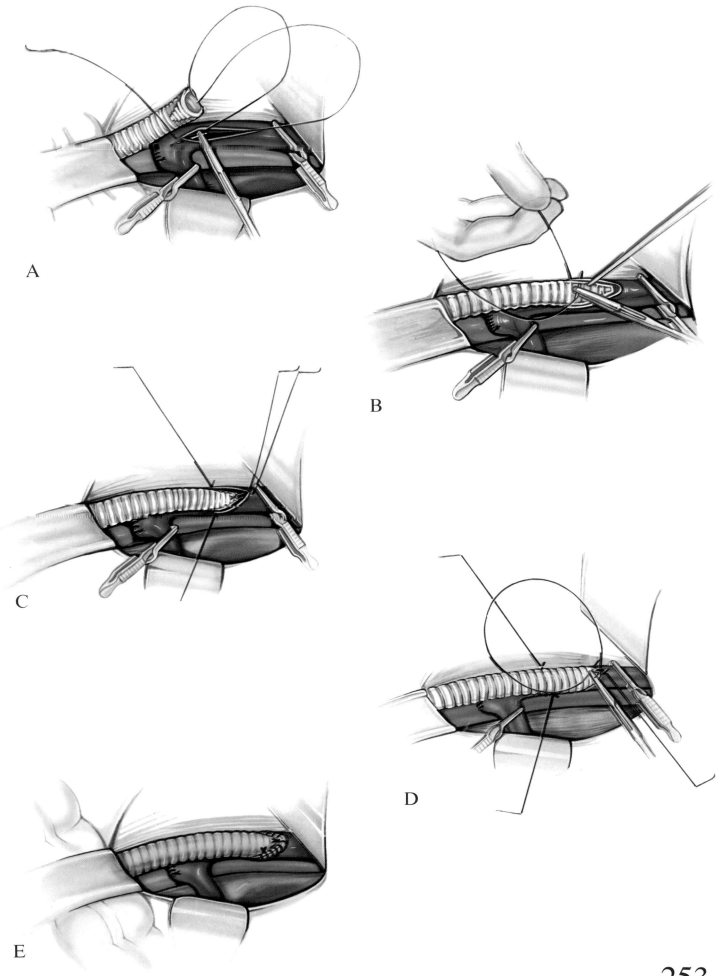

A

B

C

D

E

253

Plate 115

AN END-TO-END ANASTOMOSIS
BY THE END-TO-SIDE TECHNIQUE
OF THE RIGHT ILIAC LIMB
OF A GRAFT TO THE DISTAL
COMMON ILIAC AND A LONG
SEGMENT OF THE EXTERNAL
ILIAC ARTERIES WITH AN
ENDARTERECTOMY

A. The aortic graft which has been implanted is shown with the left iliac limb functioning. The previous techniques have all been carried out with the surgeon standing on the right side of the patient. The anastomosis between the right iliac limb of the graft and the distal end of the common iliac and the external iliac arteries, especially if a long segment of external iliac artery must be endarterectomized, can be performed much better with the surgeon standing on the left side of the patient as these illustrations demonstrate. The sigmoid colon and the mesentery are retracted to the left and downward. The hypogastric and a long segment of the external iliac arteries are exposed by retracting the peritoneum and the ureter distalward with a Richardson retractor.

B. The dissection requires sufficient of the external iliac artery to be exposed to include all of it that contains the long atheromatous plaque that can be palpated in it. A bulldog clamp is placed distal to the plaque where the artery feels soft and essentially normal.

C. A long arteriotomy is then made down the anterior part of the common and external iliac arteries, staying well away from the origin of the hypogastric artery. This can best be done with straight, fine, sharp, dull-pointed scissors.

D. The arteriotomy has been carried down to and a little beyond the long posterior atheromatous plaque in the external iliac artery. Note should be taken of the stenosed opening of the origin of the hypogastric artery caused by the large atheromatous plaque encroaching upon it.

E. The large plaque is separated from the common iliac artery with blunt dissection, and dissection is then continued to include the long posterior plaque with its tapered distal tip in the external iliac artery. The separation of the thick portion is best accomplished using fine-tipped, sharp, curved scissors, being very careful not to elevate, or leave elevated, any flap of intima lateral or distal to the plaque.

F. This shows the atheromatous plaque almost completely removed. The distal tip will usually free up and come off very neatly without its having to be cut free. Note that the ostium of the hypogastric artery has been enlarged to essentially normal size, which will mean that there will be good restoration of hypogastric arterial circulation, especially if good back bleeding is obtained on release of the bulldog clamp on it.

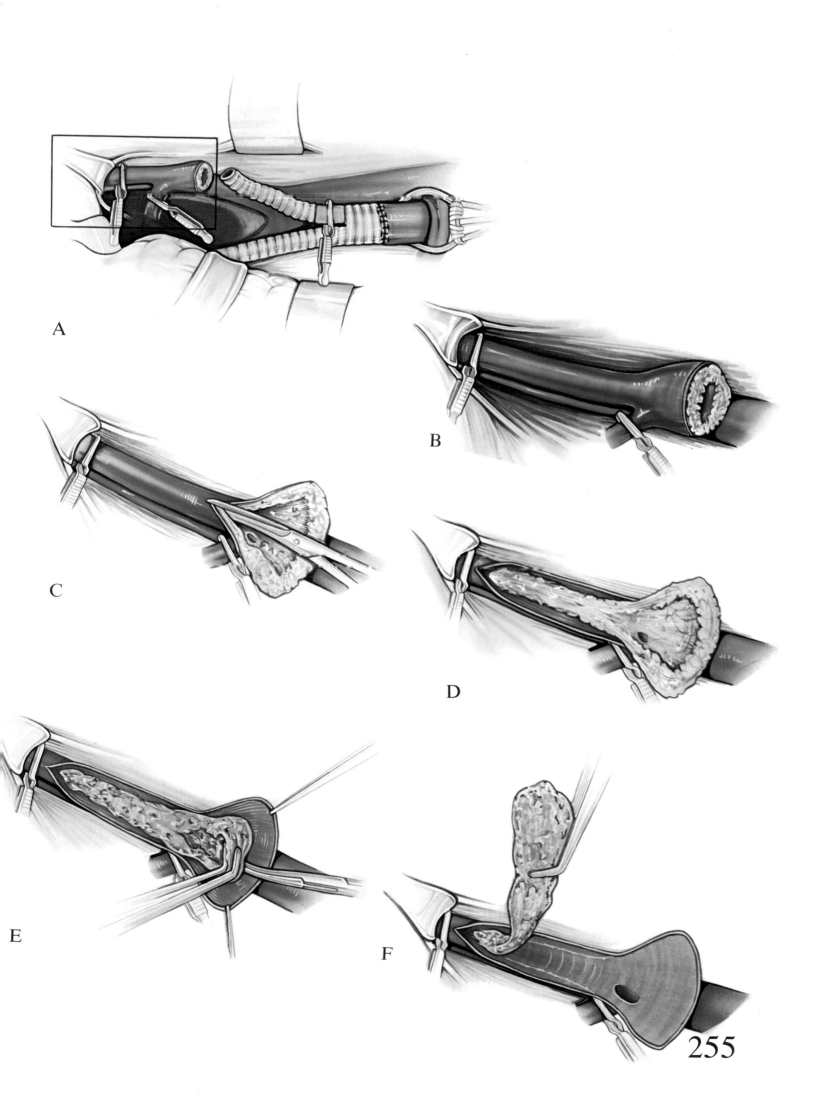

A

B

C

D

E

F

255

Plate 116

COMPLETION OF THE ANASTOMOSIS OF THE RIGHT ILIAC LIMB OF A GRAFT TO THE DISTAL COMMON ILIAC AND EXTERNAL ILIAC ARTERIES WITH AN ENDARTERECTOMY

A. It is important in reconstructing the anastomosis to make sure that its caliber is approximately the same as the normal artery. As the common iliac artery is considerably larger, some of the excess of the corners of it are trimmed away as shown; because the prosthesis will be the widest at this point, less arterial wall is necessary. Note that the posterior wall of the endarterectomized arteries is relatively smooth, and the edge of the intima where the plaque was removed is very thin, so that there is no danger that it will be dissected loose by the blood stream after the opening of the clamps. For this reason it is not necessary to suture it to the adventitia.

B. A long bevel is made in the end of the prosthesis that is longer than the arteriotomy. This is a safeguard against having it too short. If it is too long it can easily be shortened, but if it is not long enough it is difficult to complete the anastomosis without spoiling the streamlining of it. The initial posterior mattress suture is shown placed in the usual manner, first through the graft from outside in and then from inside out on the artery.

C. After this mattress suture is tied, the anastomotic suture line is continued on each side, again taking relatively large bites in the arterial wall and smaller ones in the prosthesis. It is here that one must be careful not to make too large a lumen; otherwise, it will tend to become aneurysmal. Sometimes a polyvinyl catheter of the correct size is inserted from below as a stent and is an aid in calibrating the lumen. The running over-and-over suture on each side is tied as shown to a stay suture, so that the suture line does not become loose. Constant vigilance by the surgeon with new assistants is necessary in this regard as I have learned from experience. The placing of the distal mattress suture is shown after completion of the proximal one third of the anastomosis on each side. As it is tied, the tip of the prosthesis will come down to the angle of the arteriotomy under slight tension.

D. This demonstrates the completed long end-to-end anastomosis constructed by this end-to-end technique, which revascularizes not only the limb through the external iliac artery but also the pelvis through the hypogastric artery.

E. This demonstrates the completed graft after all the clamps have been removed, with a well matched end-to-end anastomosis between the graft and the proximal aorta and the end-to-end anastomoses by the end-to-side technique of both iliac limbs to the common iliac and external iliac arteries.

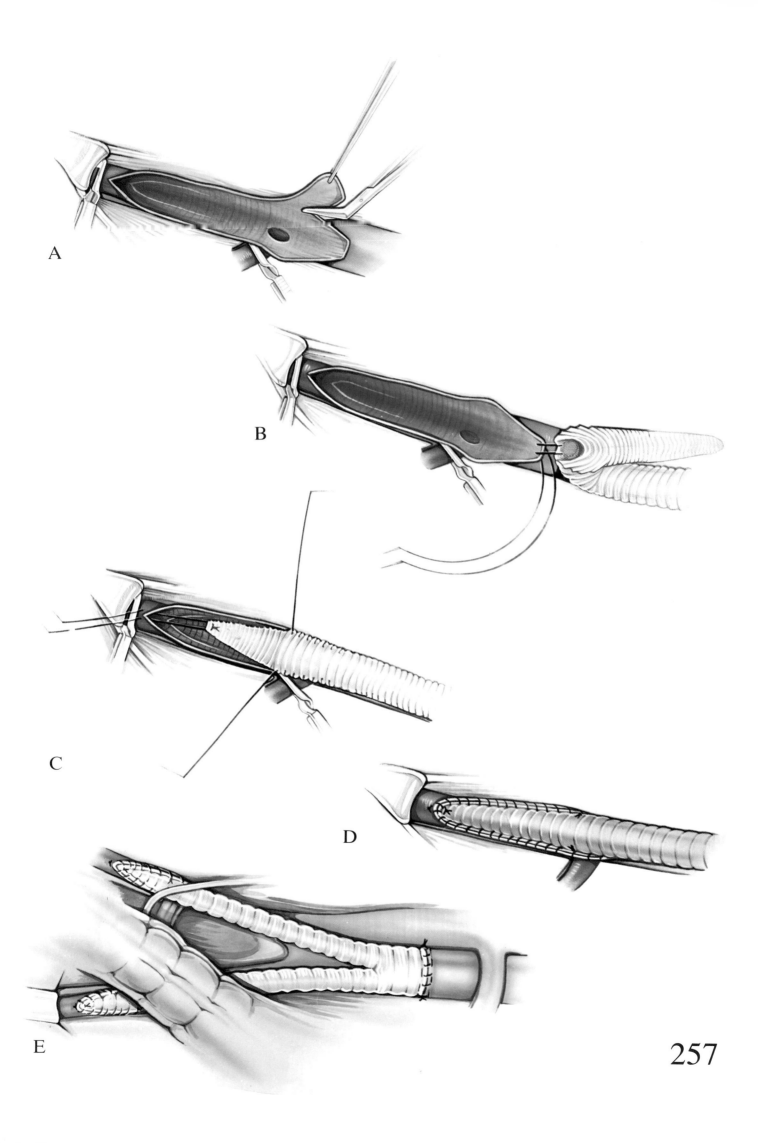

A

B

C

D

E

Plate 117

RUBBER SLEEVE METHOD OF STOPPING LEAKAGE FROM A KNITTED DACRON PROSTHESIS

A.   This demonstrates leakage from the right iliac limb of a knitted Dacron prosthesis. My technique is usually to do the left iliac anastomosis first; since this is done immediately after the preclotting, the graft seldom bleeds after completion of the anastomosis. The right one is routinely done second, so there is a longer interval between the preclotting and the completion of the anastomosis, and bleeding sometimes occurs in rather alarming amounts through the interstices of the graft because of lysis of the fibrin clot in the graft fabric.

B.   The bleeding can be controlled immediately by encircling that part of the graft with a piece of rubber sheeting, the width of it depending on how much of the graft needs to be covered. It is put on a slight stretch to squeeze the graft, but not to occlude it, and held with a clamp as shown in the illustration for about five minutes, then removed.

C.   Sometimes the clamp method of holding the rubber sheeting is cumbersome or the area of bleeding is too great; under these conditions the rubber is sewed with a catgut suture to hold it in place. It is left there for about five minutes, which is usually long enough to reclot the graft. During this short wait the surgeon can be closing the retroperitoneal tissues and the posterior peritoneum down to this level. The rubber sheeting is removed with a fine, blunt-tipped scissors as shown.

D.   This demonstrates a graft such as that shown in *A* which was leaking and now is perfectly blood tight; it is safe to proceed with closing the peritoneum over it, and one can be assured that it will not bleed again.

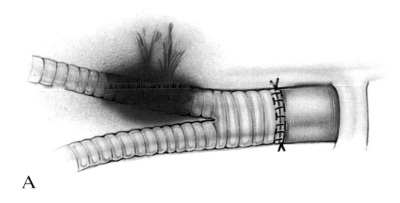

A

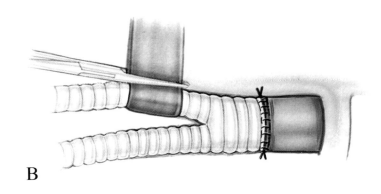

B

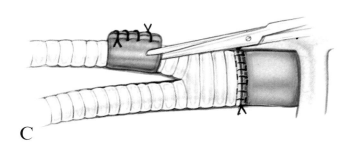

C

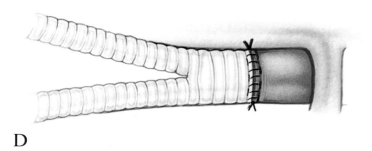

D

Plate 118

THE CLOSURE OF THE RETROPERITONEAL TISSUES AND THE POSTERIOR PERITONEUM; WITZEL GASTROSTOMY; CLOSURE OF THE ABDOMINAL INCISION

A. The posterior peritoneal incision is closed in two layers using interrupted fine silk sutures. The first layer consists of the retroperitoneal tissues sutured over the graft so that the duodenum (a) does not come in contact with it; this prevents a duodeno-aortic fistula, a most serious complication, which may develop if the duodenum lies directly over the anastomosis. It is not necessary to cover the entire iliac limbs with the first layer.

B. The posterior peritoneum is sutured as the second layer. The ureter will be seen at the lower end of the incision crossing over the distal end of the right iliac limb of the prosthesis. It may be placed either anterior or posterior to it. In most cases it is allowed to take its natural course over the reconstructed blood vessel and graft. It should *not* lie directly over the distal anastomosis as is shown in the illustration.

C. This demonstrates the construction of a Witzel type of gastrostomy for proximal gastrointestinal decompression. It is routinely performed on patients for this type of surgical procedure. It is used instead of a nasogastric tube as it is much more comfortable and equally effective. A pursestring suture of 2-0 chromic catgut is placed in the fundus of the stomach. A small incision is made in the center of this. A No. 18 Foley catheter with a 5-cc. bag is inserted into the stomach through it. The pursestring is tied snugly around the catheter.

D. The stomach is sutured over the pursestring and the catheter for a distance of about 6 or 7 cm. with a running suture of 2-0 chromic catgut. The balloon is inflated with sterile normal saline to 5 cc. The catheter is pulled downward until the balloon rests against the end of the gastric tube that has been constructed. The tube is brought out through a stab incision in the left upper quadrant. No attempt should be made to bring the stomach against the anterior abdominal wall.

E. The abdominal incision has been closed with a running suture of 0 chromic catgut to the posterior rectus sheath and peritoneum, and the same to the anterior rectus sheath with multiple stay sutures of nylon. The skin is closed with interrupted mattress sutures of silk. The long end of the gastrostomy tube comes out through the stab incision in the left upper quadrant. One pound suction is maintained for three to five days; the tube is removed on the tenth postoperative day. With this regime this type of gastrostomy has never resulted in a gastric fistula. The only complication has been a rare instance of bleeding from the gastric incision. This can be readily controlled by applying traction on it and cross-clamping it with a Kelly clamp next to the skin. This results in pressure on the bleeding vessels by the balloon in the stomach at the site of the gastrostomy. The clamp is left on for six to eight hours and then removed; then the clamp on the tube can be removed to allow it to drain again. While the drainage tube is clamped it is usual to put a nasogastric tube down so that one can check whether the bleeding has been controlled; it is then removed and the gastrostomy tube put back on suction.

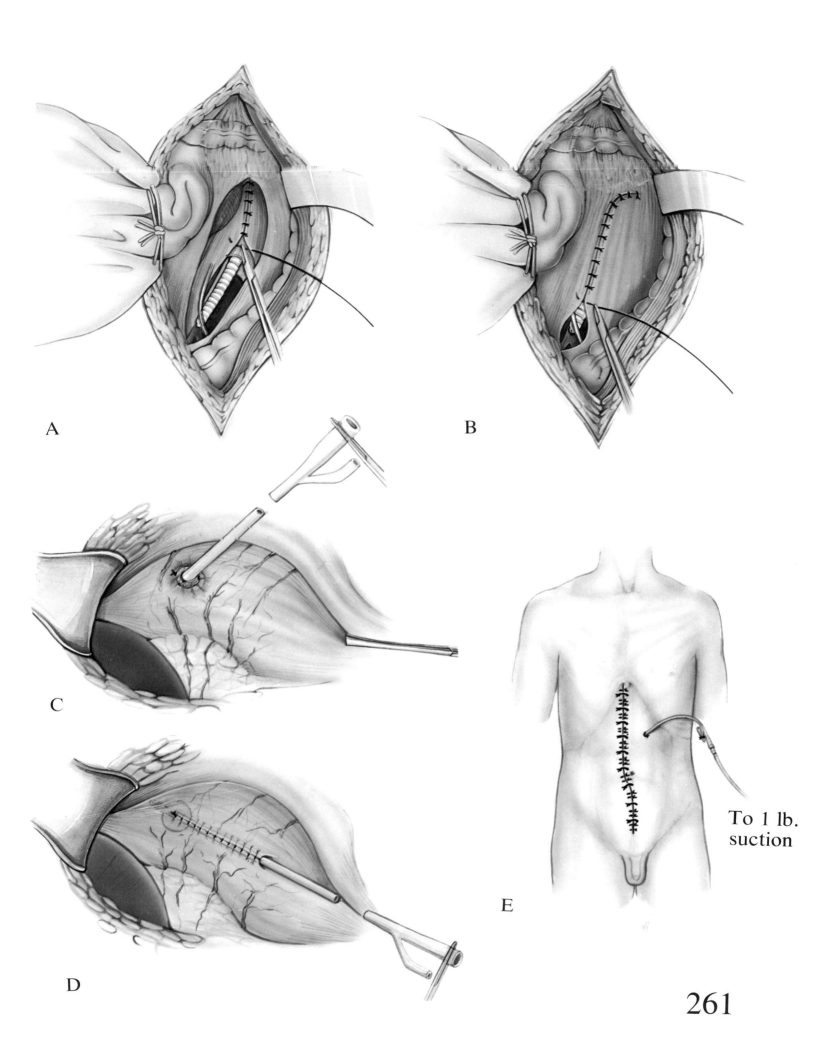

A

B

C

D

E

To 1 lb.
suction

261

Plate 119

EXAMPLES OF LARGE AORTIC AND COMMON ILIAC ANEURYSMS

A. This illustration shows an asymptomatic large abdominal arteriosclerotic aortic aneurysm measuring 10 by 14 cm. in a man, 67 years of age, as it was exposed through a long abdominal incision. The duodenum (a) is shown adherent to the proximal end, and the sigmoid and its mesocolon (b) are adherent to the distal portion. The right common iliac artery (c) is also visible. This aneurysm had eroded posteriorly into the anterior longitudinal ligament, so undoubtedly was not far from rupturing. It was removed and a knitted Dacron aortic bifurcation prosthesis implanted. The patient made an uneventful recovery and is alive and well, now 77 years of age, and still able to mow his lawn in the summertime. This is an excellent result, with the saving of the patient's life and giving him an extra 10 years and more of normal living.

B. This demonstrates a huge abdominal arteriosclerotic aortic aneurysm measuring 11 by 15 cm. and two smaller common iliac aneurysms in a man, age 66 years. The dissection has been completed to free them up. A shoestring (a) has been passed around the upper portion of the aneurysm, which extended proximally to the level of the left renal vein. This was an asymptomatic aneurysm, but at operation it seemed so large I wondered whether it would be possible to remove it safely. This was accomplished, however, and a woven Dacron Teflon graft implanted to the aortic cuff at the level of the left renal vein and distally to the left common iliac and right external iliac arteries. This patient, now age 79 years, is alive 13 years after his operation. He is suffering from coronary heart disease, but is well enough to be up and about without any abdominal symptoms. Again, an excellent result in the treatment of a huge abdominal aortic aneurysm with bilateral iliac aneurysms, all of which were removed and replaced by a prosthesis.

C. This shows a small arteriosclerotic abdominal aortic aneurysm and a very large left common iliac aneurysm in a woman, age 76 years. These aneurysms were asymptomatic, but it was thought at her age it would be advisable to remove them before she became older and the aneurysms grew larger in size. The illustration demonstrates them after they have been isolated and shows a right accessory renal artery (a) arising from the neck of the small aortic aneurysm. It was possible to remove the aortic aneurysm and the left common iliac aneurysm and to preserve the right accessory renal artery. A knitted Dacron bifurcation aortic prosthesis was implanted. The patient made a very satisfactory recovery. This patient has lived for 10 years since her operation without further symptoms from her abdominal aortic procedure, but unfortunately is suffering from progression of cerebrovascular disease, again demonstrating a 10-year follow-up from her aortic and iliac aneurysmal surgery.

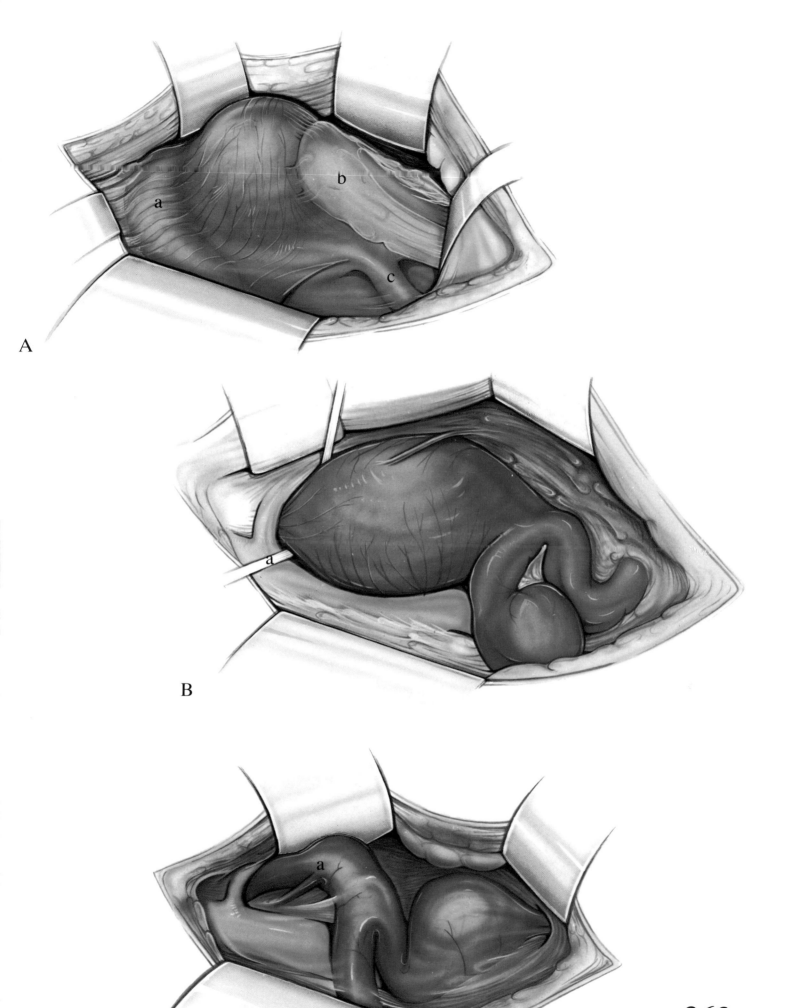

A

B

C

263

Plate 120

EXAMPLES OF LARGE
AORTIC AND COMMON
ILIAC ANEURYSMS *(Continued)*

A.   This shows a large arteriosclerotic aortic aneurysm and an aneurysmal dilatation of the common iliac arteries with an accessory right renal artery (a) rising at the distal edge of the aortic aneurysm in a woman, age 68 years. The aneurysm was asymptomatic and discovered on routine physical examination. The illustration shows the exposure of it after it has been dissected free and demonstrates a small neck at the proximal end, making it very suitable for resection. Because of the dilatation of the common iliac arteries it was thought best to remove the aneurysm, the distal aorta and the dilated common arteries. A knitted Dacron aortic graft was implanted and the accessory right renal artery was anastomosed to the right iliac limb of the graft. The patient made a very satisfactory postoperative recovery and now, 10 years since the operation, is alive and well as far as her aortic surgery is concerned, but being treated for mild congestive heart failure. The lower pole of the right kidney was exposed before and after implanting the accessory renal artery and showed a return to normal color of the lower half of the kidney, it having been very cyanotic while the artery was clamped. Postoperatively normal renal function was maintained.

B.   This shows the abdominal arteriosclerotic aortic aneurysm of a man, age 62 years. The aneurysm had been diagnosed three years prior to removal, but his physician had not advised operation. The patient complained of some epigastric discomfort and soreness for a year before he was admitted to the hospital for surgery. The illustration reveals a dark bluish black almost gangrenous area on the anterior surface of the aneurysm. The transverse colon was adherent to it, so it had to be separated very carefully to avoid opening the bowel or the aneurysm. After this was accomplished, it was possible to resect the aneurysm and implant the aortic bifurcation graft. This was performed because the distal aorta was so calcified that a sleeve graft could not be used. The patient made a very satisfactory recovery and continued to do well except for some hypertension. He died five years after the operation from a left frontal lobe infarct, secondary to thrombosis of the left internal carotid artery. Autopsy revealed that the aorta between the graft and the renal arteries had become dilated, with thrombus formation partially occluding the renal arteries; this may have played a part in the etiology of his hypertension. How much better it would have been if the local doctor had advised operation three years earlier when the aneurysm was first diagnosed. This would have permitted a more radical procedure, with resection close to the renal arteries and cleaning out of their ostia if necessary. This is another example of the fact that it is better to remove an asymptomatic aneurysm than to wait until it becomes symptomatic.

C.   This shows a moderately large abdominal arteriosclerotic aortic aneurysm in a man 71 years of age, who complained of lower abdominal pain of five weeks' duration. It has been dissected free and shows a black, almost gangrenous area on the anterior surface that would soon have ruptured. The shape of this aneurysm was unusual in that it protruded far anteriorly and was rather short in length. As a result of the increased anteroposterior diameter, the anterior wall of the aneurysm was beginning to show signs of breaking down, with a possibility of imminent rupture. This patient made a satisfactory recovery and has continued in good health now some five years since his operation. Again, an excellent result from this type of surgery for an aneurysm which, although not very large, was threatening the patient's life because of potential imminent rupture.

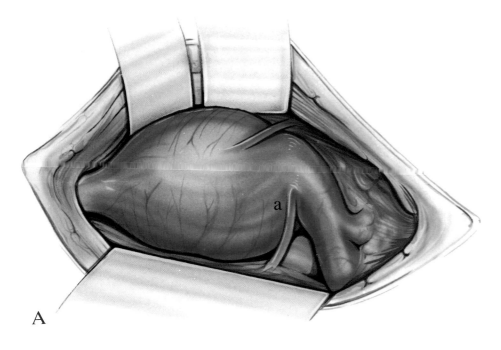

A

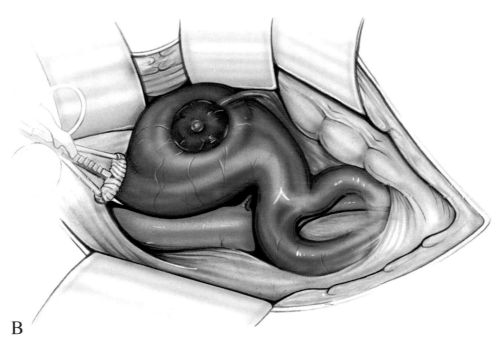

B

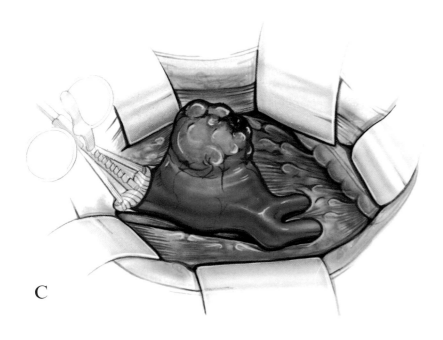

C

Plate 121

THE CREECH METHOD OF ANEURYSMECTOMY AND INSERTION OF A DACRON GRAFT FOR RUPTURED OR LARGE ABDOMINAL AORTIC ANEURYSMS

A. This demonstrates an aneurysm that has been isolated, with a tourniquet clamp placed on the aorta proximal to it and two tourniquet clamps on the iliac arteries. A long incision is made in the anterior wall of the aneurysm, carrying it down as a Y into the origin of the common iliac arteries.

B. The laminated clot has been removed from the aneurysmal sac with finger dissection. Any bleeding lumbar artery is sutured with a figure-of-eight suture to control it; then a large portion of the aneurysmal sac may be resected.

C. The posterior wall has been left in as demonstrated, still attached to the proximal aorta and the distal common iliac arteries. Incisions are made partially through the aortic and the common iliac arteries posteriorly to free up sufficient of the walls to facilitate suturing of the anastomosis. The posterior suture line is placed first, then the anterior portion of it.

D. This demonstrates another method of placing the posterior aortic anastomosis by suturing from within the graft and the aorta and then completing the anterior row as shown in the inset (a). After it is completed, the graft is preclotted; then the distal anastomoses of the iliac limbs are made to the common iliac arteries. Longitudinal arteriotomies have been made to facilitate the construction of these anastomoses. The posterior row of sutures is placed first and this is done from within the artery and the graft as demonstrated; then the posterior part of the anastomosis is completed as in inset (b). The left iliac limb is then opened to allow blood to flow down the left side. A similar anastomosis is performed to the right common iliac artery, after which the right iliac limb can be opened. This type of procedure reduces the operating time for implantation of the graft but demands great skill in accomplishing the anastomoses.

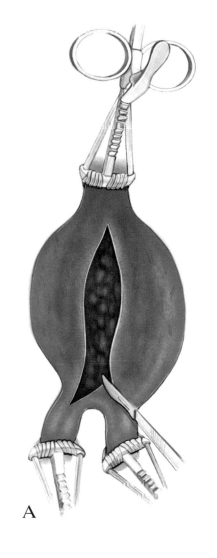

A

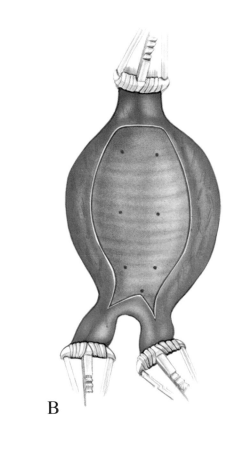

B

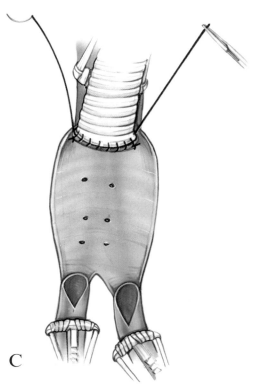

C

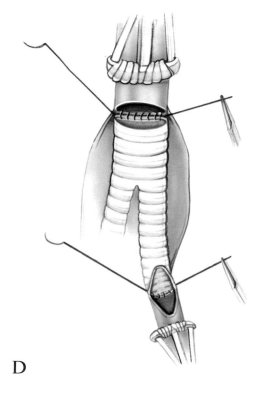

D

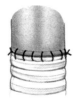

a

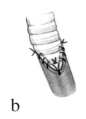

b

Plate 122

THE CREECH METHOD OF ANEURYSMECTOMY AND INSERTION OF A DACRON GRAFT FOR RUPTURED OR LARGE ABDOMINAL AORTIC ANEURYSMS *(Continued)*

A. This demonstrates the technique that I have used when it is possible to isolate the proximal aorta and divide the aneurysmal sac so that the proximal aortic anastomosis can be completed with a running everting mattress suture and an over-and-over suture outside it, as shown in Plates 102, 103, 104 and 105. The posterior wall is left in. The orifices of the lumbar arteries are secured with figure-of-eight sutures of linen or catgut. The distal ends of the common iliac arteries have also been freed up.

B. After completion of the proximal aortic anastomosis, the common iliac limbs are anastomosed to the distal ends of the common iliac arteries. Since they have been dissected free, the construction of these anastomoses is relatively easy. The left side is completed first and opened, then the right one performed in a similar manner.

C. This demonstrates the single sleeve type of aortic prosthesis which can be used when the distal end of the abdominal aorta is not involved in the aneurysmal dilatation, or if there is not too severe atherosclerotic disease in the common iliac arteries. Under these conditions it is much safer to make the distal anastomosis at some point where the arteries are less involved with atherosclerotic disease by implanting a Y type of graft rather than a sleeve type. If the latter is used, the posterior suture line of the aortic anastomosis can be placed much easier from within the aorta and the graft. The small additional Dacron within the aortic lumen at the suture line creates no thombogenic problem. From my experience, however, I have found it more satisfactory to use the Y graft almost routinely because, with this type, the distal anastomosis of the iliac limbs can be made to the common iliac or external iliac arteries, or even to the common femoral arteries if necessary.

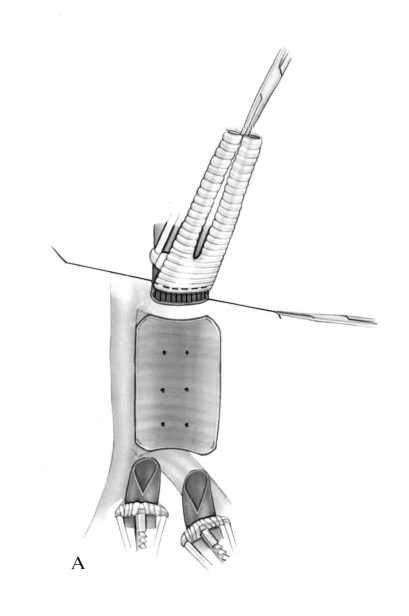

A

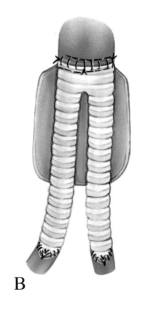

B

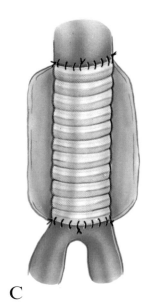

C

269

Plate 123

THE TECHNIQUE FOR RUPTURED ABDOMINAL ARTERIOSCLEROTIC AORTIC ANEURYSMS WITH INTRA-AORTIC CONTROL

Great strides have been made in the treatment of abdominal arteriosclerotic aneurysms, but unfortunately there are still too many that have ruptured before the patient comes to surgery. In many cases this is because the diagnosis is not made, since it is not until the aneurysm becomes very large that it gives any symptoms. The diagnosis is made many times when an x-ray examination of the back, the kidneys or the gastrointestinal tract is performed. Again, not all physicians recommend to the patient that the aneurysm be removed, because they believe the operative mortality rate of asymptomatic aneurysms is still too high. This certainly is not true if the operation is done by a surgeon well trained in this field. There is no question that all asymptomatic aneurysms that are 5 or more cm. in diameter should be removed unless there are contraindications such as cardiac, pulmonary, cerebrovascular or renal disease. It certainly is an error to put off the operation until the aneurysm enlarges so that it involves the renal arteries or until it has ruptured, because then the mortality rises very markedly.

There is no procedure that is a greater emergency than the sudden rupture of an abdominal aortic aneurysm. If this occurs at some distance from a large surgical center, the patient's life can sometimes be saved by placing him in a G suit and sending him to a major hospital. One of the most serious complications following rupture of an aortic aneurysm is anuria. If a patient has become anuric prior to operation, the mortality rate from renal failure is extremely high. For this reason it is imperative that the patient be operated upon as soon as possible.

A. This demonstrates a huge retroperitoneal hematoma that has formed as the result of the rupture in the anterior wall of an abdominal aortic aneurysm. In some cases this blood clot temporarily tamponades the rupture site, and the patient survives the acute hemorrhage. The abdomen is opened through a midline incision from the ensiform process to the pubis.

B. Four thousand units of heparin are injected into the aneurysmal sac. This should be done early to prevent thrombosis developing in the arteries distal to the aneurysm; if thrombosis occurs, it will complicate the operative procedure. Since the control of the ruptured aortic aneurysm will be obtained in a few minutes, heparin given early in the course of the operation does not present a hazard from excess bleeding.

C. The blood clot is removed from the aneurysmal wall with finger dissection. In this patient the site of rupture was found on the anterior surface of the aneurysm, whereas most occur posteriorly.

D. Proximal control of the abdominal aorta was then quickly obtained by the surgeon's inserting the thumb of his right hand through the fragile anterior aneurysmal wall at the site of rupture and carrying it proximally to occlude the proximal aorta from within the lumen. This procedure can also be accomplished with posterior wall ruptures. This facilitates the passage of a large right-angle clamp, as shown, around the aorta; the thumb within the aorta is an excellent guide as to where to place it. A shoestring is pulled through underneath the aorta and quickly threaded through a tourniquet clamp, with which immediate control of the proximal bleeding is obtained.

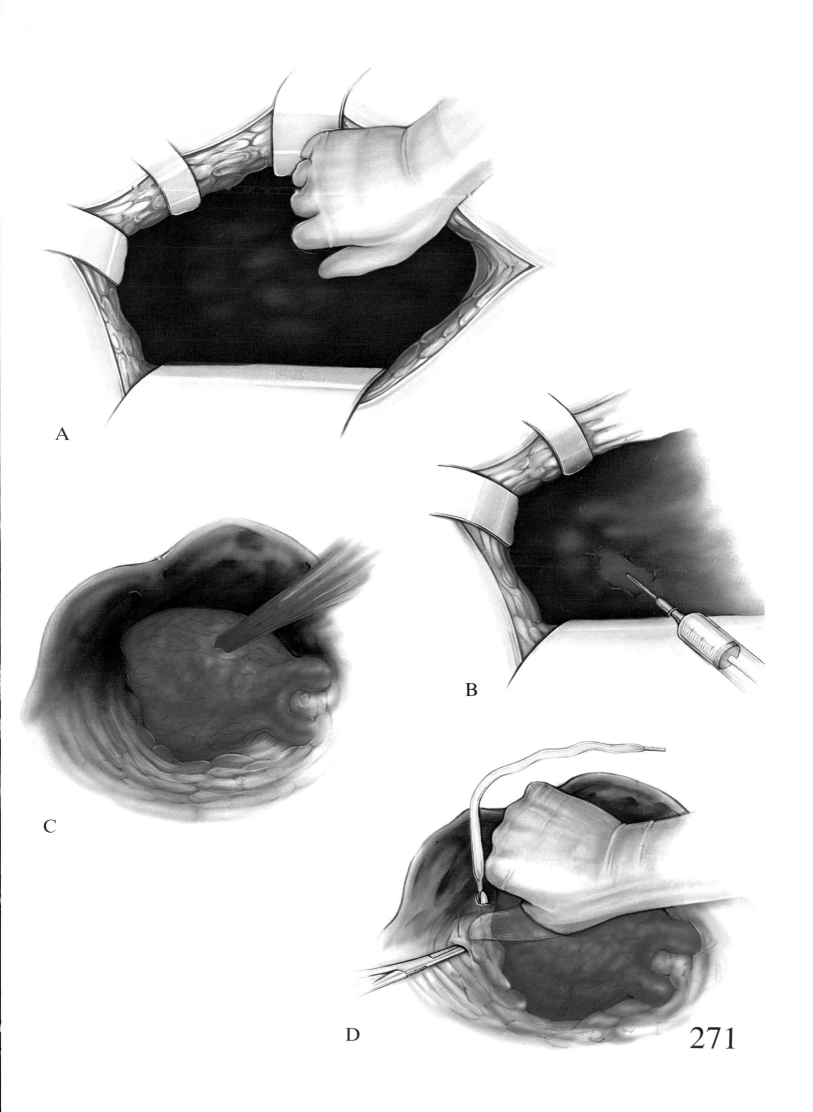

A

B

C

D

271

Plate 124

THE TECHNIQUE FOR RUPTURED ABDOMINAL ARTERIOSCLEROTIC AORTIC ANEURYSMS WITH INTRA-AORTIC CONTROL *(Continued)*

A. With the proximal aorta controlled, the next step is to isolate the common iliac arteries to control the back flow from them. This again is usually not too difficult, as one is already within the aneurysm; it is most helpful, especially in very obese patients, to use a tourniquet clamp on each of the common iliac arteries. After the arteries have been isolated and the clamps applied to them, they are temporarily opened and, with a fine polyethylene tubing, 20 cc. of dilute heparin solution containing 100 units per cubic centimeter of normal saline is injected into each common iliac artery. This will prevent distal arterial thrombosis from developing.

B. The laminated intrasaccular blood clot is cleaned out with finger dissection after making a larger incision. In addition, the inner lining of the atheromatous material of the media and intima is also removed.

C. A large portion of the aneurysmal sac can then be excised, leaving the posterior wall still attached to surrounding structures, including the vena cava.

D. There will be a few lumbar arteries which bleed; these are controlled with figure-of-eight stitches of either Dacron or catgut.

E. The proximal aorta may be completely divided from the aneurysmal sac. This makes the proximal anastomosis easier and safer to construct, preferably with a running everting mattress suture and an over-and-over suture outside this (Plates 102, 103, 104 and 105). The iliac limbs are then implanted to the common iliac arteries distally if they are not too atherosclerotic, or more distally to the external iliac arteries; occasionally it may be necessary to carry them distally to the common femoral arteries. The raw surface is then reperitonealized with a two-layer closure over the graft. A Witzel type gastrostomy is performed with a No. 18 Foley catheter; the abdominal incision is closed with 0 chromic catgut sutures to the peritoneum and fascia and multiple stay sutures of No. 22 gauge stainless steel wire going through all layers of the abdominal wall.

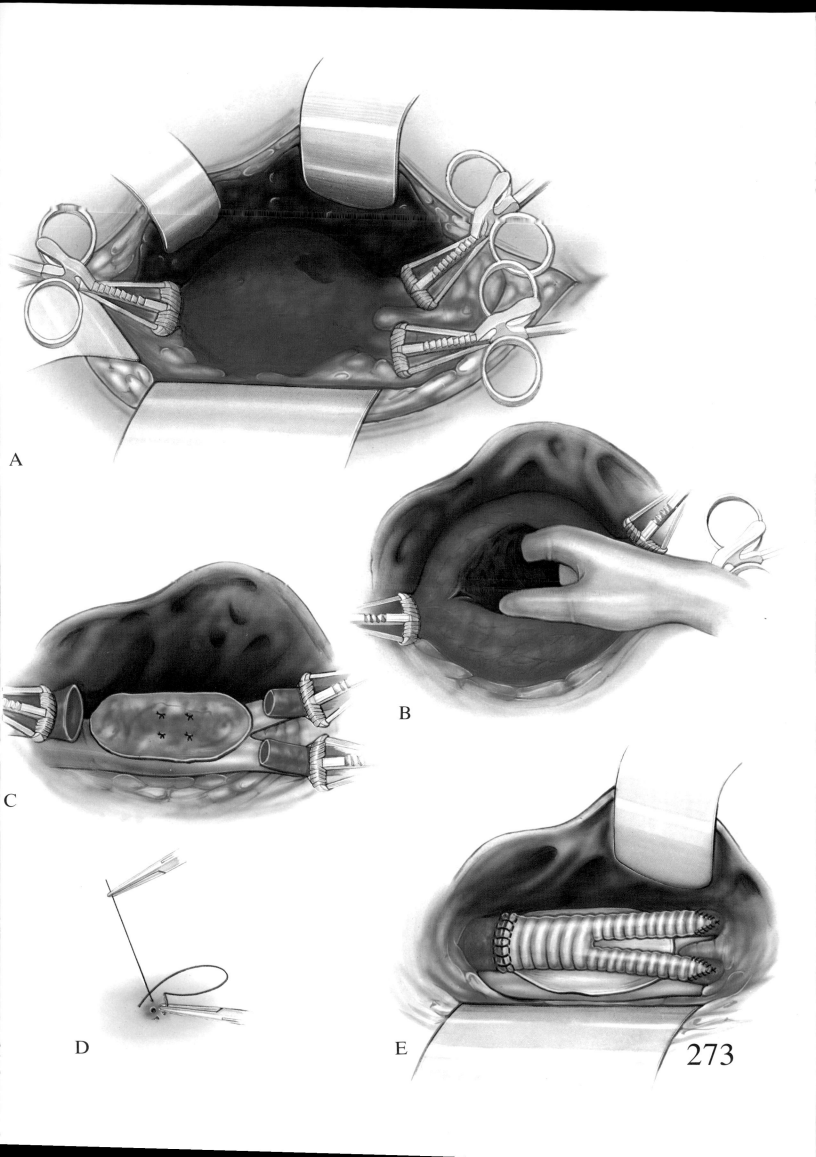

A

B

C

D

E

273

Plate 125

RUPTURED ABDOMINAL ARTERIOSCLEROTIC AORTIC ANEURYSM WITH RIGHT FEMORAL NERVE PALSY

A. This shows a large abdominal arteriosclerotic aortic aneurysm measuring 9 by 7 cm. in a man, age 58 years. He was admitted to the hospital with a chief complaint of pain and weakness in his right hip and thigh. He gave a history of a dull aching pain in his right lumbar region, which had started two months before. His symptoms increased, with more severe pain and a gradual onset of right femoral nerve palsy. The diagnosis of an abdominal aortic aneurysm was made, but he was treated primarily for his femoral neuropathy which, on admission to the Massachusetts General Hospital, had increased to almost complete paralysis of this nerve. Physical examination showed a large pulsating abdominal aortic aneurysm, with weakness and atrophy of his right quadriceps femoris muscle. The diagnosis of a ruptured abdominal arteriosclerotic aortic aneurysm with a large right-sided false aneurysm was made, and operation was performed March 3, 1966, through a transperitoneal exposure.

B. This cross-section through the region of the fourth lumbar vertebra reveals the location of the aortic aneurysm (a), the inferior vena cava (b), the false aneurysm (c), and the femoral nerve (d). Note that the blood that escaped from the ruptured aneurysm passed posterior to the inferior vena cava, between it and the body of the lumbar vertebra.

C. This demonstrates the result of the operative procedure, with removal of the aneurysmal sac, the implantation of a knitted Dacron aortic bifurcation prosthesis and closure of the central fistulous tract on the medial edge of the false aneurysm. Evacuation of the huge retroperitoneal blood clot, that was retrocecal and retrorenal, was performed and the false aneurysm area drained through a lateral incision. The patient made an uneventful recovery with return of full function of his right femoral nerve. This case demonstrates as others have that all aortic aneurysms do not succumb from exsanguination but can form large retroperitoneal false aneurysms. It was thought from the history that the aneurysm in this patient had ruptured two months prior to his operation. This type of case also demonstrates that in any patient with a large abdominal aortic aneurysm who gives a history of previous lumbar back pain and then later develops evidence of right or left femoral neuropathy, the diagnosis of a ruptured abdominal aortic aneurysm with secondary false aneurysm should be made. The patient should be operated upon to remove the abdominal aortic aneurysm and replace it with an aortic prosthesis, and to evacuate the large false aneurysm.

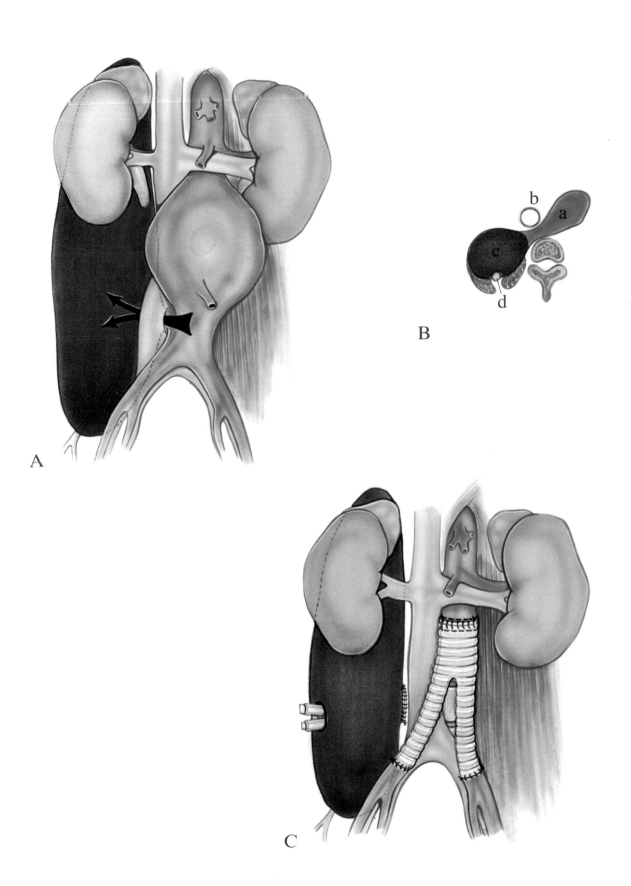

A

B

C

275

Plate 126

ABDOMINAL ARTERIOSCLEROTIC AORTIC ANEURYSMS COMPLICATED WITH SEVERE OBLITERATIVE ARTERIAL DISEASE INVOLVING BILATERAL COMMON ILIAC, EXTERNAL ILIAC, COMMON FEMORAL AND RIGHT SUPERFICIAL FEMORAL ARTERIES

A. This illustration demonstrates the aortic and peripheral arterial disease in a male, age 70 years, with a chief complaint of intermittent claudication in his right leg. The aneurysm was asymptomatic and was found when he sought help for his claudication. No pulses were present in the right lower extremity distal to the common femoral artery, whereas on the left they were all palpable. Abdominal examination revealed a readily palpable moderate-sized aortic aneurysm. Bilateral femoropopliteal arteriograms demonstrated a complete occlusion of his right superficial femoral and peroneal arteries, with some disease in the left superficial femoral arteries. The outflow tract of both popliteal arteries was slightly narrowed.

B. An aortic bifurcation graft was implanted to replace the abdominal arteriosclerotic aortic aneurysm and to bypass the external iliac arteries, with implantation in the common femoral arteries bilaterally because of the severe disease in the external iliac arteries. In order to save operative time during which the aorta must be occluded, both common femoral arteries were exposed before dissecting out the aortic aneurysm. Retroperitoneal tunnels posterior to the inguinal ligaments were made from each groin to the promontory of the sacrum. Each was marked with a Penrose tubing. The left iliac limb of the graft was implanted end-to-side to the common femoral artery. It was possible to make a more satisfactory anastomosis on the right side to the profunda femoris artery by ligating and dividing the superficial femoral artery and constructing the anastomosis to the distal portion of the common femoral and proximal end of the divided superficial femoral arteries. No attempt was made to bypass the superficial femoral block since revascularization of the profunda femoris artery, if it is in good condition, restores the blood supply quite satisfactorily in many cases. It should be noted that both common iliac arteries were interrupted proximal to the hypogastric arteries and the ends closed with a double over-and-over suture technique with 4-0 braided Dacron sutures. It is important to leave the common iliac bifurcations open to permit blood to reflux from the femoral artery anastomoses through the external iliac arteries into the hypogastric arteries. If the patient's condition is satisfactory it is advisable to perform limited bilateral lumbar sympathectomies. The operation is completed by closing the retroperitoneal tissues over the graft and the posterior peritoneum, then closing the groin incisions in layers with fine linen sutures. A Witzel gastrostomy is performed now that the Dacron prosthesis has been covered over and there is no danger that it will be contaminated by this procedure. The abdominal incision is closed in a routine manner. If the patient is still troubled with intermittent claudication and wishes this to be relieved, a saphenous vein autograft can be placed from the end of the Dacron prosthesis in his right groin down to the distal popliteal artery, but it is advisable to wait four to six months to be sure that it is really going to be necessary.

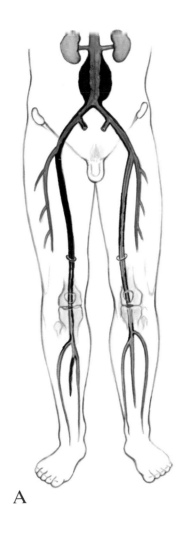

A

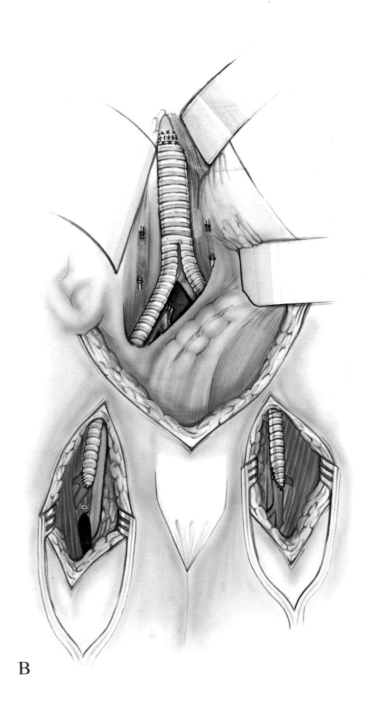

B

277

Plate 127

LARGE ABDOMINAL AORTIC ANEURYSMS WITH COMPLICATING FACTORS

A. This demonstrates a large asymptomatic abdominal aortic aneurysm measuring 8 by 13 cm. The anterior wall of the aneurysmal sac was very firm and made up of a thick layer of scar tissue. The third portion of the duodenum was intimately adherent to this, so a thin layer of the outer shell of the aneurysm had to be removed, leaving it attached to the duodenum as shown to prevent opening the duodenum. Actually it is less serious to enter the aneurysmal sac, because this can be controlled as in a ruptured aneurysm, but I have never had it occur. It was possible to place a tourniquet clamp proximal to the renal arteries and the left renal vein and distal to the superior mesenteric artery. The common iliac arteries were controlled with bulldog clamps. The aneurysm was removed, necessitating interruption of the inferior mesenteric artery and a small accessory left renal artery. The entire sac was resected up to within a half a centimeter of the origin of the renal artery.

B and C. This demonstrates the short aortic cuff with the two renal arteries and their intra-aortic orifices distal to the tourniquet clamp. Ten cubic centimeters of dilute heparin solution were injected through a fine polyvinyl catheter into them, then each was occluded with a small bulldog clamp. An aortic bifurcation graft previously preclotted was implanted to the proximal aorta with interrupted mattress sutures. Then another tourniquet clamp was placed just distal to the anastomosis but was not closed until the proximal aorta had been flushed from above. It was then closed, with restoration of the blood supply to the kidneys. It is of significance that both renal arteries were occluded for one hour and ten minutes before restoration of the circulation without later evidence of impairment of renal function, thus demonstrating that regional heparinization of a kidney is an important factor in maintaining patent blood vessels in them.

D and E. This shows a large asymptomatic abdominal arteriosclerotic aortic aneurysm measuring 9 by 14 cm. and two large iliac aneurysms in a male, age 69 years, with the right ureter coursing over the right iliac aneurysm. As the aneurysm was dissected out, a small accessory renal artery was found but was not necessary to preserve. The left renal vein passed posterior to the aorta, a rare anomaly, which is important to recognize before it is inadvertently torn or lacerated. Its presence was helpful in this case because it was possible to place a tourniquet clamp just distal to the renal arteries without interfering with the left renal vein. An aneurysmorrhaphy of the proximal part of the aneurysmal sac was performed proximally close to the renal arteries. This was accomplished by plicating the right side of the aneurysmal cuff with a running everting mattress suture going through all layers and reducing the lumen to the same size as a 25-mm. Dacron prosthesis; this was reinforced with an over-and-over type of suture. A satisfactory end-to-end anastomosis between the aorta and the prosthesis was constructed. The left iliac limb of the graft was anastomosed end-to-end by the end-to-side technique to the distal end of the common iliac artery after resecting most of the anterior portion of the iliac aneurysmal sac with an excellent streamlined anastomosis. On the right the hypogastric artery was ligated and divided and the iliac limb was anastomosed to the external iliac artery; this could have been accomplished in a manner similar to that used for the left side. A 10-year follow-up on this patient revealed that the graft is still functioning well without any evidence of further aneurysmal dilatation, demonstrating that this type of plastic procedure to the proximal portion of the aneurysmal sac stands up exceedingly well.

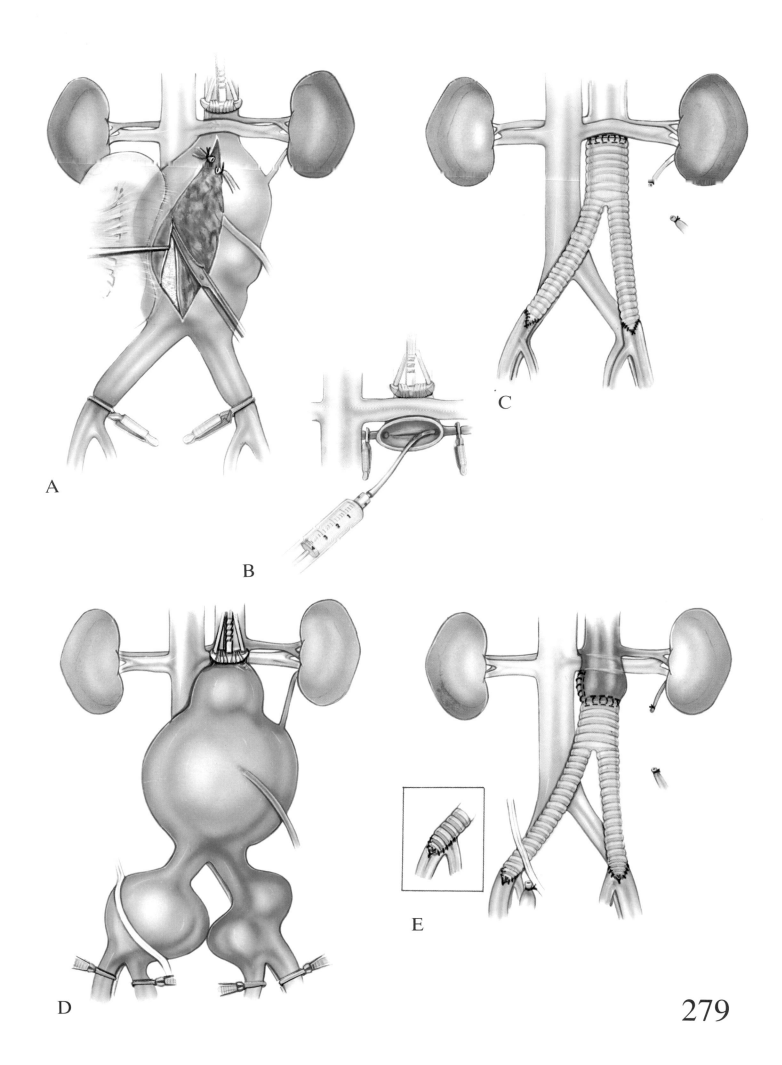

A

B

C

D

E

Plate 128

LARGE ABDOMINAL AORTIC ANEURYSMS WITH COMPLICATING FACTORS
(Continued)

A.   This demonstrates a huge abdominal aortic aneurysm measuring 9 by 14 cm. in a male, age 67 years. In addition, there is a large left common iliac aneurysm, continuous with the aortic aneurysm, measuring 5.5 by 7.5 cm. Bilateral aneurysms of the hypogastric arteries of smaller size can also be seen. These aneurysms, especially the abdominal aortic, and probably the left common iliac, had been present for a good many years but had not given any symptoms until shortly before the patient was admitted to the hospital for surgery. At that time he complained of some back discomfort, suggesting further enlargement of the aneurysm but not an actual rupture. There was a relatively long section of essentially normal-sized aorta distal to the renal arteries, so that there was no difficulty in placing the proximal occluding tourniquet clamp. The more difficult problem in this case was encountered with the iliac aneurysms because of their location, especially the hypogastric ones, and the close proximity of the ureters to them. The latter were carefully dissected free from the aneurysms and isolated by passing Penrose tubing around them so that they were readily visible and injury to them could be avoided.

B.   The portions of the posterior wall of the abdominal and the left iliac aneurysms adherent to the vena cava and the left iliac vein were not excised in order to avoid injury to these venous structures. The aortic anastomosis was performed end-to-end by the previously described techniques. The right limb of the prosthesis was anastomosed to the distal end of the common iliac artery. The hypogastric artery was preserved by performing an aneurysmorrhaphy of the small aneurysm to preserve this artery for the pelvic blood supply. The left hypogastric aneurysm was larger, so this artery was interrupted and a portion of the aneurysm removed. The distal anastomosis of the iliac limb of the graft was made to the external iliac artery. The patient made a very satisfactory recovery and continues well seven years later, with a satisfactorily functioning aortic bifurcation prosthesis and without any complications.

C.   This shows a large asymptomatic abdominal aortic aneurysm measuring 9 by 14 cm. and bilateral common iliac and hypogastric artery aneurysms in a male, age 68 years. The right hypogastric aneurysm was occluded with a thrombus. The left one was partially thrombosed. In addition, there was a thrombosed saccular aneurysm arising posteriorly from the origin of the right common iliac aneurysm. The large abdominal aneurysm was discovered on a routine physical examination; the examining doctor stated it had not been noted on a similar examination a year and a half previously, but this seems unlikely in view of its huge size.

D.   The removal of the abdominal and common iliac aneurysms was not difficult. This patient demonstrates that both hypogastric arteries and the inferior mesenteric artery may be interrupted without ischemia of the left colon or pelvic structures. The Henle-Coenen sign demonstrated that the arterial backflow from the inferior mesenteric artery was extraordinarily brisk, so that the viability of the left colon and sigmoid was assured. The patient made a satisfactory recovery and is alive and well five years after the operation.

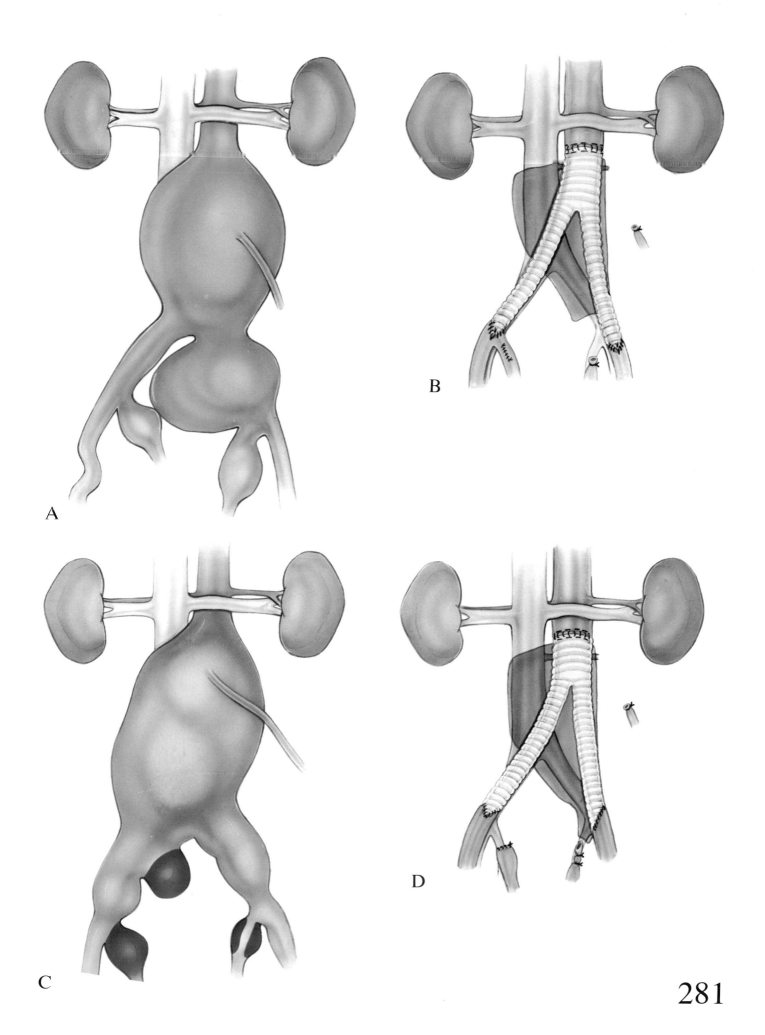

A

B

C

D

281

Plate 129

THORACOABDOMINAL
AORTIC ANEURYSMS

A. This demonstrates the thoracoabdominal incision that is necessary for the implantation of an aortic graft from the midthoracic aorta to the common iliac or the common femoral arteries. Some surgeons advocate two incisions, but the division of the costal arch gives a better exposure for the celiac axis and the superior mesenteric artery and it can be readily repaired.

B. This demonstrates a huge thoracoabdominal aneurysm extending from well above the diaphragm to involve the bifurcation of the aorta. Note that there is marked atherosclerosis of the common iliac, the external iliac and the common femoral arteries. The inferior mesenteric artery is also occluded. Both renal arteries, the superior mesenteric and the celiac axis are patent. It is important to obtain complete exposure before proceeding with the grafting procedure. Because of right iliac artery disease in this patient it was necessary to expose the right common femoral artery; on the left the common iliac artery could be used. The thoracic aorta should also be exposed so that the aortic graft can be implanted proximal to the aneurysm.

C. The first anastomoses to be constructed are the distal ones. After construction the bulldog clamps are removed and the iliac limbs of the graft are occluded with them to permit blood to flow down to the lower extremities. The graft is next anastomosed to the thoracic aorta. Just prior to opening the graft the right common femoral artery (a) and the left iliac artery (b) should be interrupted proximal to the distal anastomoses so that blood will flow through the aortic graft to the lower extremities rather than through two channels, namely, the aortic aneurysm and the graft, because, with both channels patent, the aortic graft will become occluded.

D. The aortic graft has been implanted. There is a suture line shown in the aortic portion of the graft because it was necessary to lengthen the aortic bifurcation graft. Note that the right common femoral and the left common iliac artery have been ligated proximal to the distal anastomoses.

E. This demonstrates the completed graft. The numbers indicate the sequence with which each step is done: 1 is the end-to-side anastomosis between the graft and the left common iliac artery; 2 is the anastomosis between the right iliac limb of the graft to the common femoral artery; 3 is the anastomosis between the thoracic aorta and the aortic prosthesis; 4 is interruption of the right common femoral and the left common iliac arteries; 5 is an anastomosis of a short segment of a 6-mm. Dacron graft to the aortic graft; 6, the left renal artery is ligated, the distal end anastomosed to the small side arm of Dacron from the aorta; a similar procedure is then carried out on the right side with the right renal artery at 7 and 8; 9, the celiac axis is ligated and divided and the distal end anastomosed to the Dacron side arm at 10; the superior mesenteric artery is anastomosed in a similar manner at 11 and 12; after completion of all these anastomoses, the final step is 13, the interruption of the thoracic aorta just distal to the aortic anastomosis. The proximal end is sutured with 3-0 Dacron sutures, using a running mattress suture if possible, then an over-and-over suture outside this. The distal end is closed with a running over-and-over suture. As a rule, it is not necessary to remove the entire aneurysm. These are long operative procedures, so it is probably best to limit them to patients who are in excellent physical condition from the cardiac, pulmonary and renal standpoints.

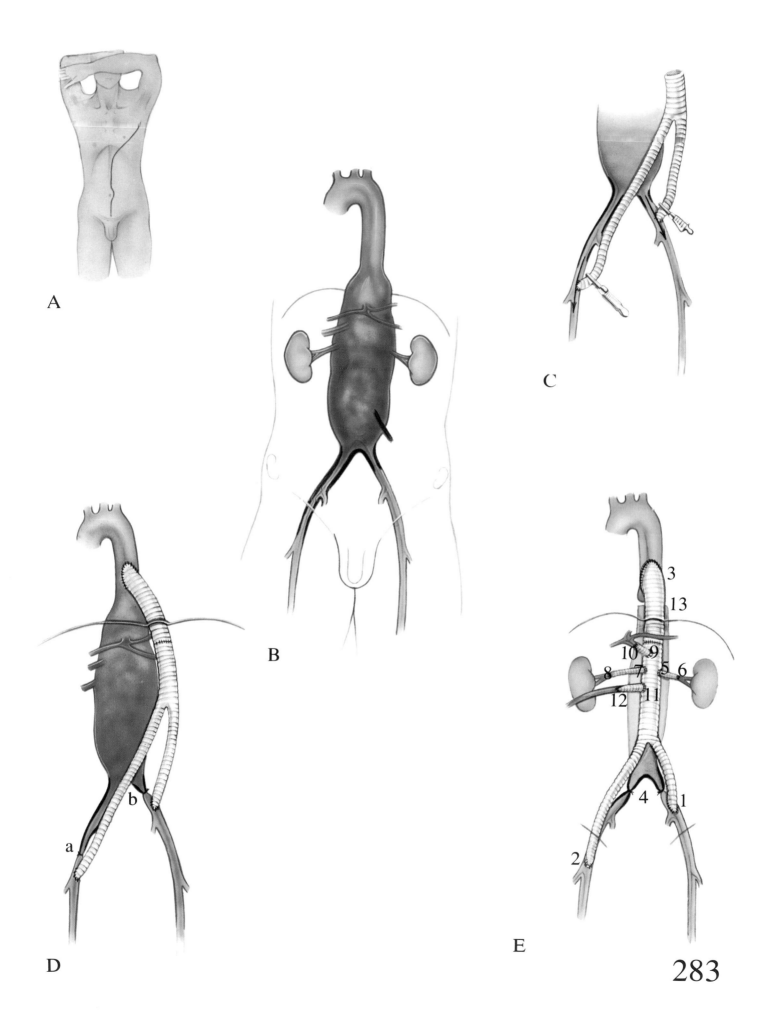

A

B

C

D

a
b

E

1
2
3
4
5
6
7
8
9
10
11
12
13

283

Plate 130

RESECTION OF ABDOMINAL AORTIC ANEURYSM WITH TRANSPLANTATION OF ACCESSORY RENAL ARTERIES

A. This demonstrates a moderate-sized, dumbbell-shaped aortic aneurysm with bilateral accessory renal arteries arising from the narrow portion of the aneurysm. The aneurysm and iliac arteries have been freed up and controlled with a tourniquet clamp on the aorta just proximal to the aneurysm and bulldog clamps on the common iliac arteries. It is not always feasible to preserve these accessory renal arteries, but when the caliber is 3 mm. it is worthwhile to save them, as it is a relatively simple procedure to anastomose them to either the iliac limbs of the prosthesis or the main aortic portion of the graft, using whichever the accessory artery lies best on without kinking or undue tension.

B. When one is dealing with a relatively small artery the anastomosis can be constructed better if a small segment of the aneurysmal wall is resected with the renal artery. It is best to do this as shown before resecting the aneurysm with a bulldog clamp on the artery to control the back bleeding from it, since there is always a little. (a) After the accessory renal artery has been isolated, 10 cc. of dilute heparin saline solution (100 units per 5 cc.) is injected into the distal end, using a small polyvinyl tubing. This amount of heparin will prevent blood from clotting in the lower portion of the kidney for at least an hour; should this develop it will prevent the artery from functioning after it has been anastomosed to the prosthesis. This is, therefore, a very important step in the procedure. While the injection is being performed, the bulldog clamp can be replaced on the renal artery more distally than the tubing has been inserted, then gently occluding the end of the artery again with one's fingers; a few cubic centimeters of the dilute heparin is injected to forcefully dilate the proximal portion of the artery to facilitate the construction of the anastomosis.

C. This demonstrates the graft being constructed without the small portion of aortic wall around the ostium of the artery; this artery was of larger size, and by incising it as shown, it is possible to make a very satisfactory anastomosis to the prosthesis. A small curved clamp, as shown, is used to pick up a portion of the side wall of the right iliac limb without totally occluding it. This is incised, making an opening in it of sufficient length to create a satisfactory ostium.

D. The anastomosis is constructed utilizing 6-0 Teflon-coated Dacron sutures. These are placed as a running over-and-over suture, taking small bites of the artery and the graft. The suture line is ligated at four points in order not to purse-string the anastomosis.

E. This demonstrates the implantation of right and left accessory renal arteries into the respective iliac limbs of the aortic bifurcation prosthesis, with satisfactory results in both instances.

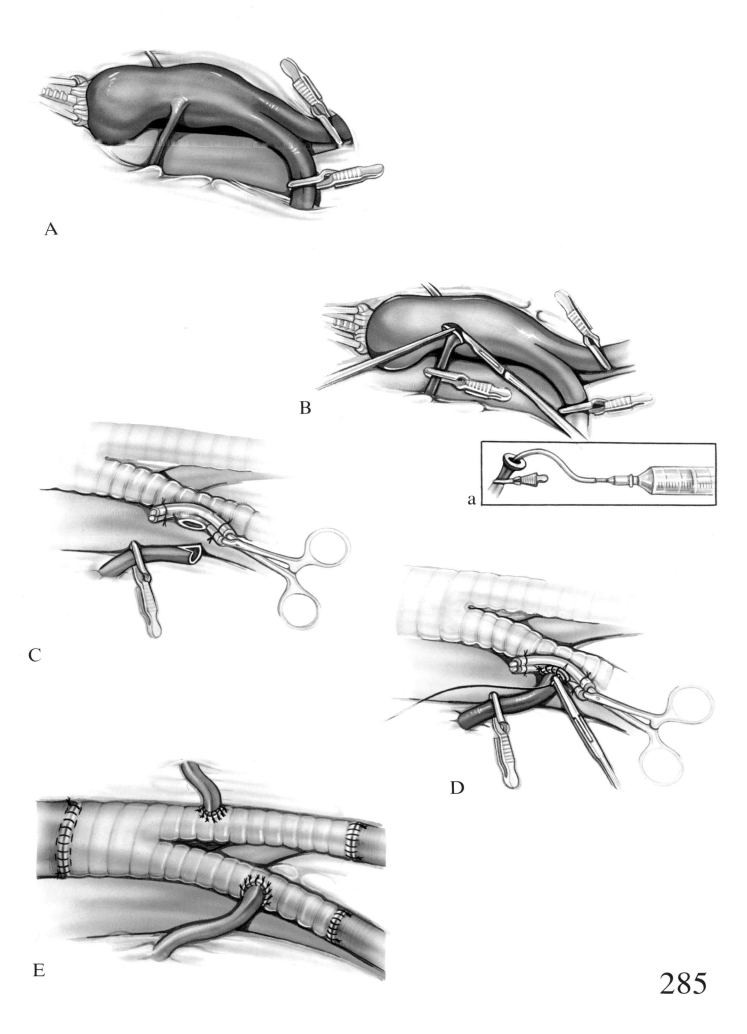

A

B

a

C

D

E

285

Plate 131

RESECTION OF ABDOMINAL AORTIC ANEURYSM WITH TRANSPLANTATION OF ACCESSORY RENAL ARTERIES *(Continued)*

A. This demonstrates a large abdominal aortic aneurysm in which two low lying renal arteries were encountered, but further dissection proximal to them revealed that these were accessory renal arteries and that the main ones were cephalad to them. It was possible in this case to place the tourniquet clamp above the accessory renal arteries and to resect the aneurysmal sac distal to them. Ten cubic centimeters of dilute heparin–normal saline solution (100 units in 5 cc.) were injected into each of the accessory renal arteries by cannulating them within the aorta. Bulldog clamps are placed on them until the aortic anastomosis has been completed; then they are removed and the aortic graft occluded after it has been preclotted, so that the accessory arteries will function during the completion of the graft implantation.

B. This shows the location of the main renal arteries just above the left renal vein, the two accessory renal arteries which were preserved and the aortic bifurcation graft implanted just distal to them, so that it was not necessary to reimplant them into the prosthesis.

C. This demonstrates another patient who had bilateral accessory renal arteries. A bulldog clamp was placed on the right accessory renal artery and after five minutes the right kidney was exposed. The illustration shows the blue cyanotic lower portion of the kidney supplied by this accessory renal artery, demonstrating the advisability of restoring the arterial blood supply to it by implantation of the artery into the prosthesis after the implantation of the graft. The left kidney was not exposed but undoubtedly would have demonstrated the same discolored area, so both accessory renal arteries were preserved.

D. Before resection of the aortic aneurysm, the renal arteries, with small segments of the aneurysmal wall, were excised from the aneurysmal sac. Ten cubic centimeters of dilute normal saline solution were injected into each accessory renal artery and they were then clamped with bulldog clamps, as shown. The aortic aneurysm was resected with the aneurysmal dilatations of the common iliac arteries and an aortic bifurcation prosthesis implanted.

E. This demonstrates the anastomoses of the accessory renal arteries to the iliac limbs of the prosthesis. This view of the right kidney shows disappearance of the cyanotic color in the lower portion, with the return to normal color indicating a reestablishment of a normal arterial circulation, thus demonstrating that the accessory renal artery functions again, so the procedure is well worth performing.

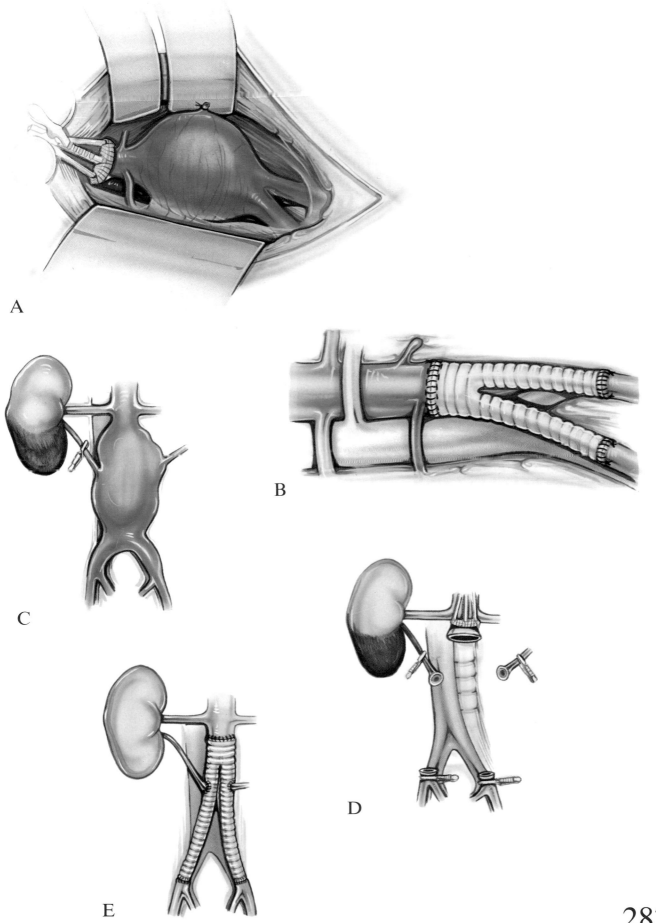

Plate 132

ABDOMINAL ARTERIOSCLEROTIC AORTIC ANEURYSM WITH HORSESHOE KIDNEY

An abdominal arteriosclerotic aortic aneurysm in a patient with a horseshoe kidney presents the surgeon with unusual difficulties in the removal of it and the implantation of a graft. One of the problems is that the renal arteries are very variable. The condition is rare, but the diagnosis should be made preoperatively with the routine intravenous pyelogram. The renal arteries should be anastomosed to the graft if they are supplying the major portion of the kidney. Aortography is of little assistance in demonstrating the abnormal renal arteries but is worth performing. The other complication is a bifid ureter. Unfortunately, intravenous pyelography does not always demonstrate this. Laceration of a ureter with a subsequent urinary leak is a serious error and may be incompatible with survival because of secondary infection involving the aortic graft.

A. This demonstrates a horseshoe kidney with bilateral renal arteries entering the superior poles of both kidneys. There is a large accessory renal artery arising from the left iliac artery and a small one from the right iliac artery. The accessory left renal pelvis and ureter are demonstrated. They have been occluded with bulldog clamps; the illustration demonstrates the marked cyanosis that subsequently occurred in a large portion of the left kidney and the isthmus. It was obvious that the accessory artery from the left iliac artery should be preserved and that the small one on the right could be sacrificed.

B. This demonstrates that a graft has been implanted. Interruption of the small right accessory renal artery permitted mobilization of the isthmus of the horseshoe kidney to facilitate the removal of the aneurysm and the grafting procedure. It was possible to preserve the large accessory left renal artery and to save the entire kidney. The procedure is facilitated by leaving the posterior wall of the aneurysm.

C. This demonstrates another horseshoe kidney, again with two accessory renal arteries coming off the aneurysm and supplying the isthmus, and also a bifid ureter. Temporary occlusion of the accessory renal arteries results in cyanosis of the entire isthmus. There is a small right common iliac aneurysm.

D. The aneurysm was removed and a graft implanted. The major right accessory renal artery was implanted into the aortic portion of the graft, with restoration of the blood supply to the isthmus of the kidneys and salvage of the entire kidney. There may be so many small accessory renal arteries that this type of surgery is not possible. In some patients the cyanotic segment may be so short that it is safe to interrupt the accessory renal artery without anastomosing it to the aortic graft. It is of extreme importance to isolate the abnormal arterial supply to these horseshoe kidneys before proceeding with excision of the aneurysm. If the major portion of the kidney becomes cyanotic in color when one or two large accessory arteries are occluded, these should be anastomosed end-to-side to the aortic graft to re-establish the arterial blood supply. Great care must also be taken to avoid injury to the ureters, which usually lie on the anterior surface of the isthmus. It also facilitates the procedure in these cases to leave the posterior wall of the aneurysm.

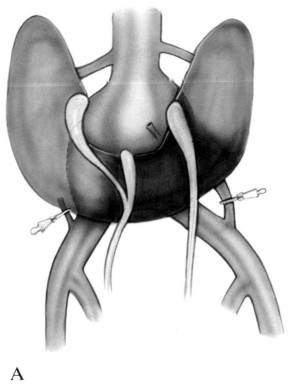

A

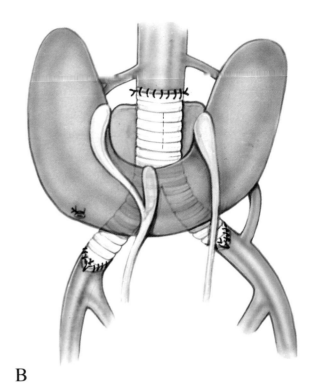

B

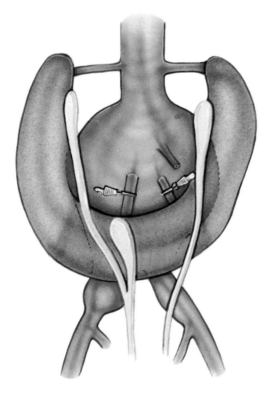

C

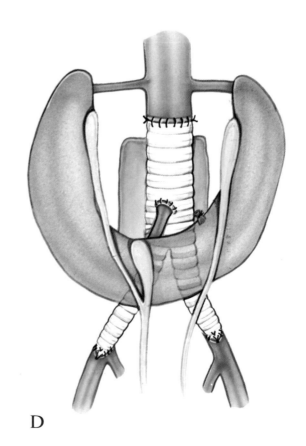

D

289

Plate 133

ABDOMINAL ARTERIOSCLEROTIC AORTIC ANEURYSM WITH AN AORTIC INFERIOR VENA CAVA ARTERIOVENOUS FISTULA

A. This demonstrates an abdominal arteriosclerotic aneurysm with an arteriovenous fistula between the aneurysm and the inferior vena cava. The patient first presented with the pulsating abdominal aortic aneurysm and a few days later reported back again because of some discomfort in her back and lower abdomen; she also reported that she had fainted three times. Examination revealed that her blood pressure had dropped between the two examinations from 140 mm. Hg to 105 mm. Hg. Her pulse had risen from 84 per minute to 120 per minute. In addition, palpation of her abdomen revealed a very marked thrill over the aneurysm. Auscultation revealed a to-and-fro murmur throughout systole and diastole which sounded very much like an angry beehive. The illustration reveals a relatively small abdominal aortic aneurysm just above the bifurcation of the aorta and some fibrous connections between it and the inferior vena cava. A tourniquet clamp has been placed around the aorta proximal to the aneurysm, and the common iliac arteries have also been isolated. The location of the A-V fistula was localized by obliteration of the thrill and bruit with finger point pressure over the distal portion of the aorta just proximal to the bifurcation of the inferior vena cava.

B. The aneurysm has been opened and this shows the inside of the aortic aneurysm after occlusion of the abdominal aorta proximal to it with a tourniquet clamp and of the common iliac arteries distally with the bulldog clamps. The blood from the inferior vena cava is shown spurting from the fistula. This drawing was made from an actual colored photograph taken at the time of operation. Once the arterial inflow has been occluded it is relatively easy to obtain control of the fistulous tract because the blood is only escaping at the pressure of the central venous system.

C. The assistant obtains this control by pressure with the fingers of his right hand to occlude the inferior vena cava and with his left hand to occlude the right and left common iliac veins. Two Allis clamps are used to grasp the edges of the fistulous tract, then it is closed with two mattress sutures of 4-0 Teflon-coated Dacron.

D. The aortic aneurysm has been removed except for the small portion of it attached to the vena cava at the site of the fistulous tract. The two mattress sutures closing it are shown. An aortic bifurcation Dacron prosthesis has been implanted, using interrupted mattress sutures of 4-0 Dacron coated with Teflon; the same type of suture is used for the iliac anastomoses. The anastomoses were direct end-to-end because the iliac arteries were of good size and the arterial walls of excellent texture.

It is recommended that this method of curing the majority of arteriovenous fistulae is the simplest. The most important thing is to first obtain proximal and distal arterial control, as has been demonstrated, then open the aorta or the artery to visualize the fistulous tract. Since venous blood comes out at a relatively low pressure compared to arterial, it is very easy to control it transarterially in this manner. If the artery or the aorta has become aneurysmal, as in this case, it is best to resect it and restore continuity with a knitted Dacron graft.

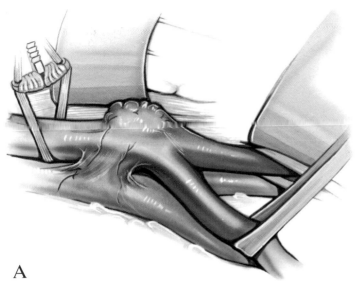

A

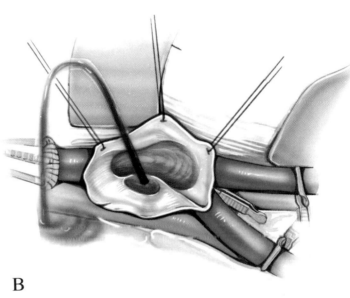

B

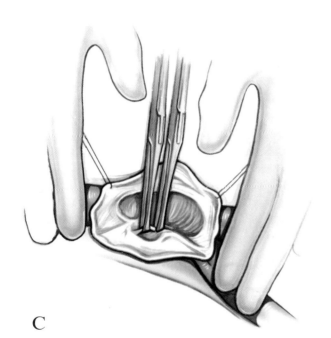

C

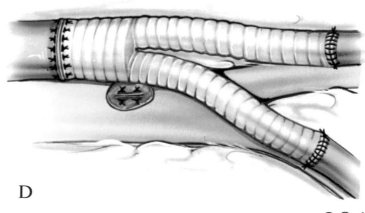

D

Plate 134

SMALL ABDOMINAL ARTERIOSCLEROTIC AORTIC ANEURYSM TREATED BY ANEURYSMORRHAPHY AND AORTIC ENDARTERECTOMY

A. This shows the distal abdominal aorta with slight aneurysmal dilatation of it and of the common iliac arteries. Palpation revealed marked atherosclerosis of the aneurysmal portion of the aorta and its bifurcation.

B. The aorta proximal to the inferior mesenteric artery, shown with a bulldog clamp on it, was of normal size and texture, so a tourniquet clamp was placed around it. The two common iliac arteries were also isolated and bulldog clamps were placed on these. A linear incision was made in the aneurysmal sac distal to the inferior mesenteric artery down to the bifurcation of the aorta. Marked thickening of the media and intima is shown. Because the adventitia of the aorta was in good condition, an endarterectomy and an aneurysmorrhaphy were performed instead of replacing the dilated aorta with a prosthesis.

C. The endarterectomy has been completed. A glass plunger of a syringe which is comparable in size to the inner caliber of the aorta above the occluding tourniquet clamp was chosen as a stent for the reconstruction of the aortic wall. The edges of the aorta were grasped with Allis clamps so that the aorta could be reconstructed snugly around the stent. A running everting mattress suture of 4-0 Teflon-coated braided Dacron was placed to form the first row of sutures, and the excess of the aortic wall was resected with scissors.

D. The suturing was continued as far distalward as possible and then the glass stent was removed. The remainder of the aortotomy was closed with a continuation of the running mattress suture then tied at the distal end of the aortotomy.

E. Since the running everting mattress suture is not hemostatic, it was necessary to place running over-and-over sutures outside the mattress sutures, thereby providing complete hemostasis.

F. This demonstrates the completed closure of the aortotomy with removal of the clamps and restoration of the blood flow. This type of aortic reconstruction, now that we have such excellent knitted Dacron prostheses, has little if any place, but the patients in whom this type of repair has been carried out have held up extremely well, some for 10 or more years, and none with recurrent aneurysms that have required excision and grafting. It is shown, therefore, to demonstrate that the technique is feasible in a very limited number of cases if the surgeon wishes to utilize this method in conjunction with endarterectomy of the aorta.

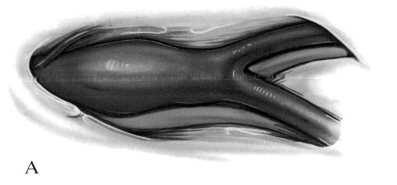

A

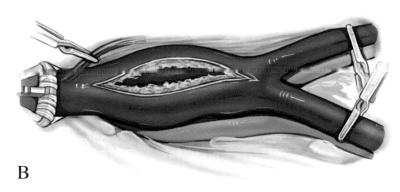

B

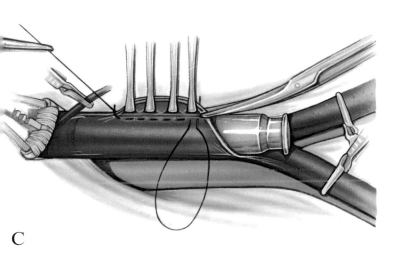

C

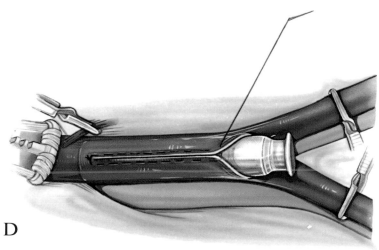

D

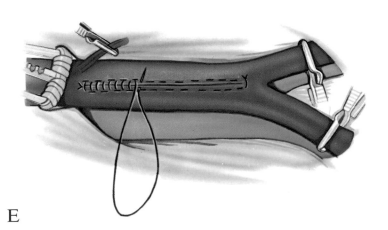

E

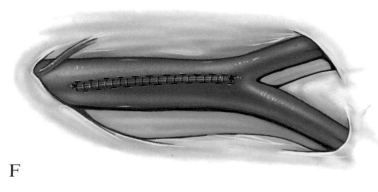

F

293

Plate 135

THE TECHNIQUE OF AN END-TO-SIDE ANASTOMOSIS BETWEEN A KNITTED DACRON PROSTHESIS AND A MAJOR ARTERY

A.   The streamlining of an end-to-side anastomosis between a Dacron prosthesis and an artery is extremely important. It should be so constructed that on auscultation with a stethoscope a bruit is not audible over it. This can be accomplished best by a relatively long anastomosis. For this reason it is recommended that the bevel at the end of the prosthetic graft be twice as long as its diameter, except for aortic grafts. A fine sharp pair of scissors, as shown, is used to cut the graft. The graft should be held under tension during the cutting so that it will be the proper length as it is sutured into place. The beveled portion should be a little longer than seems necessary since it can be shortened later to the correct length after half the anastomosis is constructed. Note that the excised portion is wedge-shaped, with the proximal end coming to a point; the distal end of the graft is 3 to 4 mm. wide.

B.   A linear incision has been made in the artery, the length of which should be approximately double the diameter of the prosthesis. A mattress suture that is knotted in the center, to make it an easy length to work with, is passed through the graft from the outside then through the artery from the inside to approximate the graft and the artery. This suturing is routinely started at the acute angle of the beveled end of the graft.

C.   This demonstrates the tying of the mattress suture as the assistant holds the graft toward him with fine forceps to facilitate the tying of the knot.

D.   The suturing is continued with straight needles that may be curved for the first few stitches then straightened. The first stitch goes through the graft from the outside and is placed close to the primary mattress suture. In order to place it at this point it is necessary to pull up on the edge of the graft as shown in the illustration.

E.   The needle and suture are pulled through the graft, then passed through the artery from inside out to complete the stitch.

F.   From then on, as a rule, the needle can be passed through both the graft and the artery together as shown without having to do them separately. Note that the assistant maintains tension with fine forceps on the edge of the prosthesis to eliminate any wrinkles in it and to make sure that there will be enough graft to reach to the distal end of the arteriotomy.

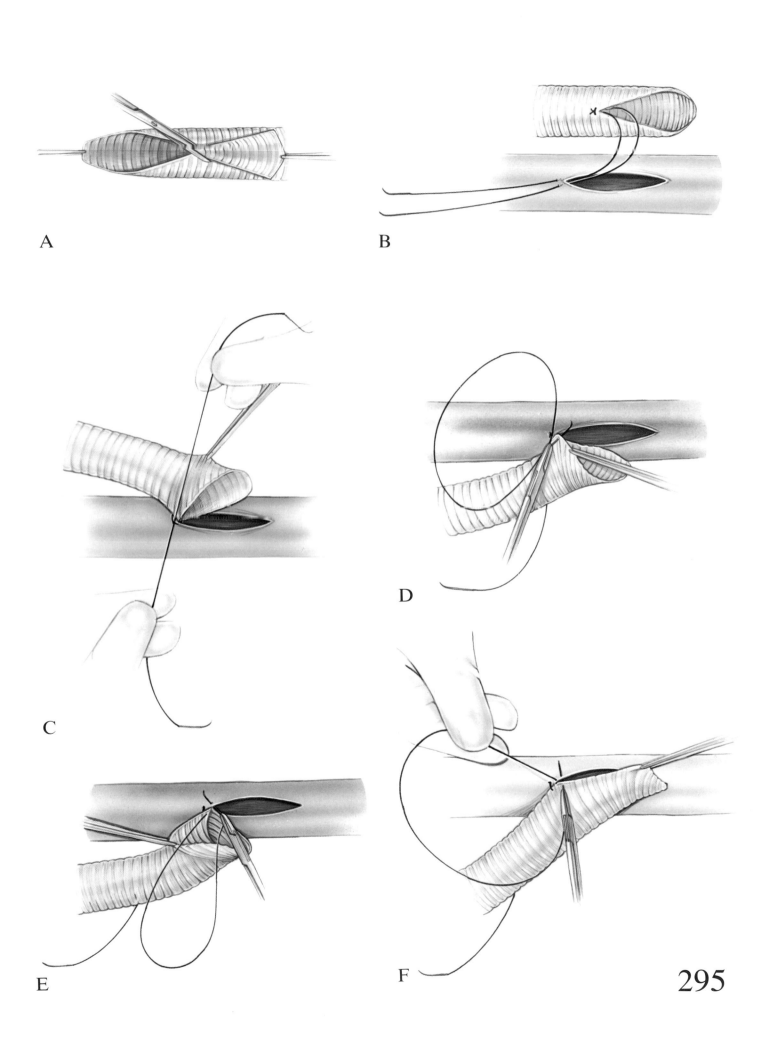

A

B

C

D

E

F

295

Plate 136

THE TECHNIQUE OF AN END-TO-SIDE ANASTOMOSIS BETWEEN A KNITTED DACRON PROSTHESIS AND A MAJOR ARTERY *(Continued)*

A. The suturing is continued as an over-and-over suture until the midportion of the anastomosis has been reached. Again, note that the Dacron prosthesis is held under tension during the suturing and that the suture is held very tightly by the assistant after each stitch is taken in order to make the suture line hemostatic.

B. This shows that the first suture has been ligated to a stay suture. The other end of the mattress suture is then passed through the near side of the graft from the outside close to the original mattress suture in exactly the same way that the other side was started.

C. The needle is put through the artery from the inside out, making an over-and-over stitch.

D. The over-and-over type of suturing is continued, again with tension on the edge of the prosthesis. The suture is held very tightly, either by the surgeon or by an assistant on the same side of the operating table, to facilitate the placing of the sutures.

E. This demonstrates what happens when the assistant holds the suture tightly from the side opposite to the surgeon. This rolls the edge of the artery and the graft so that it is difficult to see where to place the needle; as a result, the suture bites in the graft are often too large, which interferes with the streamlining of the anastomosis.

F. This demonstrates the correct method of suturing the near side of the anastomosis, with the surgeon holding the suture taut in his left hand. This brings out the edges of the graft and the prosthesis so that it is possible to place the needle very accurately, as shown, both in the graft and in the arterial wall. Again, note that the edge of the graft is still held under tension on this side.

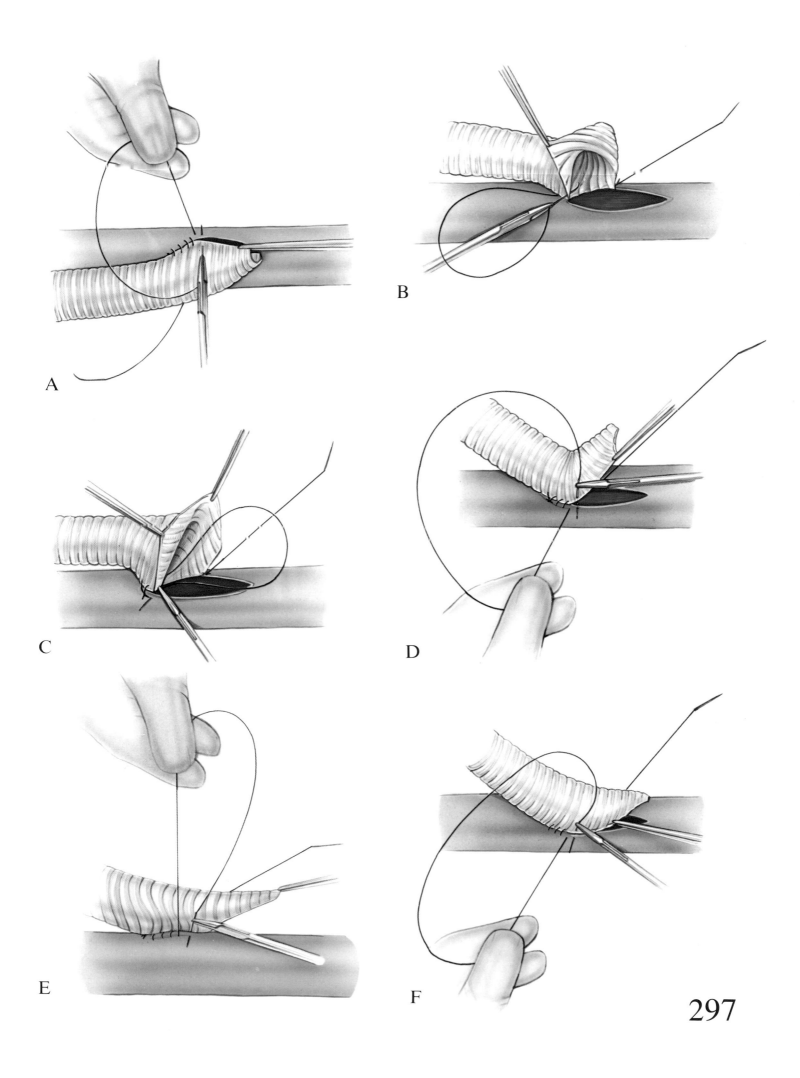

A

B

C

D

E

F

297

Plate 137

THE TECHNIQUE OF AN END-TO-SIDE ANASTOMOSIS BETWEEN A KNITTED DACRON PROSTHESIS AND A MAJOR ARTERY *(Continued)*

A. This demonstrates that the proximal half of the anastomosis has been completed, and both sutures have been secured snugly by ligating them to stay sutures placed at the midway point on each side. It is always best to cut the prosthesis a little longer than you think you may need it because it is easy to shorten it. The running type of suture tends to shorten it somewhat, and if it is measured too accurately, it may not reach the end of the arteriotomy. With moderate tension being maintained on the end of the prosthesis it is cut to the correct length with a straight pair of scissors.

B. The distal mattress suture has been placed first through the prosthesis from outside in and then through the artery from inside out. Note that a ski type needle has been used; this facilitates the suturing at the very distal end of the anastomosis. This is easily produced by bending the tip of the straight needle and then later on straightening it as one continues with the suturing.

C. The mattress suture has been tied and the suture on the far side is being passed through the edge of the graft outside in as the first step of an over-and-over suture.

D. The suture has been pulled through the graft and now the needle is being passed through the artery from within out to complete the first over-and-over stitch, still using the ski type needle.

E. The needle has been straightened and the suturing is continued as an over-and-over type of stitch, still maintaining tension on the suture after the placing of each stitch.

F. The distal half of the anastomosis has been completed, using a running over-and-over suture on each side. These are tied at the midway point to the suture that the anastomosis was started with. Note that it is a well fashioned, streamlined type of anastomosis that will not have a bruit over it, indicating good streamlining of the blood flow. The importance of using the synthetic type of suture material when one is anastomosing a synthetic graft such as knitted Dacron to a human artery cannot be overemphasized. Silk tends to disintegrate, and many late false aneurysms have developed when it has been used as the suture material; also, there is often lack of good healing between the prosthesis and the host artery. It is for these reasons that a braided Dacron suture is highly recommended; to date I have never known one to give way.

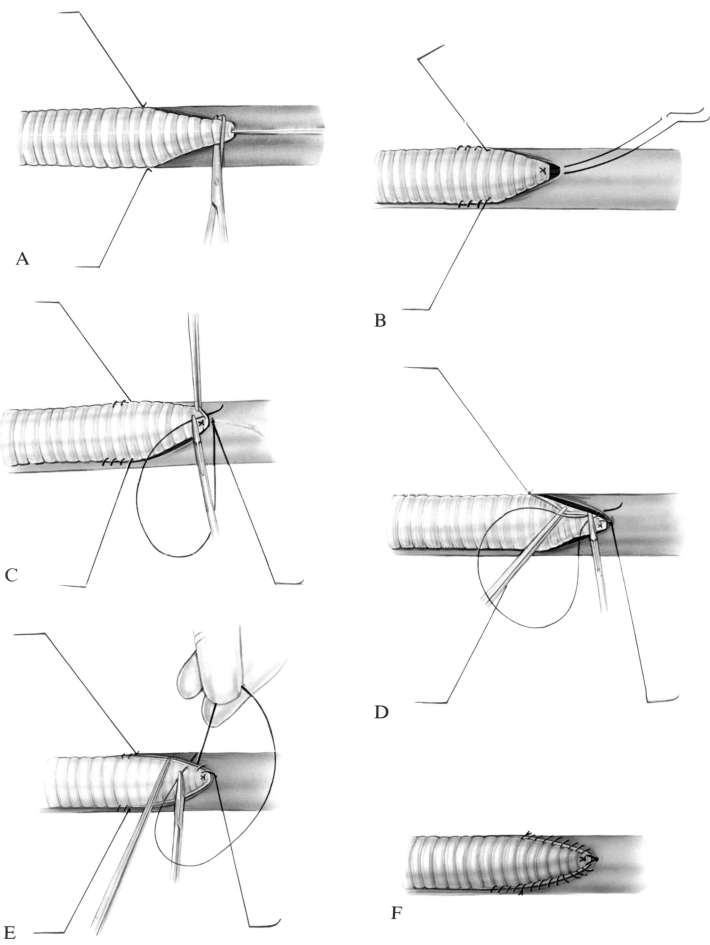

A

B

C

D

E

F

299

Plate 138

THE TECHNIQUE OF AN END-TO-END ANASTOMOSIS BY THE END-TO-SIDE METHOD BETWEEN A KNITTED DACRON PROSTHESIS AND A MAJOR ARTERY

A. This procedure is demonstrated at the bifurcation of a major artery, but the same technique may also be used for an end-to-end anastomosis. The bifurcation of a large artery such as the common iliac or common femoral is shown, where these anastomoses are most commonly constructed. The backflow has been controlled with bulldog clamps and the corners of the arterial flaps are being trimmed with fine scissors. This permits the construction of a more streamlined anastomosis. The distal end of the prosthetic graft is also demonstrated but has not been beveled.

B. This demonstrates the method of preparing the end of the prosthesis with a long bevel for better streamlining of the anastomosis. The forceps on the left are held by the surgeon and the ones on the right, holding the section of graft being removed, are held by an assistant.

C. A double needle suture of the proper length made by tying two sutures together has been passed through the graft at the narrow angle of the beveled end. This suture is a mattress type, with the knots outside the vessel wall, so the needles go from without in on the graft and then from within out on the artery.

D. The mattress suture has been ligated on the posterior aspect of the anastomosis. The first part of an over-and-over stitch is being taken by passing the suture from without in through the prosthesis. This stitch should be placed very close to the original mattress suture, as shown. The positioning of it is facilitated greatly by the assistant's pulling directly upward on the edge of the graft with a fine pair of forceps as shown.

E. This demonstrates the completion of the first over-and-over stitch, with the needle going through the artery from within out. This type of stitch is the most hemostatic to use and therefore is recommended because if there is leakage at this point after construction of the anastomosis, it may be very difficult to get at it to place further sutures to control the point that is bleeding.

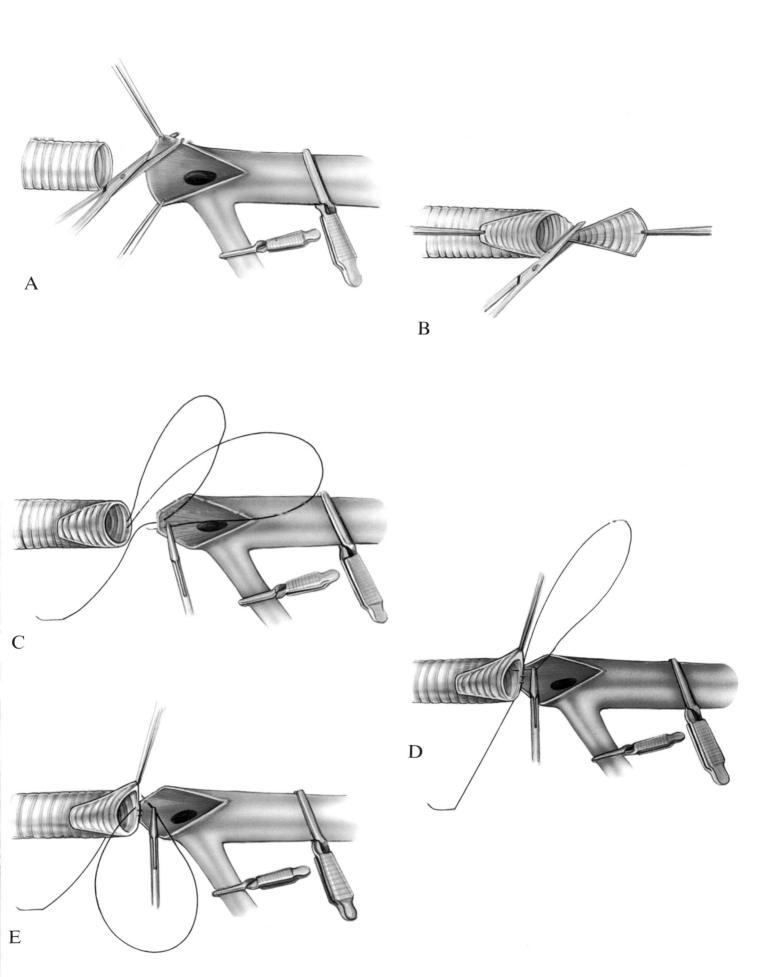

A

B

C

D

E

Plate 139

THE TECHNIQUE OF AN END-TO-END ANASTOMOSIS BY THE END-TO-SIDE METHOD BETWEEN A KNITTED DACRON PROSTHESIS AND A MAJOR ARTERY *(Continued)*

A. The running over-and-over type of suture has been continued. Note that the assistant is holding the suture very snugly after each stitch is placed, which is of utmost importance for obtaining good hemostasis of the suture line. One of the advantages of the synthetic suture is that adequate tension can be maintained without fear that the suture will break. Leakage through the suture line after construction of the anastomosis, although it can be controlled with individual stitches, may be troublesome. If the artery is a very thin and tenuous structure, the problem sometimes becomes of major magnitude, so constant vigilance in maintaining tension on the suture is of utmost importance. It should also be noted that the assistant is maintaining tension on the edge of the prosthesis with his left hand to stretch the prosthesis out so that it will be of sufficient length to reach to the end of the arteriotomy. This will also result in a much more streamlined anastomosis.

B. The suture line has been completed on the proximal half of each side and the sutures tied to stay sutures to maintain the tension on the running over-and-over type of suture. The end of the graft is grasped in a fine forceps and put on a slight amount of stretch, then cut to the exact length; the correct degree of tension is maintained so that it will fit exactly into the end of the arteriotomy. It is my custom to always make the bevel of the graft a little longer than I think is going to be necessary; it can always be shortened, as shown, whereas if it is too short it creates a difficult problem to make a satisfactorily streamlined anastomosis.

C. A second mattress suture is next placed at the distal end of the graft and the arteriotomy. Notice that a ski shape type of needle is used for placing this suture; later the needle is straightened.

D. This shows the completed anastomosis. The method of suturing is a simple over-and-over type and more details are demonstrated in Plates 135, 136 and 137. The distal bulldog clamps are always removed before removal of the proximal one. This is to permit the backflow of arterial blood to fill the prosthesis and, if leakage occurs, to control these points with individual sutures. It is much easier to place them when the blood within the vessels is at a lower pressure than at the full arterial level.

It should be noticed that most of the suturing is done with a straight needle. This has several advantages. One of the most important is that it is much easier to pass a straight needle than a curved one through a structure such as a knitted Dacron prosthesis, which is relatively tough. Another advantage of the straight needle is that it is used by pushing it away from the surgeon, so that it is easier to place it accurately for most of the suturing. The needle is readily grasped again as it projects out straight, whereas a curved needle is apt to turn over with the tip pointing downward, making it very difficult to pick it up. The straight needle also allows the surgeon to rest his needle holder on the wound edge, which steadies the end of it and allows him to place it more readily and accurately at the exact spot he wishes. (See Plate 14.)

302

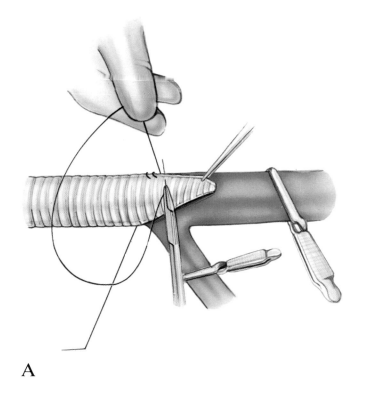

A

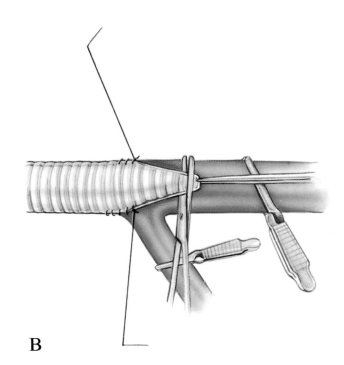

B

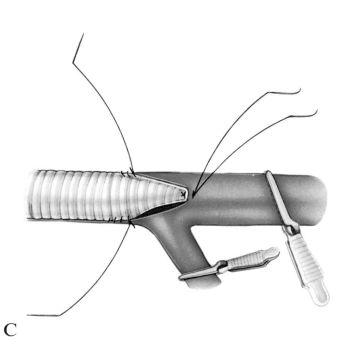

C

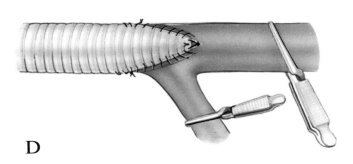

D

303

AORTOILIAC ATHEROSCLEROTIC OCCLUSIVE DISEASE

Introduction

Atherosclerosis obliterans involving (a) the arteries that carry blood to the lower extremities and (b) those that distribute the blood in the lower extremities results in an inadequate arterial blood supply of the lower extremities. The former are the infrarenal aorta, the common iliac, the external iliac, the hypogastric, and the common femoral arteries. The latter are the superficial femoral, the profunda femoris, the popliteal, the posterior tibial, the anterior tibial and the peroneal arteries. Atherosclerosis obliterans is the most common occlusive arterial lesion that afflicts the human race, and can be treated successfully by modern reconstructive arterial procedures in the majority of patients. The etiology is still not completely understood, but the individual's genes, use of tobacco, and a high cholesterol diet all play important roles of varying degrees. The surgeon cannot influence the hereditary factor but he should insist on "no tobacco" in any form, especially cigarettes, or refuse to treat the patient, and also require that the patient adhere to a low cholesterol diet. Since the advent of reconstructive arterial surgery, the cases of thromboangiitis obliterans that were so commonly diagnosed 30 years ago have disappeared. This is because operations on those afflicted with occluded arteries have demonstrated, even in patients in the 30 to 40 age group, that an inflammatory reaction involving the atherosclerotic arteries is always present. The older the process, the more marked the degree of reaction. It is believed to be the result of obliteration of the vasa vasorum and nature's attempt to develop a parasitic blood supply for the arterial walls. As a result, the diagnosis of thromboangiitis obliterans has been abandoned.

The pattern of the disease varies considerably, from simple involvement of the aorta and the common iliac arteries alone to a very extensive involvement, in severe cases including these and most of the other arteries in the body. Fortunately the disease in the lower limb is segmental in the majority of patients, so that the distal popliteal and the outflow arteries from it are usually patent. This permits restoration of the arterial circulation by means of bypass grafting procedures which are described later in this book. It has been observed that the disease arises frequently at major bifurcations, or at the origins of larger arteries, probably as a factor in hemodynamics.

It is axiomatic that before the implantation of a bypass saphenous vein autograft in the lower extremity is attempted there *must* be an adequate outflow of arterial blood from the aorta, iliac and common femoral arteries. Many failures early in the development of this type of recon-

305

structive arterial surgery were the result of implanting the grafts in the presence of marked aortic and iliac atherosclerosis obliterans. It has been learned that if the common femoral pulses are weak and the jet of arterial blood is only faintly pulsatile from the needles that are inserted into the common femoral arteries to obtain the arteriograms, instead of the normal 5 to 10 cm. or more, these observations indicate that proximal aortic and iliac artery obliterative disease is present and that reconstructive arterial procedures should be performed on these vessels before implanting a femoropopliteal bypass graft. Further confirmation of the condition can be obtained at the time of performing the femoral arteriograms by performing reflux iliac arteriograms, which often demonstrate poor caliber of the external iliac arteries and the common iliac arteries. If the femoral arteriograms also demonstrate blockage of the superficial femoral arteries, the plan in most cases should be to operate upon them at a later date.

Aortography with the above findings is considered unnecessary in the majority of patients. In fact, it may even be misleading, especially in the angiograms of the iliac arteries, because they can be demonstrated only in the anteroposterior projection, so that often the vessels may appear nearly normal in size, even when the lumen is very small and ribbon-like, since most of the plaque formation lies on the posterior wall of the arteries. I have also learned that the obliterative disease is invariably much more extensive than the angiograms show. The surgeon must learn that if the femoral pulses are weak, with a poor flow from the arteriogram needles, and there is disease in the external iliac arteries, a transperitoneal abdominal exposure must be carried out. The type of procedure and the extent of it will depend on what the conditions are in these arteries after they have been exposed.

Aortography is definitely indicated if renal or mesenteric artery disease is suspected. It is also of value if secondary operations have to be performed on patients who develop trouble with their circulation several years later because of failure of the previous aortoiliac procedure.

Aortoiliac disease involving only the infrarenal abdominal aorta and common iliac arteries can be treated successfully by endarterectomy down to the bifurcation of the latter, into the hypogastric and external iliac arteries. It is possible by this type of procedure to preserve the male sex function by saving the pre-aortic and presacral sympathetic nerve plexuses that control ejaculation. If endarterectomy is performed as described here, using a transverse incision (rather than performing a longitudinal aortotomy), it is much easier to implant a Dacron prosthesis later in life if the disease recurs. Implantation of an aortic bifurcation graft from the abdominal aorta to the distal ends of the common iliac arteries is also satisfactory if the surgeon prefers this procedure.

For these procedures limited to the aorta and common iliac arteries, the surgeon must be certain that the external iliac arteries are normal and not involved in serious atheromatous plaque formation. If they are diseased, the operation of choice is to implant an aortic bifurcation graft from the distal abdominal aorta and the limbs of the graft to the common femoral arteries. This is because even though endarterectomies of the external iliac arteries can be accomplished, late failure of them is much higher than for the common iliac arteries, owing to their smaller caliber and the difficulty of obtaining complete endarterectomy. It has also been found that it is very difficult to endarterectomize the external iliac arteries if they are still patent but diseased. This is because the atheromatous plaques do not encompass the entire arterial lumen but lie chiefly on the posterior wall; the anterior wall is thin, with normal intima and media. Endarterectomy of this type of artery always leaves long rough edges of media and intima where the plaques have been removed, causing early failure as a result of clot formation and thrombosis. The distal end of the external iliac artery may also be difficult to endarterectomize where the deep epigastric and circumflex iliac arteries arise, beneath the inguinal ligament. Endarterectomy of the common femoral arteries may also be difficult because of their extremely thin and friable anterior walls. Under these conditions it is better to implant the limb of an aortic graft by a long, streamlined end-to-side anastomosis, usually without performing endarterectomy. However, if the ostium of the profunda femoris artery is narrowed by a thick posterior plaque, resulting in poor backflow, the plaque should be carefully removed; this will enlarge the ostium, thereby increasing the outflow into this artery after completion of the graft implantation. Not only is this procedure important to give the limb a better blood supply, but it also improves the outflow from the graft and reduces the incidence of occlusion from thrombosis. The lumina of the superficial femoral arteries are frequently narrowed as a result of plaque formation that extends far distally. It is best to leave these arteries undisturbed and to implant the graft limbs to the common femoral artery with a long streamlined anastomosis as far distally as its bifurcation.

The implantation of an aortic graft to the aorta by the end-to-side technique is not recommended for several reasons. The most important is that the aortic blood will still flow out through the distal aorta and iliac arteries in most cases, since both common iliac arteries are seldom totally occluded. As a result, the graft and the patient's own aorta will be in competition and will have to share a reduced outflow of blood from the diseased proximal aorta. One of these may then occlude—usually the graft, especially if there is a poor outflow tract from the common femoral artery. It is axiomatic, therefore, in arterial reconstructive surgery that when a bypass graft is being implanted for atherosclerosis, the diseased portion of the artery that is being bypassed must be interrupted. Another serious defect of the end-to-side type of anastomosis is that it makes it much more difficult to endarterectomize the diseased aorta, even impossible if a Statinsky side-biting type of clamp is used to control the aorta in order to construct the anastomosis. This may cause the outflow from the proximal aorta to be less than it would be after endarterectomizing it. There is also the danger that trauma from the clamp on the aortic wall will cause the breaking off of thrombi, which will be carried distally to produce peripheral emboli.

The best method for the implantation of an aortic bifurcation graft is complete division of the abdominal aorta so that the aortic anastomosis to the graft is constructed end-to-end. (See Plates 164 and 165.) This is performed either proximal or distal to the inferior mesenteric artery, depending on whether or not the artery is occluded. If it is patent, it is best to preserve it and construct the anastomosis distal to it, to help prevent ischemic lesions of the left colon. The proximal end of the aorta, if its lumen is compromised by atheromatous plaques, should be endarterectomized to restore the aorta to its normal caliber, leaving only the adventitia of the aorta (which may be extremely thin), to which the graft is anastomosed. The procedure can be accomplished safely by following the technique described here. Fortunately the aorta rarely, if ever, becomes dilated or aneurysmal. Using the end-to-side technique, the limbs of the aortic graft are anastomosed end-to-end (see Plates 138 and 139) to the distal ends of the common iliac arteries, provided the external iliac arteries are essentially normal and the surgeon selects this method instead of endarterectomy of the aorta and common iliac arteries. However, if there are obliterative plaques in the external iliac arteries, the graft limbs in most cases are best anastomosed to the common femoral arteries by the end-to-side technique (see Plates 135 to 137) just distal to the inguinal ligament.

The main advantage to this method of implantation of an aortic bifurcation graft is that the total aortic outflow must pass through it and as a result will supply a better blood flow to the common femoral and the profunda femoris arteries, and sometimes to the superficial femoral artery, thereby delivering blood at a high degree of arterial pressure into the limb. In addition, there will be a reflux of arterial blood back through the common femoral and external iliac arteries to the hypogastric arteries, provided they are patent. In fact, this flow may even be better postoperatively than it was preoperatively because of the increased outflow of blood from the iliac limbs of the aortic graft, which are anastomosed to the common femoral arteries. Furthermore, there is much better assurance that the graft will remain patent because of this increased outflow tract from the limbs of the aortic graft.

The majority of patients with aortoiliac and femoral atherosclerosis obliterans have involvement of the superficial femoral and popliteal arteries, and usually of one or more of the outflow arteries from the latter into the lower leg. The arteries that are involved can usually be determined by the examination of the limb pulses, the oscillometric determinations at the ankle, calf and lower thigh, and the color of the foot and toes. The exact extent and location of the arterial involvement should always be determined by angiography. If the patient has occlusion of the superficial femoral arteries or involvement of the distal outflow arteries in the lower leg, it is worthwhile to perform bilateral lumbar sympathectomies before heparinizing the patient and implanting the graft (see Plate 144). This is especially true of patients under 70 years of age who still have vasomotor innervation in the feet and toes because it is important to obtain as rich an arterial blood supply as possible to the integument of these most distant parts of the extremity. In the younger male patients between 40 and 55 years of age, bilateral lumbar sympathectomies done in conjunction with aortic surgery may increase the chance of interference with the sex functions. For this reason it is best not to perform them in this age group of males unless there are already serious obliterative arterial lesions in the distal part of the extremity.

Early in the development of the procedure of implanting aortic bifurcation Dacron grafts to the femoral arteries in the groin, there was fear that the limbs of the graft would occlude because they cross the groin creases in a manner similar to the femoropopliteal Dacron grafts that are carried across the knee joint, which involve high occlusion rates. Fortunately this has not occurred. However, sepsis involving an aortic femoral bifurcation graft has been reported and is one of the most serious of all complications. According to the literature it usually develops in the groin incisions and then involves the entire graft. It is best treated with bilateral axillary profunda femoris grafts with excision of the aortic graft, and later, if successful, implantation of a new aortic bifurcation graft from the thoracic aorta to the distal portions of the axillary grafts. Septic infections have not occurred in my own cases because the strictest aseptic conditions have been maintained. The most common source of operative wound contamination is the skin of the patient's abdomen, groin, and extremities. Therefore, to maintain operative asepsis, it is of vital importance to cover these areas with a self-adherent transparent thin plastic sheet called Steridrape. This *must* remain adherent to the skin throughout the entire operation. In order to prevent it from separating at the edges of the incisions, the skin must be absolutely dry when the plastic sheet is applied; the skin should be wiped with ether after having first been prepared with an alcohol hexachlorophene solution. It is my opinion that the Steridrape is absolutely useless if it becomes separated from the skin edges of the incision, especially in the groin, because it is through these incisions that most of these grafts become infected. It should be the rule of all vascular surgeons, as it is mine, that the skin at all the sites of the operative incisions must never become uncovered during the operative procedure, especially when implanting a Dacron vascular prosthesis. In addition, prophylactic antibiotics are an absolute necessity and should be started when the patient leaves his room to go to the operating suite. My routine is to give 500,000 units of penicillin and 250 mg. of streptomycin by intramuscular injection. These injections should be repeated in six hours if the operation has not been completed. In addition, one gram of Ilotycin is added to 1000 cc. of dextrose and water and given as a slow intravenous drip throughout the operation. These same antibiotics are continued for five to seven days postoperatively in those patients in whom a synthetic graft has been implanted. If a patient is allergic to penicillin, one of the other antibiotics is substituted.

Since the mortality rate from infected aortic grafts is so high, every possible precaution should be taken. The above regimen of asepsis and prophylactic antibiotics has so far avoided this dreadful catastrophe for my patients.

309

Plate 140

AORTOILIAC ENDARTERECTOMY

A. The artist's drawing demonstrates severe atherosclerotic occlusive disease involving the infrarenal abdominal aorta and both the right and left common iliac arteries. The lumens of the aorta and the iliac arteries are demonstrated by the cross-section views. That of the aorta is markedly narrowed. The inferior mesenteric artery is still patent, and the left common iliac artery has a small lumen. The right common iliac artery is totally occluded, with atherosclerotic plaques and a relatively fresh thrombus filling the small channel. The renal arteries are not seriously affected, nor is that portion of the aorta from which they arise. The external iliac, common femoral, superficial femoral and profunda femoris arteries are also relatively free of disease. Endarterectomy of the infrarenal abdominal aorta and the common iliac arteries has given excellent results in this type of case, and so it is preferred to the resection of the aorta and insertion of a synthetic bifurcation prosthesis in this type of case.

B. This demonstrates the position of the patient on the operating table. The arms are suspended, as shown, to a metal hoop at the head of the table. It is extremely important that the fixation is of the forearms only and rather loose. The upper arms *must not* be fixed in any way to the uprights of the hoop because this will result in a brachial palsy in a high percentage of patients. This position is advantageous for the surgeon in that it provides more room for him and his assistants to perform these operative procedures. A central venous catheter is inserted, usually into the jugular vein. This may be used also for intravenous fluid administration. In addition, another intravenous cannula is placed in a vein in one of the forearms. A Foley catheter is in the bladder so that throughout the operation the urinary output can be checked in the collection bottle hanging from the head of the table. One of the radial arteries is cannulated for constant recording of the blood pressure. The skin of the abdomen and legs is prepared with an antiseptic solution and then the skin is cleaned with ether; a thin, transparent, self-adhering plastic sheet is placed over the abdomen and the legs. The draping is then completed with the usual towels and sheets.

C. This demonstrates the operative exposure that is planned. The incision is usually a right paramedian muscle retracting one. The distal abdominal aorta, both common iliacs and the origins of the external iliac and hypogastric arteries are exposed by incising the posterior peritoneum in the mid abdomen and the left iliac fossa. The inferior mesenteric artery, the large veins and the right ureter are shown. The sigmoid, its mesocolon and the ureter are isolated with a large Penrose tubing.

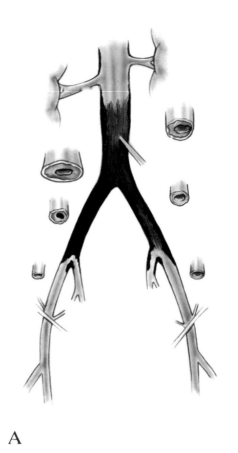

A

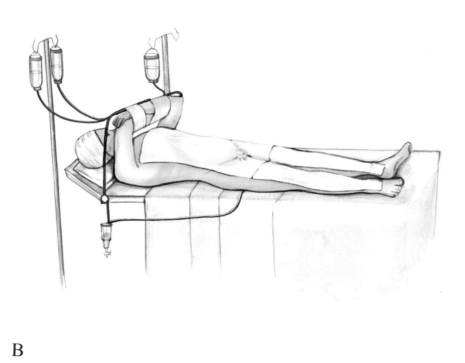

B

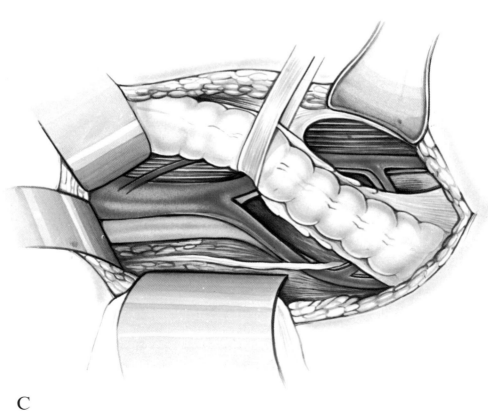

C

311

Plate 141

AORTOILIAC ENDARTERECTOMY
(Continued)

A. This shows the abdominal aorta and its bifurcation distal to the origin of the inferior mesenteric artery (a), the inferior vena cava and the common iliac veins. The presacral sympathetic nerve plexus is demonstrated arising from both sides of the aorta and crossing the proximal portions of the common iliac arteries. These nerves play an important part in the ejaculatory mechanism of sexual intercourse in the male. If they are ablated the semen refluxes into the bladder instead of being ejected from the penis. This results in what patients call "a dry run." It is important, therefore, to preserve these nerves if it is at all possible, especially in men in the younger age group. In some instances patients will be impotent when first seen because of the marked obliterative disease involving the aorta, iliac and hypogastric arteries, which interferes with the erection mechanism because of insufficient arterial blood supply. It is possible in doing aortoiliac endarterectomies to preserve these nerves, whereas resection of the aortic bifurcation usually means they are interrupted. In view of this fact, it seems worthwhile, if possible, to perform the endarterectomy type of procedure rather than to replace the aorta with a bifurcation graft, in an attempt to preserve, and in some to improve, sexual function.

The aorta has been freed up and a large right-angle clamp has been passed behind it. The plastic tip of a white shoestring is grasped in the clamp and pulled through to the other side.

B. This demonstrates an angled tourniquet clamp, showing the back side of it with the shoestring threaded through it. This clamp is used to occlude the abdominal aorta. It has been found superior to any other method of occlusion because it is relatively atraumatic. It can be released and reapplied at various stages of the operation as becomes necessary without danger of injuring the aorta, or actually visualizing it, once it has been placed. The presacral nerve plexus has been omitted from the remainder of the illustrations for simplicity, but it is to be pointed out that these nerves are left intact for the most part. The right ureter (a) is shown crossing the right common iliac artery.

C. This demonstrates the completion of the preparation of the tourniquet clamp with the shoestring tied in a square knot.

D. A relatively long loop of shoestring is shown just distal to the inferior mesenteric artery; the tourniquet clamp is threaded on but is not shown. The clamp is left open until all the arteries have been isolated. This illustration also demonstrates the utilization of ring forceps to retract the right common iliac artery, the inferior vena cava and right iliac vein as the common iliac artery is separated with scissors from the venous structures.

312

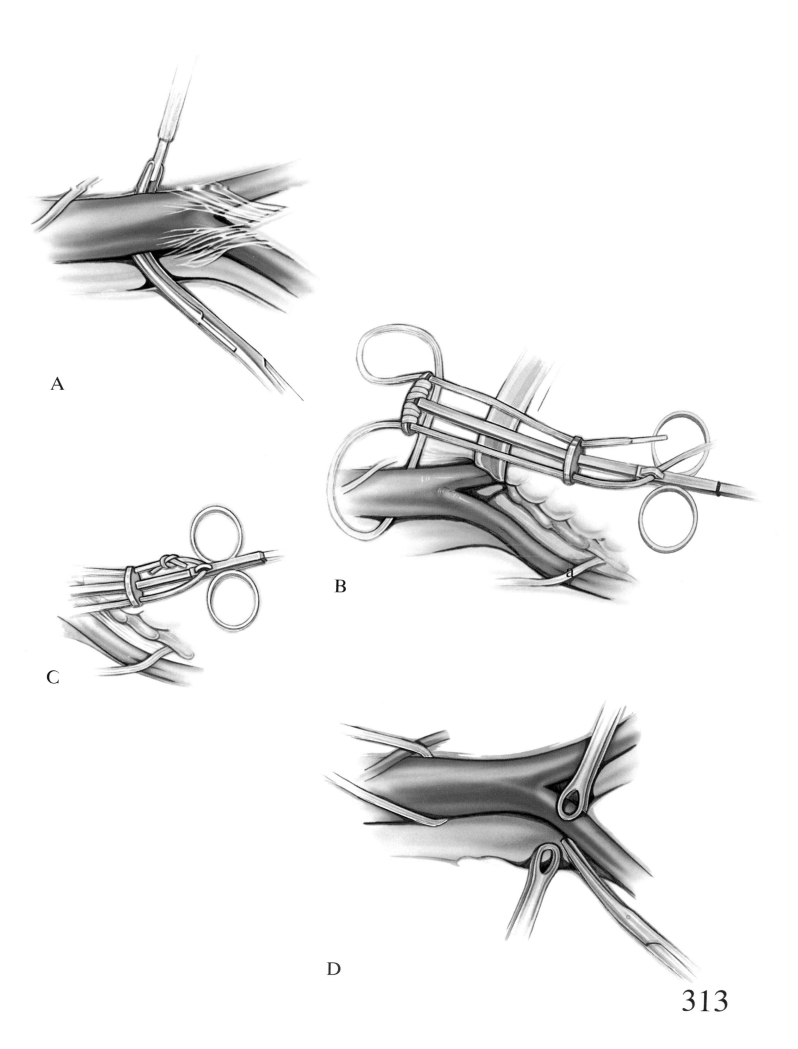

A

B

C

D

Plate 142

AORTOILIAC ENDARTERECTOMY
(Continued)

A. This shows a one quarter inch thin-walled Penrose tubing being pulled through underneath the right common iliac artery with a right-angled clamp to further aid in the separation of the artery from the inferior vena cava. This is important to aid in the exposure of the mid sacral artery and the distal lumbar arteries. Note that the Penrose tubing has a wick of gauze in it. This is important because, when traction is applied, this prevents the tubing from stretching, and the dissection is much more easily performed.

B. The right common iliac artery has been freed up sufficiently; a similar freeing of the left common iliac artery is carried out by scissor dissection. It is not unusual to find a small branch of the iliac vein arising in this location; this should be looked for and carefully ligated and interrupted to avoid injury to the common iliac vein if the branch is inadvertently torn loose.

C. This demonstrates the utilization of the Penrose tubing to help in the dissection of the left common iliac artery; it also aids in the separation of the bifurcation of the aorta from the inferior vena cava in order to visualize the mid sacral artery.

D. This demonstrates the aorta separated from the inferior vena cava, showing the right distal lumbar artery (a) and mid sacral artery (b). It is very important to isolate these, and the distal left lumbar artery on the other side of the aorta as well, before making the incision in the aorta because, in some patients, there is a tremendous backflow from them which makes it difficult to dissect them out and obtain control once the aortotomy is performed.

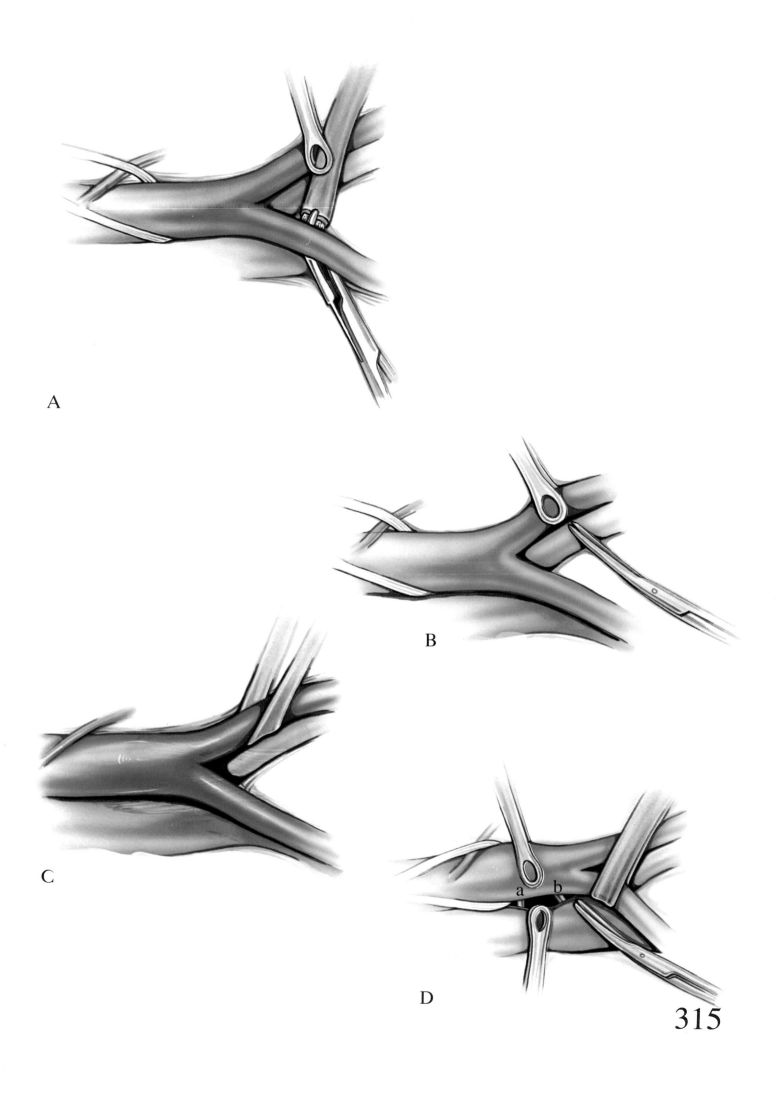

A

B

C

D

315

Plate 143

AORTOILIAC ENDARTERECTOMY
(Continued)

A. This demonstrates, in addition to the distal abdominal aorta with the tourniquet clamp in place but not closed, the exposure of the bifurcation of the left common iliac artery and the origins of the left external iliac and hypogastric arteries. This is accomplished by retracting the sigmoid colon cephalad and opening the peritoneum in the left lower quadrant over these blood vessels. As always, care should be taken in separating them from their corresponding veins.

B. The sigmoid, the sigmoid mesocolon and the left ureter (a) are lifted up readily from the left common iliac artery with finger dissection.

C. After obtaining this passageway a one-inch Penrose tubing with gauze in it is passed underneath the sigmoid, the mesosigmoid and the left ureter to isolate them and to protect them, especially the left ureter, during the remainder of the operation. It is usual to wait later in the operative procedure to isolate the right common iliac bifurcation and the origin of the external iliac and hypogastric arteries.

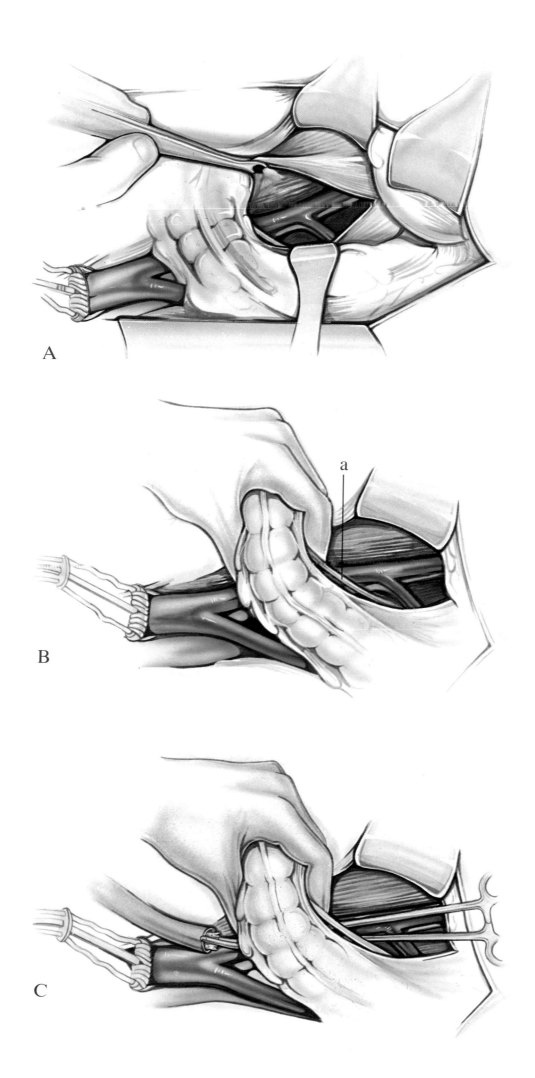

A

B

a

C

317

Plate 144

AORTOILIAC ENDARTERECTOMY
(Continued)

A. This demonstrates the most satisfactory method of general heparinization, which is recommended for all patients in this type of surgery. It is done by the surgeon so that he is sure that the heparin has been injected in the amount that is necessary. It is recommended to use 4000 units or 40 mg. of heparin for the average-sized individual; this will maintain good anticoagulation for approximately four hours. It is always given into the inferior vena cava, which has already been exposed; since it is the largest vein available, one can be absolutely certain that the heparin gets into the blood stream. It is usually injected with a small syringe and a 22-gauge needle.

B. My routine is to allow 15 minutes to elapse after injecting the heparin before occluding the abdominal aorta and the iliac arteries to commence the endarterectomy, so it is well worthwhile to leave some part of the operative procedure to do during this short period that does not require occlusion of aorta and iliac arteries. This demonstrates the performance of a left lumbar sympathectomy, which can be readily accomplished in most individuals. It is a rather limited ablation but it does result in a good response in the distal part of the extremity and the foot. As a rule, about 2 cm. of the chain, including at least one ganglia, is removed; one silver clip is left on the distal and the proximal ends of the chain.

C. After completion of the left side, the right sympathetic chain is then exposed by retracting the inferior vena cava to the left and picking the chain up with a nerve hook and resecting a short length of it. It should be pointed out that in younger individuals in the fifth and sixth decades, sympathectomies are usually not done since they tend to increase the interference with sexual function that may occur after aortic bifurcation surgery. It is advisable to perform them, however, especially in those patients who, in addition to the aortoiliac disease, have occlusive atherosclerosis of the superficial femoral arteries. Just how much this procedure increases the blood flow to the extremity is somewhat questionable, but it definitely does improve the circulation of the integument of the foot and toes.

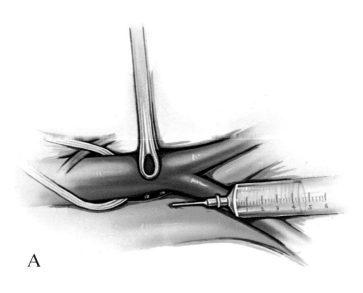

A

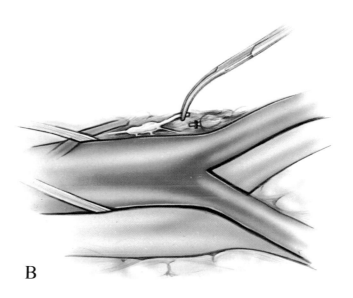

B

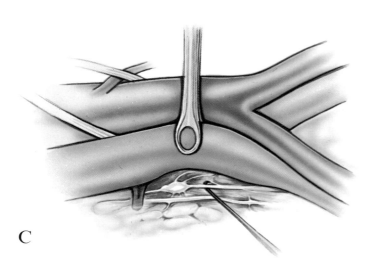

C

319

Plate 145

AORTOILIAC ENDARTERECTOMY
(Continued)

A. This demonstrates the control of the aorta with closure of the tourniquet clamp and of the inferior mesenteric artery (a), the distal lumbar arteries (b) and the middle sacral artery (c) with bulldog clamps. The middle sacral artery is exposed best by lifting the crotch of the abdominal aorta and the two common iliac arteries as shown. The distal lumbar arteries are exposed by raising the aorta and retracting the vena cava. Control of both the right and left arteries can frequently be obtained with this one clamp. Sometimes, however, it may be necessary to expose the left artery from the left side of the aorta.

B. After these proximal arterial controls have been completed, bulldog clamps with cloth covering on the blades to prevent them from slipping are placed on the origins of the left external iliac artery (a) and the hypogastric artery (b). On the right side, because the arteries will be occluded for a longer period as it is operated upon after restoring the blood flow on the left, the bulldog clamp is placed on the common iliac artery (c) to permit the collateral blood from the hypogastric artery to flow down the external iliac artery to prevent distal arterial thrombosis. The right ureter (d) is also shown.

C. The most satisfactory arteriotomy incision for an endarterectomy of the abdominal aorta is a transverse one just proximal to the carina. The beginning of this incision is shown, with the use of a small knife blade. The right common iliac bulldog clamp is temporarily released to fill the aorta and common iliac arteries with blood. This helps to avoid incising the posterior wall of the aorta.

D. After the initial opening in the aorta is made, the transverse incision is increased by the use of an angled pair of fine scissors. The aortotomy should be equal to one half the circumference of the aorta. Less than this makes it difficult to perform a satisfactory endarterectomy; a longer one is unnecessary and is more difficult to close. It is at this point in the procedure that control of the lumbar, middle sacral and any other accessory arteries that sometimes are encountered arising from the common iliac arteries is so essential to prevent blood from welling up into the aortic lumen. The aortic lumen must be free of any blood in order to do a satisfactory endarterectomy procedure. The control of these vessels is much more difficult after making the aortotomy, especially when there is large backflow which spills over and obscures the location of the source, so again it is stressed that control should be obtained before incising the aorta. Control is readily determined, after applying all the various bulldog clamps and occluding the aorta with a tourniquet clamp, by forcing the blood out of the aorta and its iliac branches by pressure on them while temporarily releasing one of the bulldog clamps and then reapplying it. If the aorta remains collapsed one is sure that control of the accessory arteries has been obtained, whereas if the aorta fills up with blood a further search should be made for an anomalous tributary that has been missed. Some vessel arising from these main arteries may not have been controlled, or one of the bulldog clamps may have failed to completely occlude the artery on which it had been placed. This type of bleeding is seldom caused by incomplete closure of the tourniquet clamp.

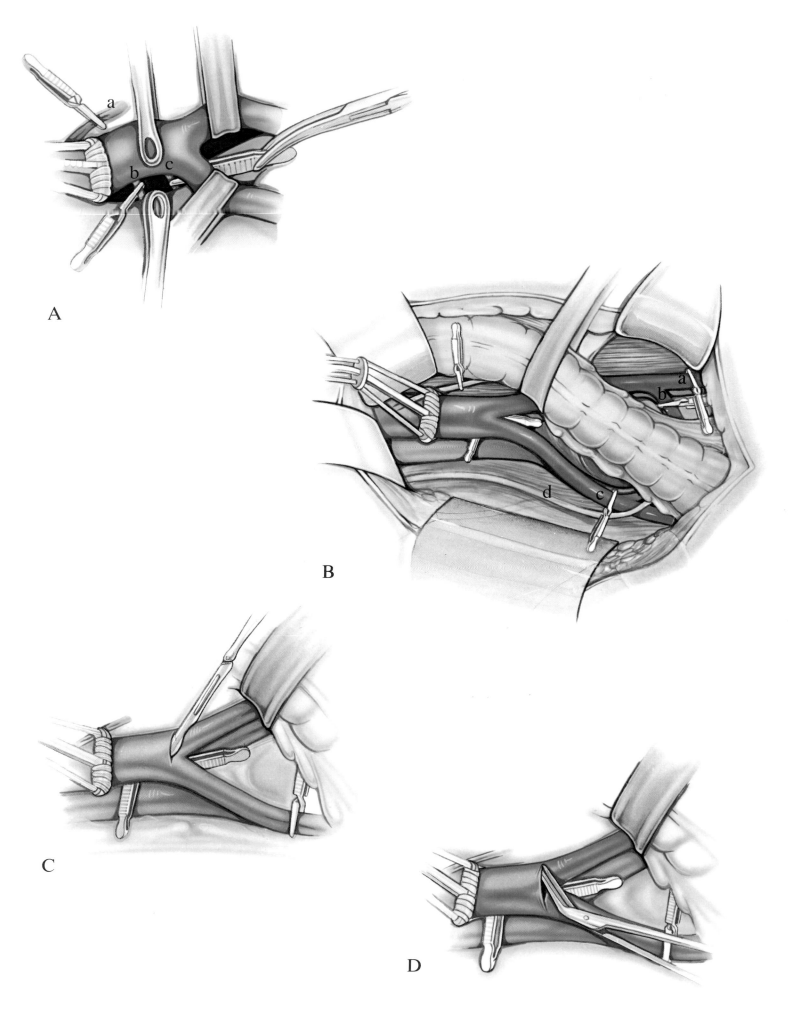

A

B

C

D

321

Plate 146

AORTOILIAC ENDARTERECTOMY
(Continued)

A. This demonstrates the aortotomy that has been made through the thin outer adventitial layer of the aorta and the thickened atheromatous media and intima that have caused a markedly reduced lumen of the aorta.

B. The proximal and distal edges of the aortic adventitia are elevated with fine forceps and a right-angled clamp is used to separate the media and intima from it, starting from the far side of the aorta. The tip of this instrument should be dull and not too pointed.

C. After freeing up the opposite side, the instrument is then brought around and inserted from the near side and passed behind the thickened tube of media and intima.

D. The blades of the right-angled clamp are then separated slightly and the aortic core of media and intima is readily divided with a fine pair of dull-pointed scissors.

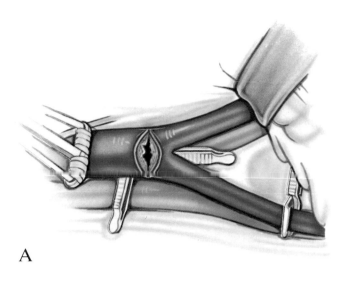

A

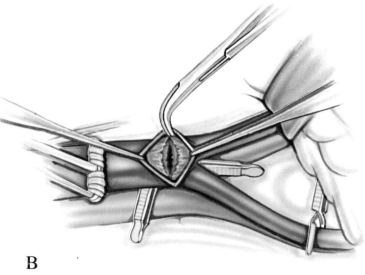

B

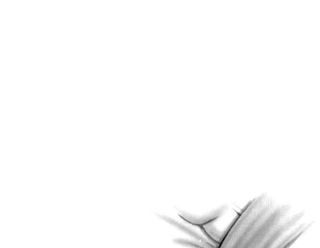

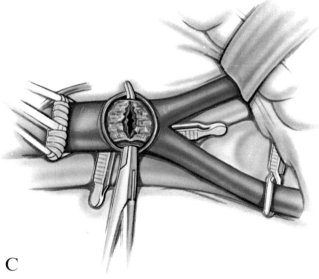

C

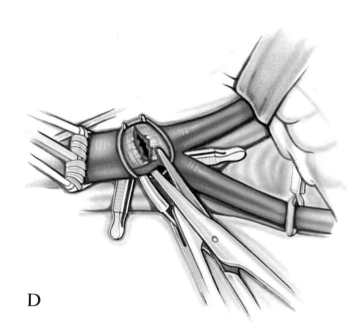

D

323

Plate 147

AORTOILIAC ENDARTERECTOMY
(Continued)

A. The atheromatous core is separated from the adventitia of the aorta, using a slightly curved, blunt-tipped instrument such as a Schnitt clamp. It is always surprising how readily this separation can be accomplished with the most gentle of maneuvers. It is first carried out on the anterior side of the aorta.

B. The clamp is then moved posteriorly behind the atheromatous core, freeing it up from the posterior wall of the aortic adventitia; the sides are freed by sweeping the clamp around in a circular motion.

C. With the third and fourth fingers of the left hand the aorta is compressed against the bodies of the lumbar vertebrae proximal to the occluding tourniquet clamp. A bulldog clamp is placed on the inferior mesenteric artery if it is patent and pulsating. The tourniquet clamp is released and brought caudad, as shown. A longer curved clamp such as a hysterectomy type clamp that has a dull point is then inserted proximally and the end of it is swept around circumferentially from side to side to free up the aortic core as the arrows show. It is of extreme importance to use a dull-pointed instrument for this to prevent perforation of the thin adventitial aortic wall.

D. After freeing up the aortic core to the point where pressure is being maintained with the fingers of the left hand it is then possible to pull out this core, sometimes in one piece, usually in several pieces. The fingers of the left hand are also utilized to determine whether the aorta has been cleared of the atheromatous plaques as far proximal as they extend. If some remain, they can be removed by directing the tip of the curved instrument to these residual pieces of the core.

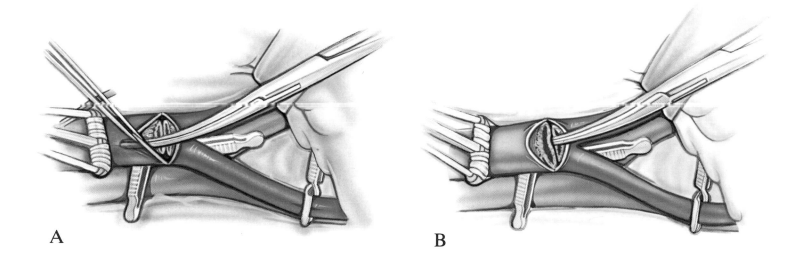

A

B

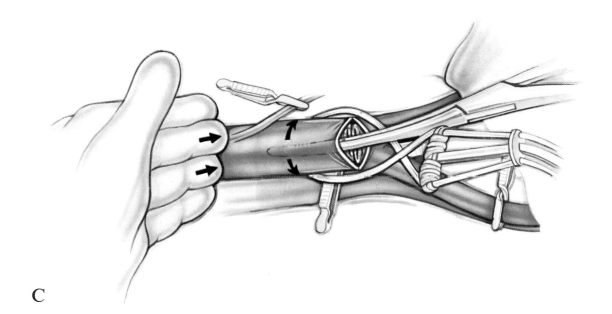

C

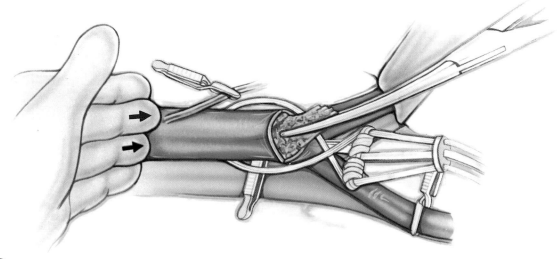

D

325

Plate 148

AORTOILIAC ENDARTERECTOMY
(Continued)

A. This demonstrates the proximal part of the core removed as a single piece, which is possible if the core has been freed up sufficiently before attempting to remove it. Sometimes a few additional areas may need to be cleared out at the level of the finger control or slightly above it, in which case the compression of the aorta is obtained in the same way by moving the hand more proximally.

B. This demonstrates the removal not only of the atheromatous plaques in a completely occluded aorta, but also the very tip of a proximal thrombus which has extended almost to the origin of the renal arteries. Again, if done carefully, this can be accomplished without danger of embolizing renal arteries, providing pressure control is maintained by placing the fingers proximal to the level of the renal arteries. It should be pointed out that the tourniquet clamp has been placed, but it is never closed until the aorta is cleared of thrombi, otherwise it might fragment the proximal portions of them and embolize the renal arteries. Since the aorta is completely occluded, there is no danger of bleeding from the proximal end while making the aortotomy and freeing up the atheromatous plaques and the proximal thrombus, until blood begins to find its way out; then proximal pressure control of the aorta with the fingers of the left hand is obtained while completing the thromboendarterectomy.

C. After a thorough cleaning out of the proximal aorta it is advisable to flush out this portion of the aorta by releasing the finger pressure on it, which permits blood to gush out through the aortotomy, carrying with it the loose particles of the media, intima and thrombus that may have been left behind. In some cases the flow will not be as adequate as expected, and further search will reveal that there are additional plaques higher up that should be removed. After this has been accomplished the flush becomes much more impressive. The total loss of blood from these maneuvers probably is about 200 cc., although actually it appears to be a great deal more. It is essential, however, to carry out this maneuver to prevent embolization of the renal and distal arteries.

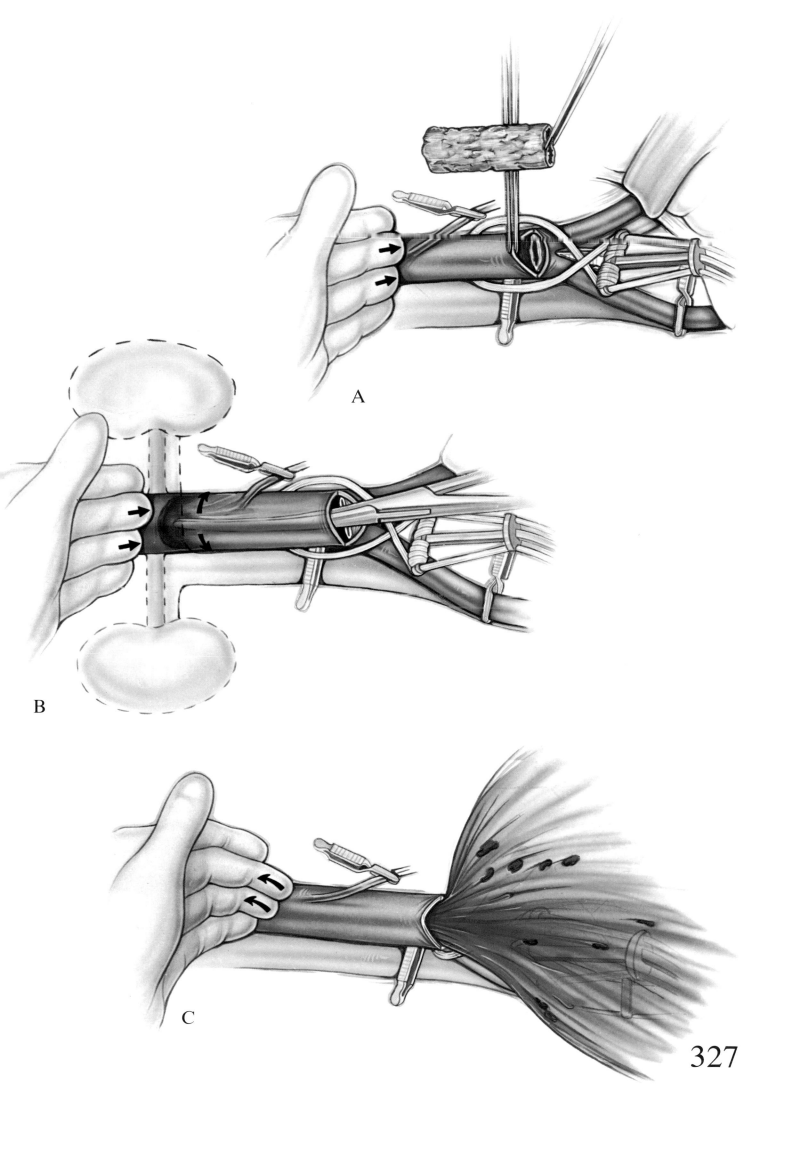

A

B

C

327

Plate 149

AORTOILIAC ENDARTERECTOMY
(Continued)

A. The tourniquet clamp has been closed again and the bulldog clamp removed from the inferior mesenteric artery, which as a rule has an improved pulsation and blood flow through it following the aortic endarterectomy. The next step is to endarterectomize the left common iliac artery. It is necessary to separate the atheromatous cores of the right and left common iliac arteries at their origins. This is readily accomplished by inserting a small curved clamp between them, as shown.

B. The plaques at the carina must be divided so that each can be freed up at the proximal end of the common iliac arteries. This is accomplished, as shown, by lifting up the adventitia of the aortotomy and inserting a curved Schnitt clamp to separate the adventitia of the common iliac arteries from the plaque.

C. This demonstrates the bifurcation of the left common iliac artery and the origin of the external iliac and hypogastric arteries. They always go into a state of vasoconstriction from the trauma of dissection, which makes it more difficult to perform a satisfactory arteriotomy endarterectomy and closure of the arteriotomy. This demonstrates the hydrostatic method of dilating short segments of these vessels, especially the proximal portion of the external iliac artery, because this is the main outflow tract to the lower extremity. This is done by placing a bulldog clamp on the common iliac artery. The clamps on the external iliac and hypogastric are already in place. Then with a 26-gauge needle on a small syringe a weak solution of heparin in normal saline solution is injected under pressure, which will dilate the artery if it is not calcified. It is of interest also that once it has been distended by this means it maintains its state of vasodilatation for hours. This facilitates greatly the operative procedure of endarterectomy and closure of the arteriotomy, which is always carried out at this point. Great care must be taken, of course, to make sure the needle is well within the lumen of the artery before injecting the fluid to prevent separation of the media and the intima. Another method of dilatation, if the common iliac artery is patent, is demonstrated in Plate 153 *C.*

D. The endarterectomy is then performed by using a ring stripper made of 20-gauge stainless steel wire. The ring should be slightly larger in diameter than the common iliac artery. The atheromatous plaques separate from the adventitia very readily with this blunt-edged ring stripper, especially those in the common iliac arteries. A pin vise is placed on the end of the stripper as a handle for ease of manipulation. A slight curve is made in the wire between it and the end ring to make it easier to insert and push forward through the artery.

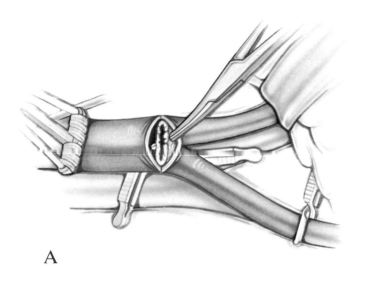

A

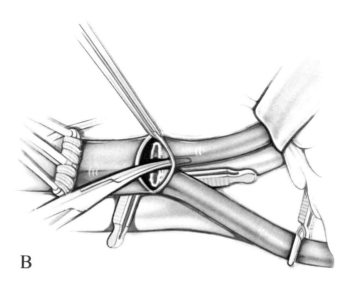

B

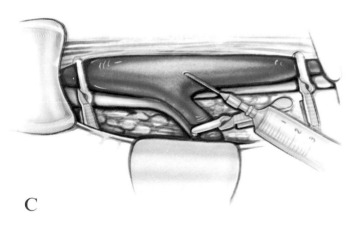

C

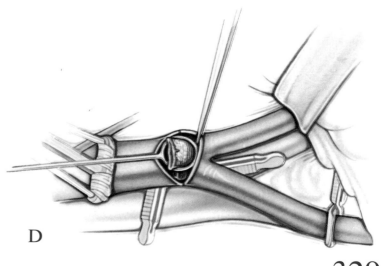

D

Plate 150

AORTOILIAC ENDARTERECTOMY
(Continued)

A. The ring stripper has been passed down through the common iliac artery to its distal end and then drawn back a short distance. An arteriotomy incision is made in the common iliac artery on the anterior surface, well away from the junction of the hypogastric with the common iliac artery. If the arteriotomy goes too close to the hypogastric artery it is very difficult to close the arteriotomy without a patch graft.

B. The stripper is then pushed on a little farther to the origin of the hypogastric artery, where it usually stops; it may be necessary to increase the length of the arteriotomy incision by carrying it into the external iliac artery.

C. This demonstrates the atheromatous core that has been removed from the proximal end of the common iliac artery distally into the external iliac artery. The arteriotomy incision has been lengthened a short distance in the external iliac artery to demonstrate the tapered distal end of the plaque. This is a very welcome sign because, beyond this, the external iliac artery is relatively normal and so it is possible to make a very clean-cut smooth removal of the entire plaque without any trouble from loose distal intimal edges.

D. Sometimes it is necessary to extend the arteriotomy incision with fine blunt-pointed scissors still farther down the external iliac artery, because the plaque may continue for another centimeter or two beyond the origin of the hypogastric artery. It is usually possible to determine how far the plaque extends by careful palpation of the external iliac artery. If other plaques are palpable more distally, endarterectomy of the external iliac and the common femoral arteries should be performed, or a bypass Dacron tube graft inserted between the common iliac and common femoral arteries if the endarterectomy does not go easily.

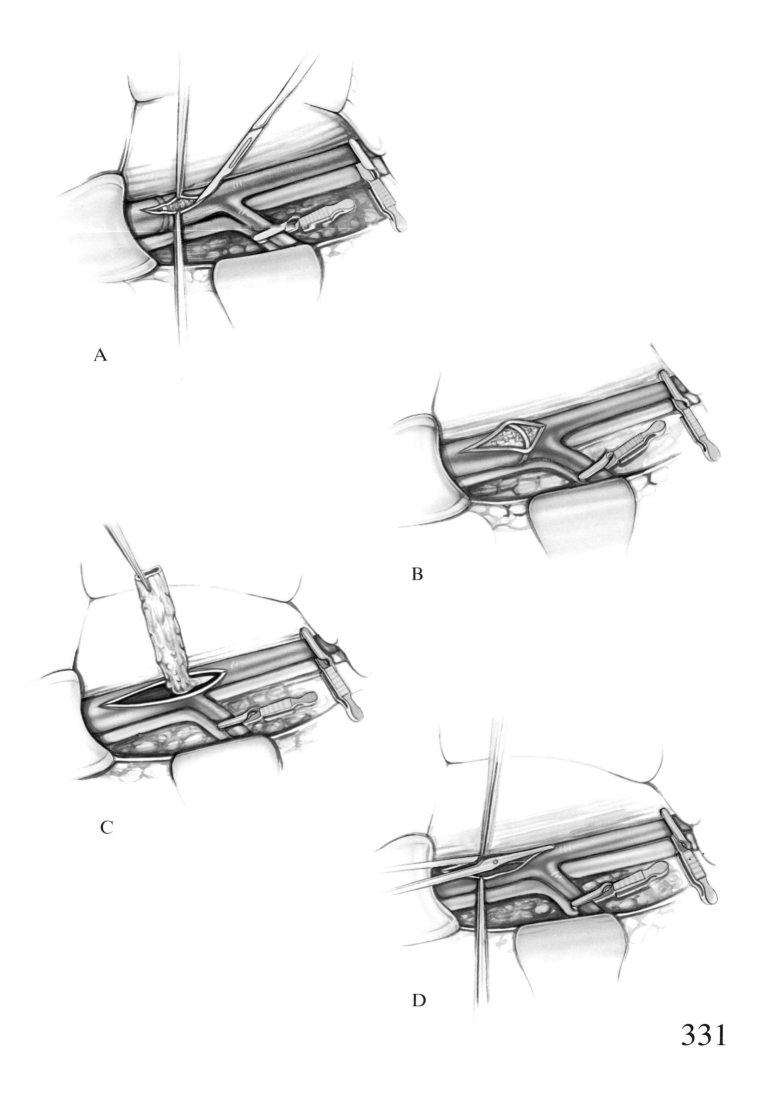

A

B

C

D

331

Plate 151

AORTOILIAC ENDARTERECTOMY
(Continued)

A. This demonstrates the use of an angled Potts' type of scissors to lengthen the arteriotomy in the external iliac artery. This type of instrument is most useful when one is operating in a deep narrow pelvis; otherwise, a straight pair with dull points is preferable.

B. The arteriotomy is continued far enough to expose the entire length of the posterior atheromatous plaque, which is the one most commonly encountered. It is readily removed using sharp-pointed scissors, leaving a very smooth edge to the distal arterial intima. This is considered a safer method of removing these plaques than doing it blindly, especially when they extend for several centimeters beyond the origin of the external iliac artery.

C. This demonstrates the removal of the atheromatous plaque from the hypogastric artery, which can be accomplished readily by using a fine-tipped curved instrument such as a Schnitt type of clamp. Care must be taken not to push the tip of the clamp through the arterial wall. If this happens it is usually necessary to ligate the artery. As a rule, the procedure is facilitated by placing the forefinger of one hand against the hypogastric artery to palpate the atheromatous plaques and guide the tip of the clamp with it.

D. After removing the plaque in the hypogastric artery it is very important to instill a weak solution of heparin in a normal saline solution (100 units per 5 cc.) beyond the bulldog clamp, as shown, using a fine polyvinyl tubing. If this is not done the hypogastric artery may become occluded by a blood clot that may develop because of the rough inner lining of the vessel following the endarterectomy, with stagnation of the blood in this portion until the blood flow is established in the iliac arteries.

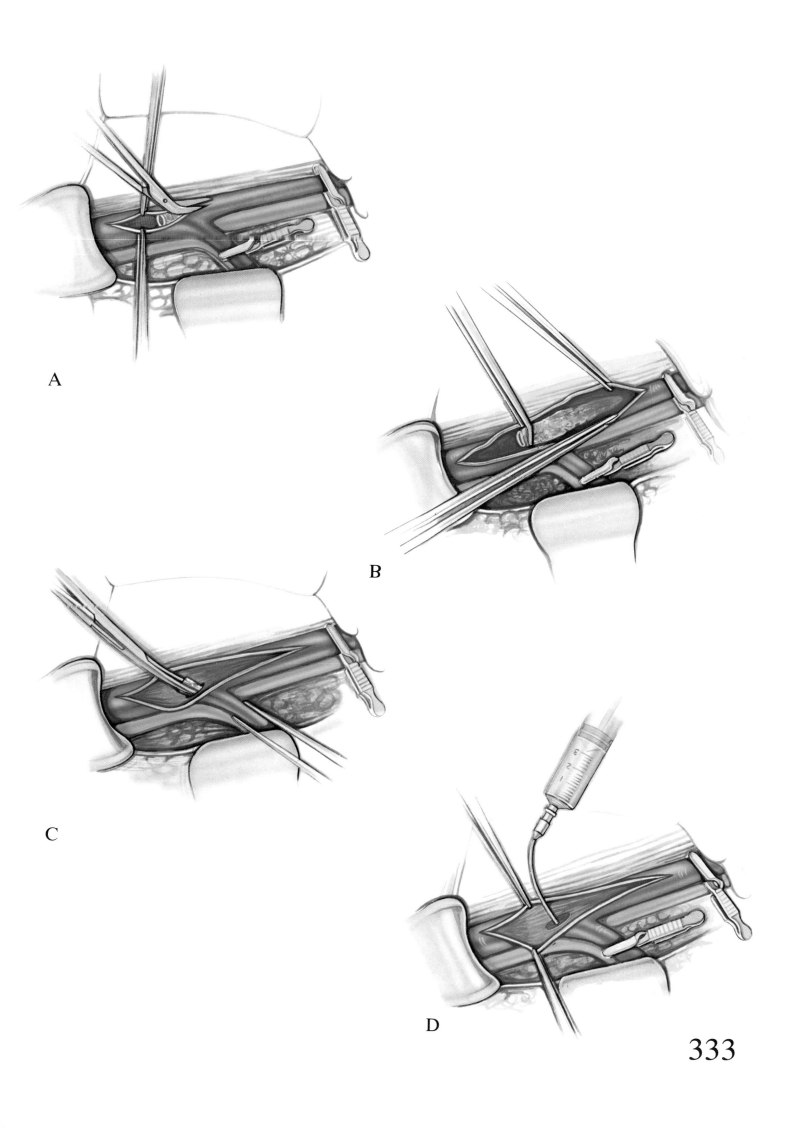

A

B

C

D

333

Plate 152

AORTOILIAC ENDARTERECTOMY
(Continued)

A. Loose fragments of intima may remain after removal of the main obstructing atheromatous core with the closed type of endarterectomy of the common iliac artery. It is therefore necessary to have some means of clearing out these fragments. One method of doing this is by the use of a gauze pledget which is pulled through the previously endarterectomized artery. A sufficient amount of gauze is chosen so that when it is tied at one end, as shown, it will fluff out and fit the inner lumen of the vessel snugly. After the end is tied with a silk ligature, the long end of the ligature is passed through the ligated end of the pledget as shown; this prevents the ligature from slipping off as it is pulled through the vessel. Different sized pledgets are made, depending on the diameter of the arteries.

B. In order to pass the pledget through the vessel, the end of the long silk ligature is passed through the end of a small polyethylene catheter and secured by a knot.

C. The polyvinyl catheter has been passed through the left common iliac artery from the lower arteriotomy to the aortic one; the ligature is attached to the catheter at one end and to the gauze pledget at the other. The two edges of the distal arteriotomy incision are picked up with fine forceps by the first assistant and the small ligated end of the pledget is directed into the lumen of the vessel by the surgeon as he pulls on the silk ligature at the aortotomy.

D. The pledget should come through with moderate resistance, indicating a tight fit. As it comes out through the aortotomy, fragments of the partially detached intima and media that were not previously removed come out on it. My rule is to pass this pledget through a sufficient number of times until it comes through without bringing any additional fragments with it. This sometimes necessitates passing it four or five times.

E. This shows three pledgets that have been pulled through different arteries, one without any fragments on it, and the other two with large fragments which actually are circumferential segments of the media and intima. Sometimes, in addition, to make sure that no loose partially adherent fragments are still present, a large-caliber polyvinyl catheter that fits the lumen quite snugly is passed through and the vessel wall palpated against this. By this means it is possible to detect fragments that may not have been removed; by additional passage of the gauze pledget they can be removed, or sometimes picked out with a fine, curved, pointed instrument passed through the aortotomy or the iliac arteriotomy.

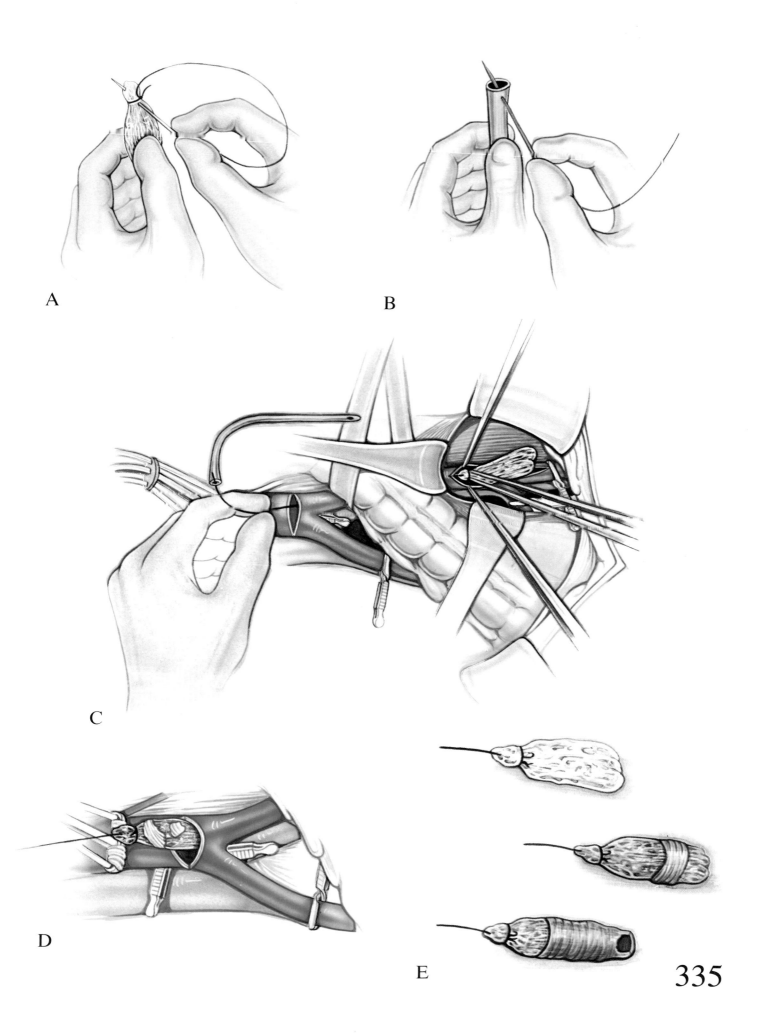

A

B

C

D

E

335

Plate 153

AORTOILIAC ENDARTERECTOMY
(Continued)

A. This demonstrates the atheromatous core that has been removed from the common iliac artery; the tapered distal portion has come from the origin of the external iliac artery.

B. The surgeon has moved to the left side of the patient in order to facilitate exposure and working on the right common iliac, external iliac and hypogastric arteries. This illustration demonstrates one method of dilating hydrostatically the distal end of the common iliac and the proximal portions of the external iliac and hypogastric arteries by injecting dilute heparin in normal saline solution with a 26-gauge needle on a 2-cc. syringe. The three arteries are isolated with bulldog clamps to prevent the heparin solution from escaping from the entrapped arteries. When this method is used one must make certain that the needle is in the arterial lumen by aspirating blood before injecting the solution; this will insure against separation of the intima and media from the adventitia.

C. This demonstrates another method of dilating these arteries if the common iliac artery has a slightly larger lumen. A 12-gauge polyvinyl catheter is passed distally from the aorta through the common iliac artery to its bifurcation. A 0 silk ligature is passed twice around the common iliac artery to use as proximal control during the injection of the heparin solution. The catheter is first filled with dilute heparin in normal saline solution to evacuate the air in it, then the solution is injected under moderate pressure. It is a pleasing sight to see the external iliac artery, especially, dilate under these conditions because this is the important outflow tract. It will not, of course, do so if it is calcified. Either of these methods of arterial dilatation completely reverses the arterial vasospasm and leaves the artery widely dilated for several hours, so that there is more than ample time to complete the reconstructive arterial procedure with the assurance that it can be accomplished without stenosis at the origin of the external iliac providing the suturing is done to perfection.

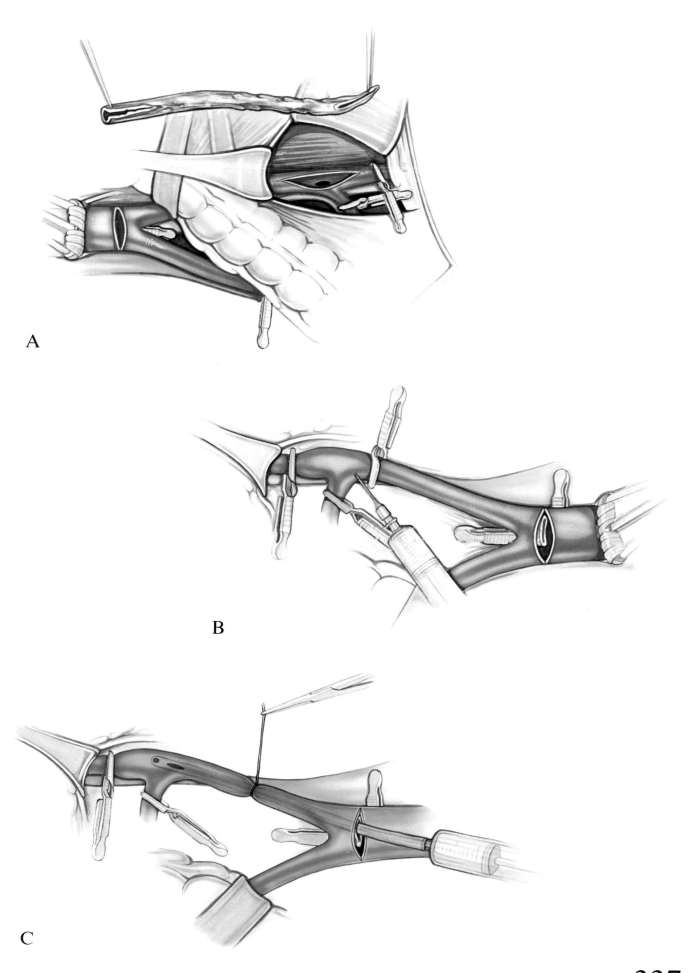

A

B

C

337

Plate 154

AORTOILIAC ENDARTERECTOMY
(Continued)

A.   The proximal portion of the atheromatous core in the right common iliac artery is freed up with a relatively sharp, curved type of clamp similar to a Schnitt. The tip of the instrument is swept around between the core and the adventitia, being careful not to perforate the latter.

B.   A stripper with a ring made of the same wire as the handle is preferred; it has a rounded (not a cutting) edge slightly larger than the common iliac artery, and it is passed distalward to the bulldog clamp. Occasionally there will be a hard, calcified plaque that is larger in diameter than the ring, in which case the next larger size ring must be used. The blunt type of ring seldom tears or lacerates the adventitia, separating the atheromatous core much more easily than the ring with a cutting edge.

C.   An arteriotomy is then made in the distal portion of the common iliac artery proximal to the bulldog clamp in order to remove the detached atheromatous core.

D.   This shows that the core has been lifted out through the distal arteriotomy. The major portion is being removed after division with scissors. When this has been accomplished, a gauze pledget is pulled through the common iliac artery in order to clear it completely. The pledget should be pulled proximally from the iliac arteriotomy rather than the reverse because of the danger of tearing the aortotomy, which will make it difficult to close, sometimes even requiring a patch graft of saphenous vein or Dacron. The plan is not to endarterectomize the right external iliac and hypogastric arteries at this stage of the procedure even if they need it, but to complete the left side and close the aortotomy so that the blood may be allowed to flow down the left side.

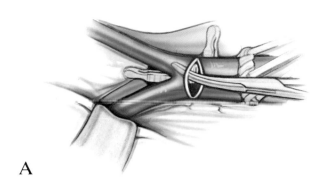

A

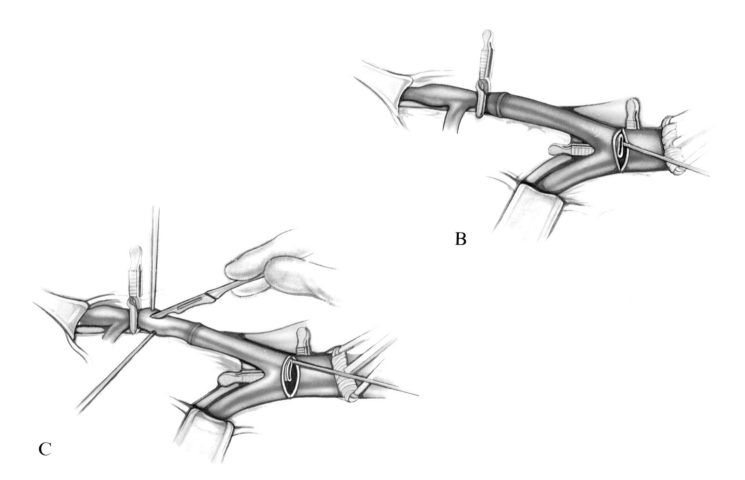

B

C

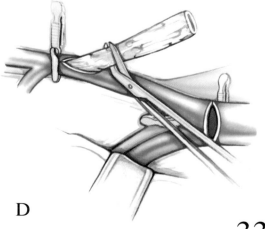

D

339

Plate 155

AORTOILIAC ENDARTERECTOMY
(Continued)

A.   The surgeon has now returned to the right side of the patient. The bifurcation of the aorta and the common iliac arteries is shown and the suturing of the left iliac arteriotomy is being performed. Note that a polyvinyl catheter has been inserted through the aortotomy distally into the external iliac artery as a stent. This is very important in order to obtain an accurate, smooth closure of the external iliac artery portion of the arteriotomy and so leave it with the widest possible lumen. The use of the stent is the best way to prevent wrinkling and narrowing of the artery at its take-off from the common iliac artery unless one uses a vein or prosthetic patch to close it.

B.   This is a closer view to demonstrate the technique of closing the iliac arteriotomy. The use of the stent cannot be overemphasized; it is also very important that the artery be dilated before incising it, as shown in Plate 149 *C*. Guy sutures are first placed at (a) and (b). Suturing is commenced at each end of the arteriotomy and continued as a running over-and-over type of stitch. It has been carried from the distal end to guy suture (a), to which it is ligated. The type of suture that has been found most useful is a Teflon-coated Dacron rubbed thoroughly with bone wax to make it smoother so it does not pick up the adventitia, and with a swaged-on, taper-pointed straight needle. After commencing the suture from each end it is completed either at guy suture (a) or suture (b).

C.   This demonstrates the arteriotomy completely closed. It is recommended that the suture line be tested after isolating the section of the artery with the three bulldog clamps as shown. A weak solution of heparin in normal saline is injected through a small caliber needle into the lumen of the common iliac artery. Not infrequently one finds a sizable leak in the suture line, which can readily be closed with a single stitch. It is much easier and safer to correct the suture line leaks at this stage of the procedure instead of waiting until the blood flow is re-established through the arteries.

D.   The next step in the procedure is the closure of the transverse aortotomy. This is accomplished with mattress sutures of 4- or 5-0 arterial type of suture. Silk is often used because it is more thrombogenic than the synthetic sutures, so that there is less leakage from the suture line holes in the thin adventitia. As a rule, a curved taper-pointed needle is more satisfactory than the straight or the cutting-pointed one. I prefer to make my own two-needle mattress sutures by tying two of them together. (See Plate 189.) This type has the advantage that it leaves a knot in the middle of the two-needle sutures, which acts as a buttress against the thin aortic adventitia which is less apt to pull or tear through it. It is customary to place the middle mattress suture first, as shown.

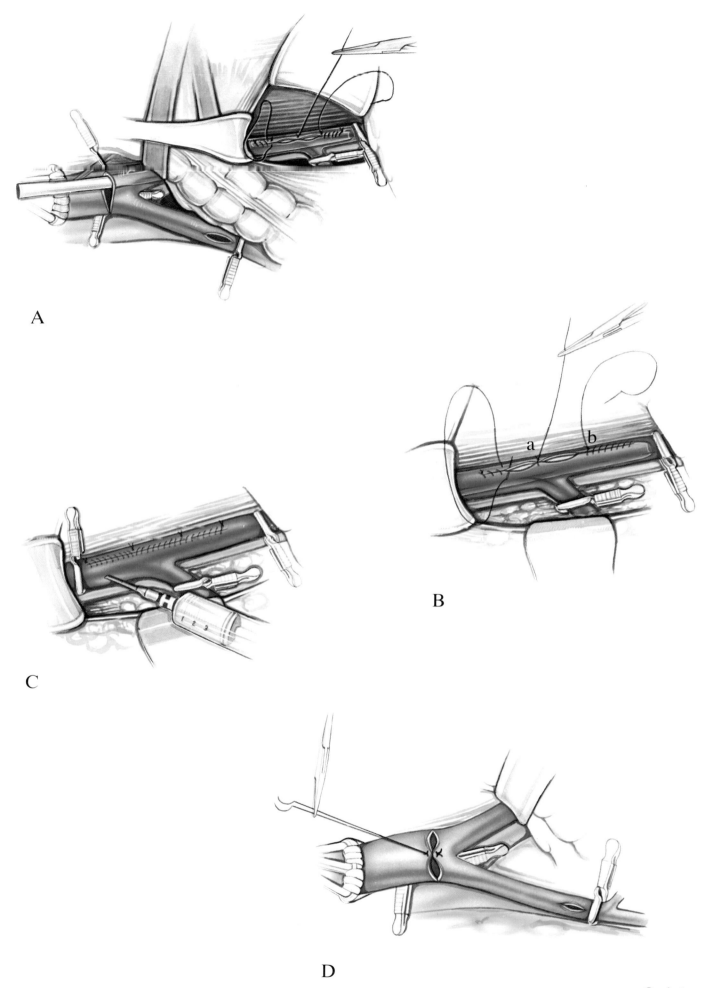

A

B

C

D

341

Plate 156

AORTOILIAC ENDARTERECTOMY
(Continued)

A. This shows one half of the aortotomy closed. Note that it has been accomplished with interrupted mattress stitches with knots on both ends of them. The usefulness of this method of closure cannot be overemphasized, because it is the most secure method of closing this thin-walled adventitial tube of aorta. This type of suture line has never been known to give way. If a running suture is used, it tends to tear the tissue and is much more apt to leak as a result. In addition, it tends to constrict the aorta to a greater degree at the aortotomy because a running suture must be pulled very snug to be hemostatic.

B. The closure has now been completed. Note that it is not necessary to interlock the interrupted sutures or even to place them exactly next to each other. Bulldogs (a) and (b) are placed on the common iliac arteries to isolate this segment of the aorta. The suture line is then tested before releasing the aortic tourniquet clamp by injecting a dilute solution of heparin and normal saline solution through a 22-gauge needle inserted at the carina of the aorta. There may be an occasional leak between one or two of the sutures which can be readily closed with interrupted stitches.

C. After determining that the suture line of the aortotomy and the left iliac arteriotomy are secure and tight, the proximal aorta is flushed out through the right common iliac arteriotomy by releasing the aortic tourniquet clamp, after removing the proximal bulldog clamp on the right common iliac artery. After the flushing, the aortic tourniquet clamp is closed, then all the bulldog clamps are removed except the one on the distal end of the right common iliac artery. This permits the surgeon to determine whether there is good backflow from the left hypogastric and external iliac arteries, as the blood will escape through the arteriotomy of the right common iliac artery. If this is observed, a strong bulldog clamp is then placed on the origin of the right common iliac artery and the tourniquet clamp is released again but not removed.

D. This shows the two remaining bulldog clamps on the right common iliac artery, the proximal one to control the blood flow from the aorta and the distal one the backflow from the hypogastric and the external iliac arteries. Blood now flows down through the left iliac artery to re-establish the arterial blood flow to the left lower extremity.

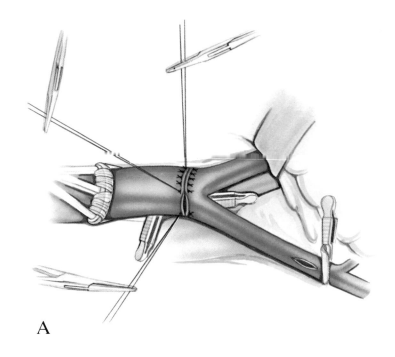

A

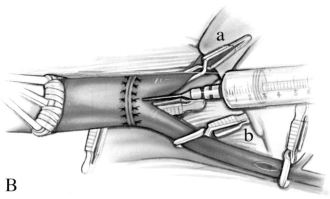

B

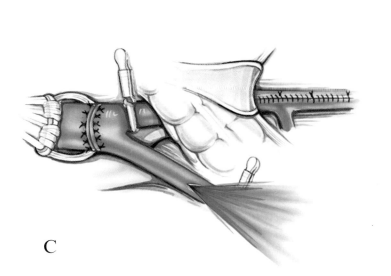

C

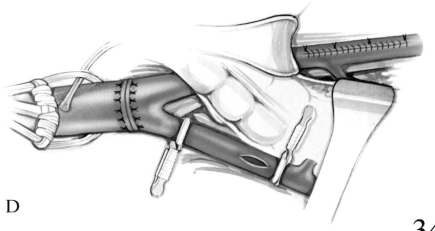

D

Plate 157

AORTOILIAC ENDARTERECTOMY
(Continued)

A. The surgeon has returned to the left side of the patient. This demonstrates another method of dilating the proximal end of the right external iliac artery if it was not done before making the arteriotomy in the distal end of the common iliac artery. The bulldog clamp on the latter is removed, and clamps are placed on the proximal ends of the hypogastric and external iliac arteries. A fine, polyvinyl, 18-gauge tubing is then inserted through the arteriotomy and connected to a 5-cc. syringe filled with dilute heparin and normal saline solution. The common iliac artery is encircled twice with a 0 silk suture and held firmly while the solution is injected. Note the dilatation of the proximal part of the external iliac artery compared to that distal to the bulldog clamp, indicating how much easier it will be to close the arteriotomy incision. Additional dilute heparin solution may be injected down the external iliac artery by temporarily releasing the bulldog clamp on it.

B. The arteriotomy incision in the common iliac artery is then extended distally across its bifurcation and the proximal portion of the external iliac artery with fine, angled scissors.

C. This demonstrates a posterior plaque which ends with a tapered distal tip. Through the center of it one can see the small orifice of the hypogastric artery.

D. The remaining portion of the atheromatous plaque is readily removed by cutting it out with very fine-tipped, curved scissors. Sometimes it comes out without the necessity of using the scissors but, as shown, it can be done neatly with them, leaving the intima smooth and firmly attached, without loose edges that need to be sutured to the arterial wall.

E. This shows the thin, unsutured edges of the intima where the plaque was removed and the proximal end of the partially occluding atheromatous plaque in the hypogastric artery.

344

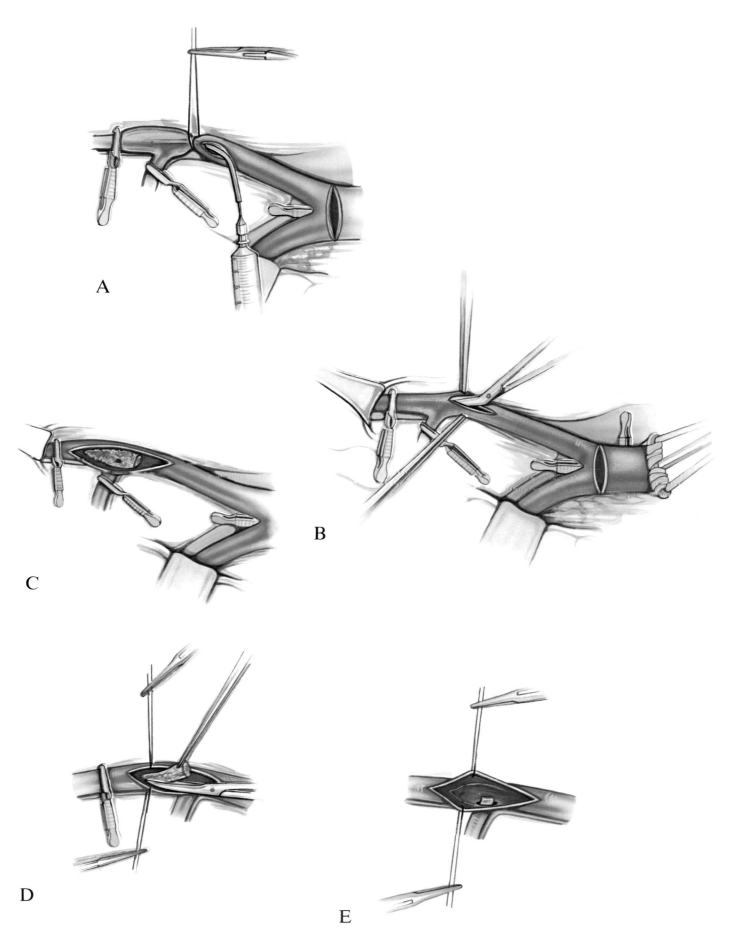

A

B

C

D

E

345

Plate 158

AORTOILIAC ENDARTERECTOMY
(Continued)

A. Additional dilute heparin in normal saline solution is injected into the external iliac artery through the fine polyvinyl tubing. This is another check and safeguard against distal thrombosis in the arterial system of the right lower extremity, since it has been occluded longer than the left one. The endarterectomy of the hypogastric artery, using a curved Schnitt clamp, is also shown. The bulldog clamp on the artery has been removed and the bleeding from it controlled readily with a pair of angled forceps (a), which is released as the instrument is passed distally through the lumen to perform the endarterectomy.

B. It is important to instill dilute heparin in normal saline solution into the hypogastric artery also, as shown, after it has been endarterectomized to prevent it from becoming thrombosed during the remainder of the procedure.

C. This demonstrates the method of closure of the iliac arteriotomy by the use of a venous patch graft. This is occasionally necessary when the external iliac artery cannot be dilated, or if in performing the endarterectomy it has been damaged at the site of the arteriotomy, so that it cannot be sutured without narrowing the lumen of the proximal end of the external iliac artery. The most satisfactory vein for obtaining this patch graft is the distal end of the long saphenous vein at the ankle because the walls of it are very strong and will withstand arterial blood pressure. The removal of this portion does not jeopardize the later use of the long saphenous vein as a bypass graft, if it becomes necessary. Note that there is a short segment of a polyvinyl catheter within the vessel lumen as a stent while the graft is being implanted.

D. The stent is being removed after completion of all but a short segment of the suture lines, which is just large enough to allow removal of the stent.

E. The vein patch graft implantation has been completed. The bulldog clamps have been removed, permitting blood to flow through the right iliac system into the lower extremity. Although not shown, the suture lines were tested before opening the arterial inflow by injecting dilute heparin solution in normal saline with the bulldog clamp still in place.

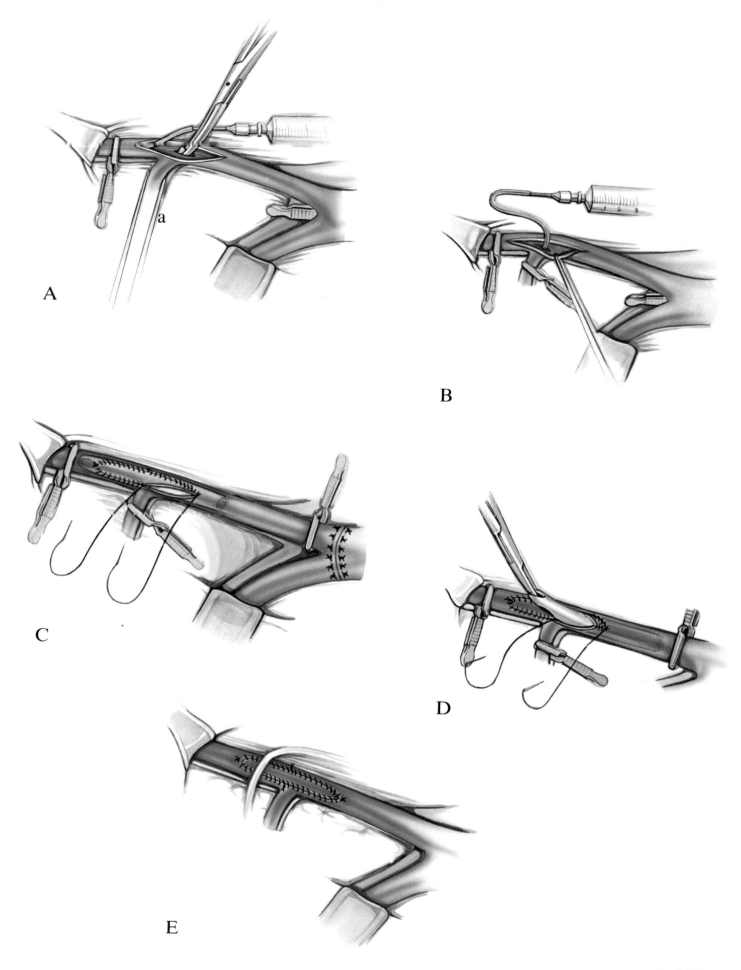

Plate 159

AORTOILIAC ENDARTERECTOMY
(Continued)

A. Since it was learned that it is possible to dilate the origin of the external iliac artery without damage to it, the necessity of implanting a venous or synthetic patch graft to the arteriotomy is much less common than it used to be. This illustration demonstrates the closure of the arteriotomy of the external and common iliac arteries using a stent of a short segment of a polyvinyl catheter. Two guy sutures have been placed at (a) and (b), which stabilizes the stent and also helps to maintain a tight suture line by dividing it into segments.

B. The stent is being removed after most of the suturing of the arteriotomy has been performed. It is best to complete the suture line of the external iliac artery first with the stent in place because it is at this site that the vessel is smaller and every effort needs to be made to obtain a smooth, streamlined closure without stenosis or wrinkling. Although the same rule holds for the larger common iliac artery, it is not so vital, and the last short segment of the common iliac arteriotomy can be sutured without the stent.

C. The suture lines have been completed and the blood flow restored after testing with dilute heparin in normal saline solution. Note that the ureter (c), which has been displaced distalward, is still intact.

D. This demonstrates the operative field as seen from the right side of the patient after completion of the aortic and bilateral common iliac artery endarterectomy and suturing of the aortotomy and the arteriotomies and restoration of the arterial blood flow to both the lower extremities.

The hemostasis is checked, the tourniquet clamp is removed, and the posterior peritoneum is closed over the aorta and the iliac arteries above the sigmoid in a single layer with interrupted fine silk sutures; the same procedure is followed in the left lower quadrant. This is another advantage of the endarterectomy type of procedure, because the closure can be done in one layer, whereas with the prosthesis it should be in two layers over the aortic part of the prosthesis to separate it from the third portion of the duodenum.

Follow-up studies have revealed that this type of operative procedure stands up extraordinarily well for many years when the external iliac and femoral arteries are patent and in good condition and is equally as good as the implantation of an aortic bifurcation prosthesis. This method has the advantage that it maintains the circulation through the inferior mesenteric artery in many instances, and also revascularizes the pelvis by the endarterectomizing of the hypogastric arteries. It also leaves the patient with autogenous tissues which, in a young individual especially, has an advantage since as yet we do not know how long the synthetic prostheses are going to last. It is easier to reoperate on patients treated in this manner, especially when the aorta is not dissected free proximal to the inferior mesenteric artery, if occlusion of the iliac artery should develop at a later date and a prosthesis becomes necessary at a second procedure. It also has the definite advantage that, as a rule, the presacral nerves can be preserved and the sexual life of the younger male patient is less apt to be interfered with and in some cases may even improve.

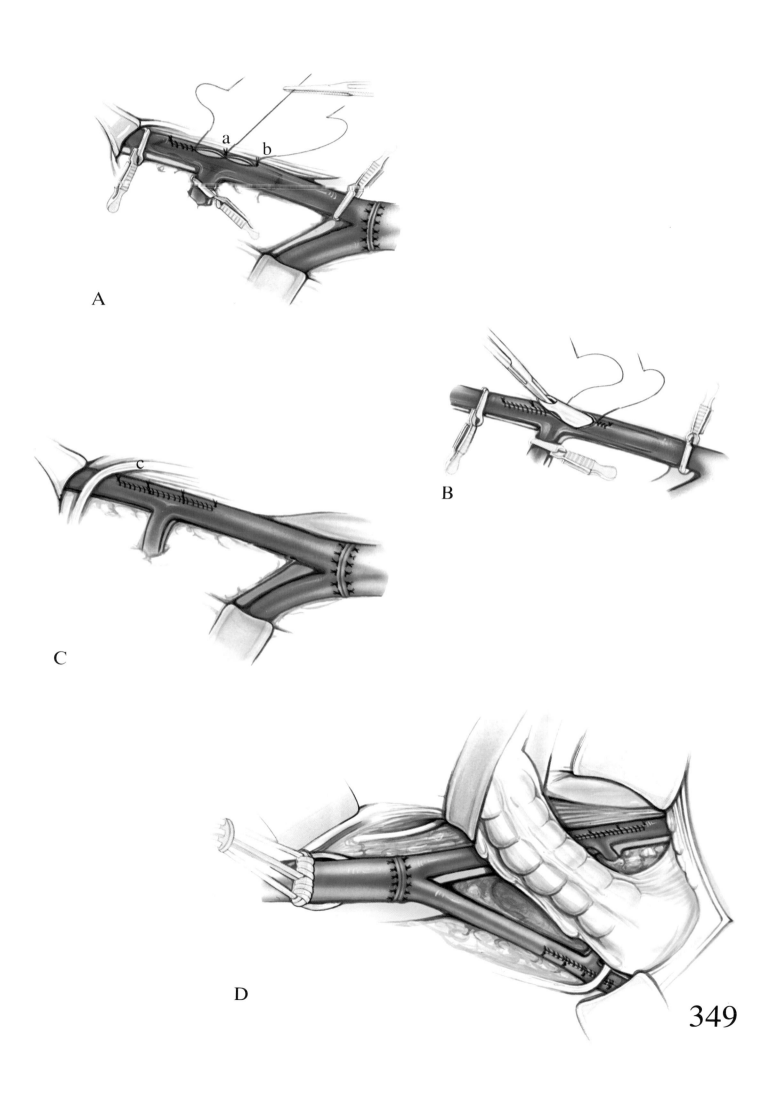

A

B

C

D

349

Plate 160

AORTOILIAC FEMORAL
ENDARTERECTOMY

A. It is necessary in some patients, because of involvement of the external iliac and common femoral arteries, in addition to endarterectomizing the aorta and common iliac arteries, to also endarterectomize the external iliac and common femoral arteries, and occasionally the proximal portion of the profunda femoris. Palpation of the groins in these patients will usually reveal hard, firm, cord-like femoral arteries. This explains the advantage of exploring the groins prior to opening the abdomen to determine the condition of these arteries and their outflow tract. Examination of the common femoral arteries will frequently determine whether it is advisable to do an endarterectomy of them and the external iliac arteries, in addition to the aorta and the common iliac arteries, or whether a bypass aortic bilateral femoral type of prosthesis is necessary. This illustration shows the completed endarterectomy of the aorta and common iliac arteries, and exposure of the femoral arteries in the groins.

B. This is the area outlined in black of *A* to show the left common femoral, profunda femoris and superficial femoral arteries. Dural clips have been placed on the lateral circumflex iliac artery (a) and the deep epigastric artery (b) for temporary control of them, as they will be removed after completing the procedure. The superficial external pudendal (c) has been ligated and divided. A bulldog clamp is on the profunda femoris artery (d) and another on the superficial femoral artery (e). This usually controls the blood flowing into these major vessels, although there may be other tributaries. It is vital to control all of them to prevent clot formation in the arteries after they have been endarterectomized. A large posterior plaque is seen with a small orifice of the profunda femoris showing in it.

C. The distal portion of the plaque has been removed. This results in enlarging the orifice of the profunda femoris artery. The proximal part of the plaque is then separated from the adventitia with the tip of a Schnitt clamp. It is important to sever the connections of it from the origins of the deep epigastric and the lateral circumflex iliac arteries with this clamp because, if not, the stripper will be held up at these branches and the adventitia may be torn in trying to pass the stripper beyond if the plaques have not been freed up first with the curved clamp.

D. A wire type of stripper is then chosen with a loop that is a little larger than the lumen of the common femoral and external iliac arteries. The handle is bent as shown because the course of the external iliac artery posteriorly is at about a 45-degree angle. A pin vise is placed on the stripper to help in manipulating it.

E. The stripper is passed proximally. It frequently passes very readily from this arteriotomy to the common iliac one. It is important not to be too vigorous in pushing it if resistance is encountered, because it may be forced through the adventitia under these conditions. Gentle pressure with a little rotation of the handle will usually free up the atheromatous material.

F. This shows the distal end of the abdominal incision and the left groin incision. A wire loop stripper with a pin vise as a handle can be seen projecting out from the arteriotomy of the femoral artery, as well as the ring end of the stripper that is encircling the proximal end of the atheromatous core of the external iliac artery. It can be seen presenting in the arteriotomy of the left common iliac artery. The atheromatous core is then readily removed, usually in one piece. After its removal, gauze pledgets are pulled through these arteries, usually from the common femoral proximally because if it is done in the reverse direction, the origin of the external iliac artery may be seriously damaged or even evulsed.

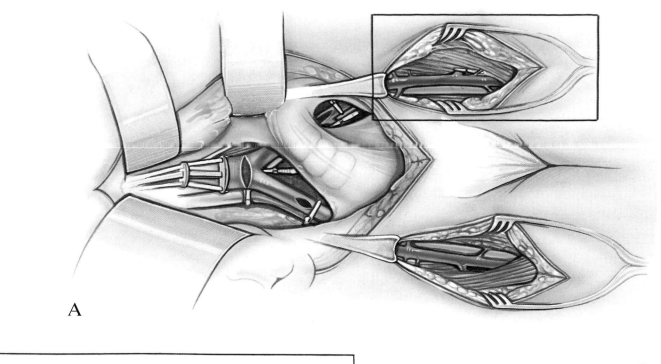

A

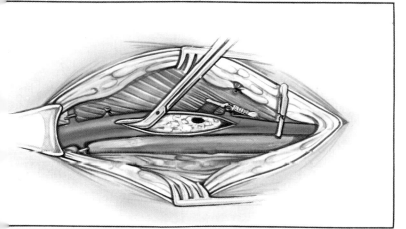

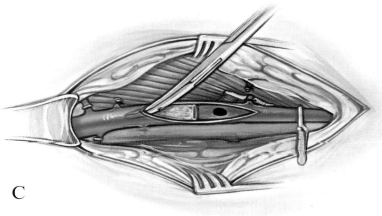

C

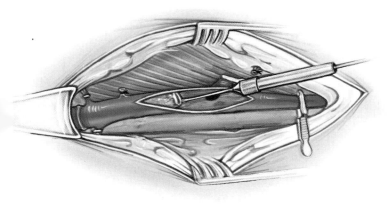

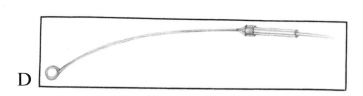

D

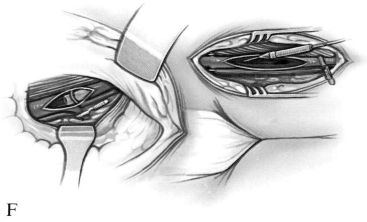

F

351

AORTOILIAC FEMORAL
ENDARTERECTOMY *(Continued)*

A. This demonstrates the completion of the endarterectomy of the abdominal aorta, bilateral common iliac, external iliac and common femoral arteries. The arteriotomies of the left common iliac and common femoral arteries have been closed with a running over-and-over type of stitch, using 5-0 Teflon-coated Dacron sutures. A strong bulldog clamp is placed on the right common iliac artery near its origin; the tourniquet clamp has been released to restore the blood flow to the left pelvis and the lower limb. Bulldog clamps are still in place on the right hypogastric, superficial femoral and profunda femoris arteries. The small branches of the common femoral and superficial femoral arteries are controlled with dura clips which will be removed later, as has been done on the left side.

B. This demonstrates the completed procedure with all the occluding clamps removed except the tourniquet clamp, which is the last one to be taken off just in case one of the suture lines should leak and it becomes necessary to take a few additional stitches at the points of leakage. It is readily removed by simply cutting the shoestring near the aorta, after which it slips out easily. It was necessary to use a vein patch graft to close the right femoral arteriotomy because the edges of it were so thin and frayed that suturing it would have resulted in marked constriction of the common femoral artery. (See Plate 162.) A short section of the long saphenous vein (removed at the ankle level) was used for the patch graft. The posterior peritoneum over the aorta and in the left lower quadrant is closed as a single layer, using interrupted fine sutures of silk. One of the advantages of the endarterectomy procedure is that the closure of the posterior peritoneum can always be accomplished in one layer. It is not necessary to make a two-layer closure, as must be done when a Dacron graft is implanted. The groin incisions are closed in layers, using fine linen or cotton. The abdominal incision is closed in the routine manner, usually with 0 chromic catgut and stay sutures of nylon. The skin in all three incisions is closed with interrupted mattress sutures of silk. If the patient has atherosclerotic occlusive disease of the superficial femoral arteries, it is customary to do lumbar sympathectomies before closing the posterior peritoneum over the aorta. (See Plate 144.)

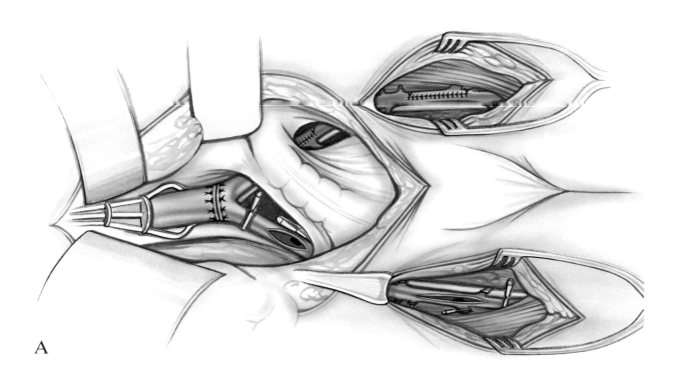

A

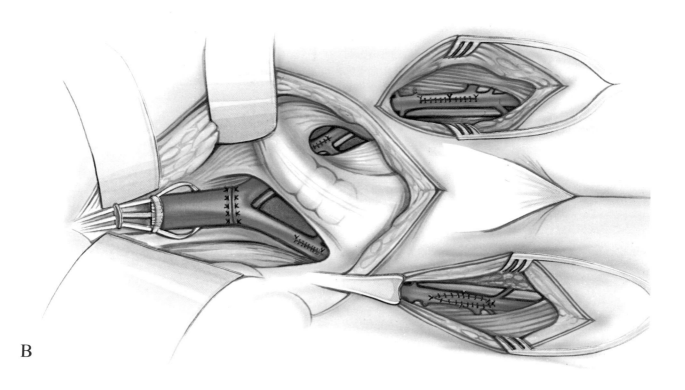

B

353

Plate 162

TECHNIQUE OF CLOSURE
OF AN ARTERIOTOMY
WITH A VEIN PATCH GRAFT

A. This illustration demonstrates an arteriotomy made in the distal end of the common femoral and the proximal end of the superficial femoral artery opposite the origin of the profunda femoris artery. Note the ragged edges to the arteriotomy, which occurs if the atheromatous core of the artery is difficult to separate from a very thin adventitia.

B. Closure of this arteriotomy with a running over-and-over stitch will result in marked stenosis, as demonstrated. This will interfere with the outflow to both the profunda femoris and the superficial femoral arteries and, therefore, should be avoided.

C. A small section of the long saphenous vein is usually removed from either ankle, providing the arterial blood supply is adequate; if not, it can be removed from the saphenous vein higher in the lower leg just distal to the knee. It is best not to take a portion of it in the groin incision, because this might mean the loss of the main saphenous trunk, which might be needed later for a bypass graft in the leg. The vein segment should be reversed if one is not certain there is no valve in the section removed. It is then implanted as shown, with mattress sutures at each end and stay sutures in the middle. The ends of the patch graft should be left square as shown rather than cut to a point. A short segment of a polyvinyl catheter the same size as the internal lumen of the femoral artery is used as a stent to maintain the same size lumen as the main portion of the artery. If this is not done, the graft may result in a dilatation of the artery which later will become aneurysmal.

D. Most of the suturing has been accomplished and the stent is being removed, leaving only a small section of the suture line that must be completed without the stent; care should be taken to make it as streamlined as possible.

E. This demonstrates a correctly implanted saphenous vein patch graft without constriction at either end of the graft or dilatation of the arterial lumen.

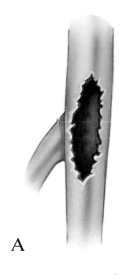

A

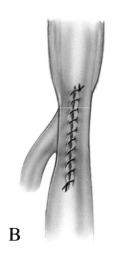

B

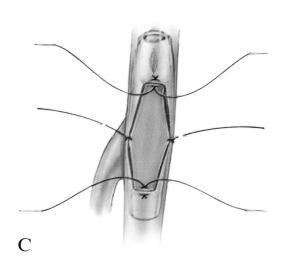

C

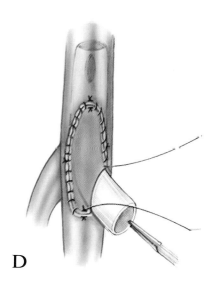

D

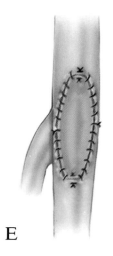

E

355

Plate 163

AORTOILIAC FEMORAL
ENDARTERECTOMY WITH
RIGHT ILIOFEMORAL PROSTHESIS

A. This shows a completed aortic bilateral common iliac, left external iliac and common femoral endarterectomy. It was necessary, however, because of difficulty encountered in endarterectomizing the right external iliac artery, to implant a Dacron prosthesis from the right common iliac artery to the right common femoral artery. This complication occurs infrequently, but when the endarterectomy on the left has gone very well and difficulty is encountered on the right side, it seems worthwhile to use an iliofemoral Dacron graft rather than implant a bifurcation aortic prosthesis from the aorta to both common femoral arteries. When it is realized after examining the external iliac arteries that there will be difficulty in endarterectomizing them, the insertion of the bifurcation Dacron prosthesis to the common femoral arteries is the treatment of choice. (See Plate 164.)

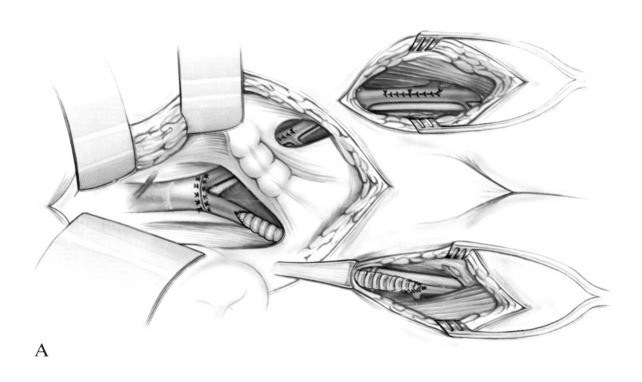

A

Plate 163 (Continued)

AORTIC BILATERAL COMMON ILIAC DACRON PROSTHESIS

B.   This illustration demonstrates the localized nature of aortoiliac disease in some patients, unfortunately too few. This type can be treated either by endarterectomy, which is the method of choice providing the external iliac arteries are in good condition, or by the implantation of an aortic bifurcation prosthesis.

C.   This demonstrates the method of implanting a bifurcation Dacron prosthesis consisting of excision of the distal abdominal aorta and all of the common iliac arteries except the very distal 1 cm. of each. The proximal abdominal aorta and the distal portions of the common iliac arteries are then endarterectomized. On the left side the arteriotomy is carried distally in the external iliac artery a short distance to permit removal of the plaque at the origin of this vessel and also from the hypogastric artery. An aortic prosthesis is then anastomosed end-to-end to the abdominal aorta, and the left iliac limb of the prosthesis to the distal end of the common iliac and proximal portion of the external iliac arteries by a long end-to-end anastomosis by the end-to-side technique (Plates 138 and 139). The anastomosis on the right side is more readily accomplished as it is a shorter end-to-end anastomosis by the end-to-side technique and because the endarterectomy of the external iliac artery did not have to be carried as far distally.

358

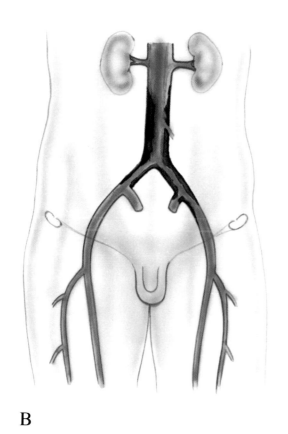

B

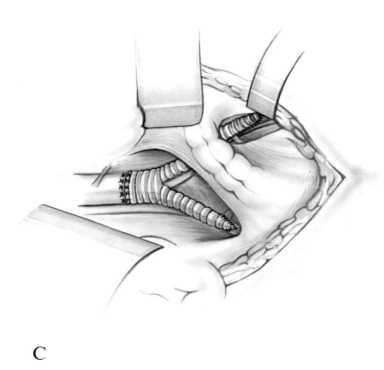

C

359

Plate 164

DIVISION OF ABDOMINAL AORTA WITH PROXIMAL ENDARTERECTOMY AND INSERTION OF A DACRON AORTIC BILATERAL FEMORAL PROSTHESIS

A.   This illustration shows severe infrarenal abdominal aortic and bilateral common iliac, external iliac and common femoral atherosclerotic disease. It is unusual not to see more involvement of the superficial femoral, popliteal and outflow vessels, but even if they are involved the same type of procedure would be performed as a first stage and later, if the patient still complains of claudication, a saphenous vein bypass graft could be carried down from the femoral limb of the aortic graft to the popliteal artery. Not infrequently, however, even with the superficial femoral artery occluded, many patients obtain sufficient relief from the implantation of a graft from the abdominal aorta to the common femoral arteries. Under rare circumstances it may be necessary to implant a femoropopliteal graft at the same operative procedure. In most patients, however, to attempt to do this routinely will result in a poor long-term patency rate for the bypass graft in the lower extremity.

B.   The abdominal aorta has been dissected free and two tourniquet clamps have been placed around it and closed; the proximal one is placed well below the renal vein and the distal one just proximal to the bifurcation of the aorta. A transverse incision is made in the aorta between them. The atheromatous core demonstrated has been partially freed up. It is important to endarterectomize the proximal abdominal aorta. This can be done more satisfactorily by not completely dividing the aorta at this stage of the procedure.

C.   This demonstrates the technique of endarterectomy of the proximal aorta. The proximal tourniquet clamp has been released and aortic control is obtained with the third and fourth fingers of the left hand of the surgeon by compression of the aorta against the lumbar vertebrae. This enables an adequate removal of the atheromatous plaques well up to the level of the renal arteries, if necessary, with a blunt, pointed, curved clamp.

D.   The endarterectomy of the proximal aorta has been completed. The aorta has been divided. It is advisable to inject 20 cc. of dilute heparin into each common iliac artery prior to closing the distal aorta. This is in addition to the 4000 units of heparin that was given intravenously before occluding the proximal aorta.

E.   The next step is to anastomose the Dacron prosthesis to the proximal aorta. This is done either with interrupted mattress sutures or, as shown, with a running everting mattress suture and then, in addition, an over-and over running suture. The suture closure of the distal end of the aorta and the common iliac arteries with a 3-0 Dacron suture is also demonstrated, using a double row of over-and-over stitches.

F.   In some patients it is advisable to explore the groins first before making the abdominal incision to make sure that there is an adequate outflow tract from the common femoral arteries to implant a graft at this level, and if not, to determine whether there is one more distal that can be used. This illustration demonstrates the completed insertion of a bifurcation aortic Dacron prosthesis from the abdominal aorta to both common femoral arteries. For the technique of the latter anastomoses, see Plates 135, 136 and 137.

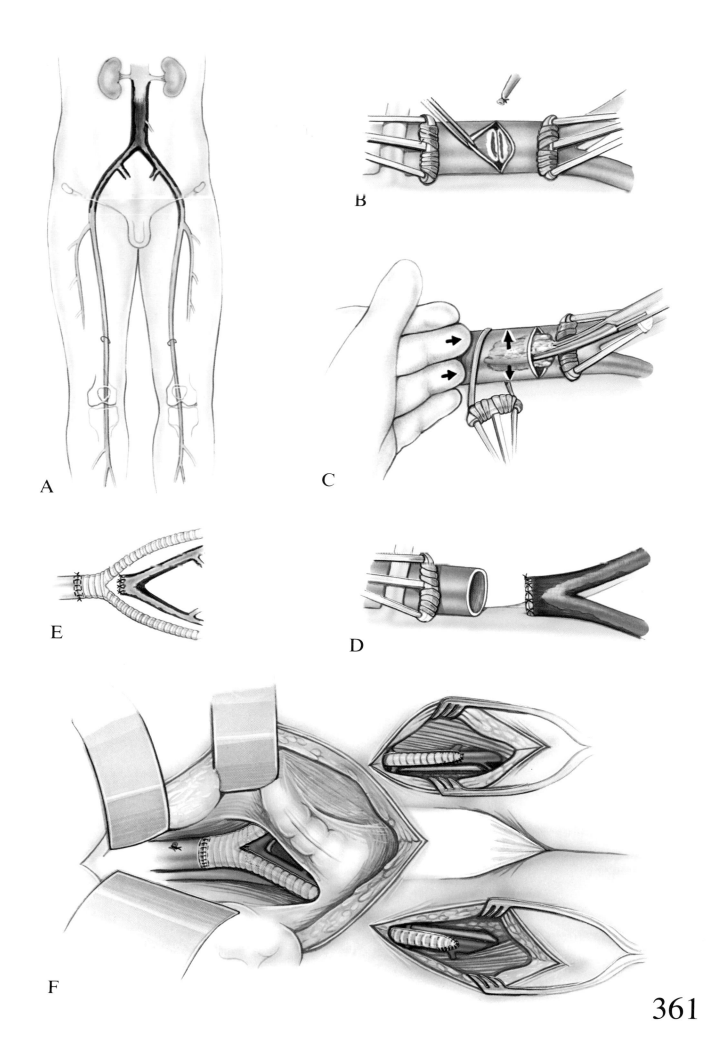

A

B

C

E

D

F

361

Plate 165

THE CORRECT AND INCORRECT METHODS OF IMPLANTING AN AORTIC BIFURCATION GRAFT BILATERALLY TO THE COMMON FEMORAL ARTERIES

A. This demonstrates atherosclerotic disease involving the infrarenal abdominal aorta, bilateral common iliac, external iliac and common femoral arteries, with symptoms of intermittent claudication.

B. This demonstrates the correct method of implanting an aortic bifurcation graft from the abdominal aorta to the common femoral arteries bilaterally by resection of the abdominal aorta and its bifurcation with interruption of the common iliac arteries, or it can be performed similarly to the procedure described in Plate 164. The advantage of these techniques is that the aortic outflow is entirely through the graft. Some blood will reflux retrograde up the external iliac artery to the hypogastric arteries, and the remainder will flow into the superficial femoral and profunda femoris arteries.

C. This demonstrates the technique of leaving the abdominal aorta in continuity and anastomosing the aortic bifurcation graft end-to-side to the abdominal aorta, using a Statinsky clamp to isolate a portion of the aorta in order to construct the end-to-side anastomosis of the graft to the aorta.

D. This demonstrates the bifurcation aortic graft implanted end-to-side to the abdominal aorta with the iliac limbs end-to-side to both common femoral arteries. The chief disadvantage to this method in such a case as the one shown in *A*, in which the aorta and iliac arteries are not totally occluded, is that the aortic blood flow will be divided between the prosthesis and the abdominal aorta. This may result in early closure of the graft if the degree of obstruction in the patient's blood vessels is not too marked, or the reverse may also take place. It has another disadvantage in that there is considerable turbulence at the site of the aortic anastomosis, which tends to produce platelet deposition and thrombus formation. It is a cardinal principle in reconstructive vascular surgery utilizing bypass grafts that the diseased arterial system should be interrupted distal to the proximal anastomosis so that the blood flow will be entirely through the graft. If a surgeon performs the proximal aortic anastomosis end-to-side, he should interrupt the common iliac arteries by ligation proximal to the hypogastric arteries. The better procedure, however, is that demonstrated in *A* and *B*.

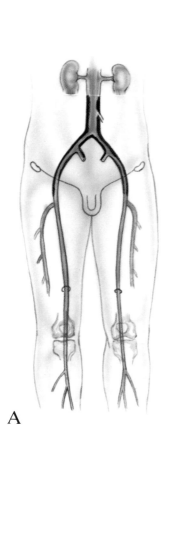

A

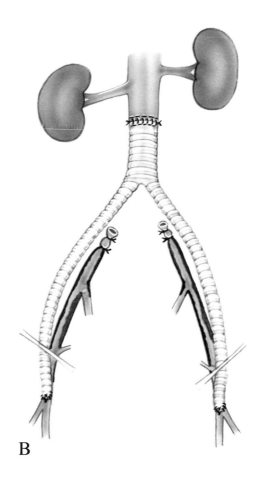

B

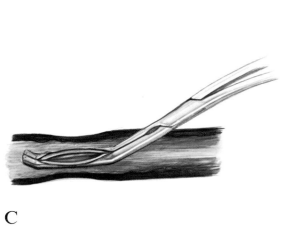

C

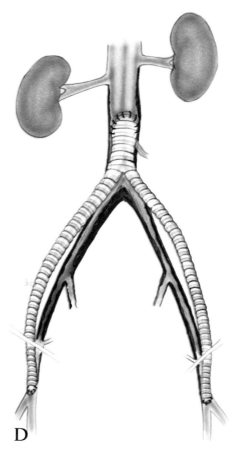

D

363

Plate 166

SUPRAPUBIC ILIOFEMORAL
AND FEMOROFEMORAL
CROSS-OVER GRAFTS

A. This demonstrates a previously implanted Dacron bifurcation graft to the right common femoral artery and the left common iliac artery. Angiographic studies revealed that the aortic graft, the left iliac limb, external iliac, common femoral and profunda femoris were open, with occlusion of the superficial femoral artery but patent popliteal and outflow vessels. On the right side the iliac limb anastomosed to the common femoral artery had become occluded. In addition, the external iliac, the origin of the profunda femoris, the superficial femoral artery, the distal popliteal and outflow vessels were occluded. The patient had extreme pain in the right foot, with beginning ischemic lesions of the toes. As he was 80 years of age and not a good surgical risk, it was elected to implant a cross-over, 6-mm., knitted, tubular, velour Dacron graft from the left external iliac artery to the profunda femoris artery of the right leg.

B. The proximal anastomosis was made by the end-to-side technique to the left external iliac artery through an extraperitoneal approach above the inguinal ligament, which is a simple and easy exposure. The graft was preclotted, then brought through a subcutaneous suprapubic tunnel to the incision in the right groin. The common femoral artery was so diseased it could not be used. For this reason the profunda femoris artery was isolated, a thrombectomy of the proximal end performed and a long end-to-end oblique type of anastomosis was made between it and the graft. The external iliac artery is preferred for the take-off of these cross-over grafts because they come off more nearly parallel to this artery and so are more streamlined than the ones that are anastomosed to the common femoral artery. They may be placed also by preference in the prevesical space.

C. This demonstrates the arterial tree in a patient with complete occlusion of the right common iliac, external iliac and superficial femoral arteries. The common femoral artery is diseased but is still patent and connected with a patent profunda femoris artery. The distal popliteal and posterior tibial arteries are patent.

D. The patient was a man age 78 years who was a good operative risk but was suffering considerably from ischemic symptoms in his right foot and so needed a reconstructive arterial procedure to save his extremity. For that reason it was elected to implant a 6-mm., double velour, knitted Dacron cross-over graft from the left common femoral artery to the right common femoral artery, the external iliac artery being too sclerotic. The left anastomosis was end-to-side off the common iliac artery. On the right side it was made to the distal portion of the common femoral artery and carried a short distance down the first portion of the profunda femoris, making a very satisfactory anastomosis. The superficial femoral artery which was occluded was ligated and divided, which made it possible to make a more streamlined anastomosis.

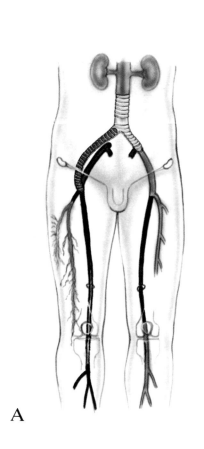

A

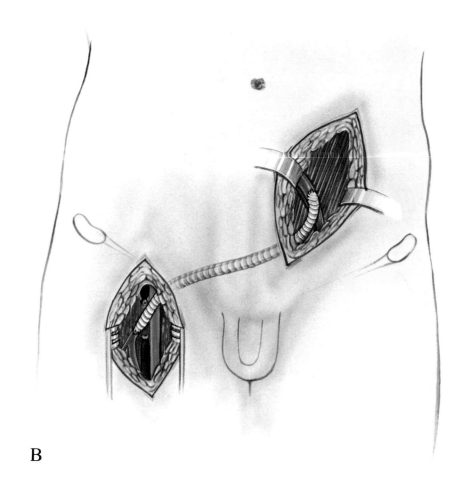

B

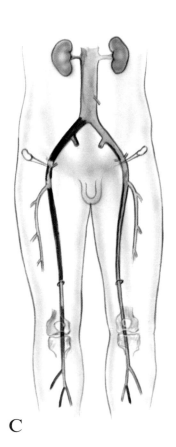

C

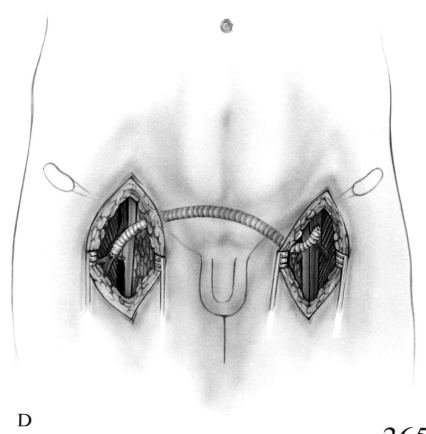

D

365

Plate 167

AXILLOFEMORAL BYPASS
DACRON GRAFT

A. This demonstrates an 8-mm., single velour Dacron graft implanted from the left axillary artery to the left common femoral artery with the outflow tract, the profunda femoris artery. There was complete occlusion of the left common iliac and superficial femoral arteries, with marked atherosclerotic disease of the right iliac and femoral arteries, so that a cross-over suprapubic graft could not have been implanted. Also, the patient's general condition, because of age and poor cardiac condition, did not warrant a transabdominal aortofemoral procedure. The femoral artery is always exposed first to make sure that this is a suitable site for implanting the graft. In some instances it may be necessary to carry the graft down to the mid portion of the profunda femoris artery because of severe disease in both the superficial femoral and the proximal end of the profunda femoris. The tunnel is also made between the two incisions before performing the proximal anastomosis, being developed between the pectoralis major and pectoralis minor muscles and carried down the mid axillary line. A small incision is made below the tenth rib to facilitate making the tunnel. The tunnel is then continued on to the femoral incision.

B. This demonstrates the exposure of the first portion of the axillary artery below the clavicle. The arm is placed at right angles to the body. The exposure is carried between the clavicular and sternal heads of the pectoralis major muscle. The coracoclavicular fascia is opened. The medial edge of the pectoralis minor muscle is exposed and is retracted laterally. The dissection is then carried down to expose the first portion of the axillary artery and vein. There may be a few venous branches and a small arterial branch that need to be interrupted. An 8-mm., single velour, knitted Dacron graft, which had been previously preclotted, is anastomosed to the axillary artery by the end-to-side technique. After completion of the anastomosis, the bulldog clamps are removed from the axillary artery and one placed on the prosthesis just distal to the anastomosis to restore blood flow to the left arm.

C. The graft is then brought down through the tunnel to the femoral incision and anastomosed either to the common femoral artery as shown with only the outflow tract to the profunda femoris or, in some instances, carried down to the mid profunda if the proximal portion is too severely involved with atheromatous plaques. The construction of the anastomosis is performed by any of the different methods shown in Plate 169. The incisions are closed in layers with fine interrupted sutures of linen and cotton and with mattress stitches of silk to the skin.

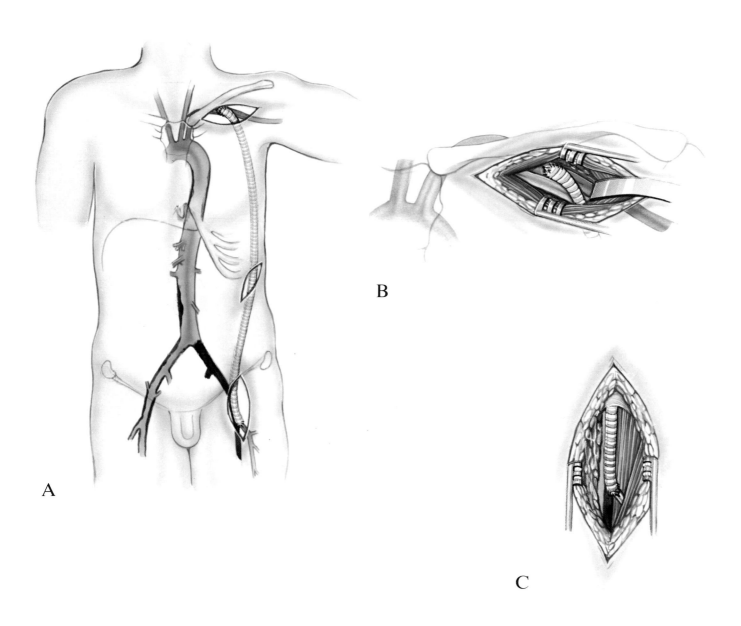

A

B

C

367

Plate 167 (Continued)

AORTOFEMORAL BYPASS
DACRON GRAFT

D. This demonstrates a knitted Dacron tubular graft implanted from the abdominal aorta to the common femoral artery in a patient with severe atherosclerotic disease whose right iliac and femoral system were patent; however, the arteries were too calcified to perform a satisfactory iliofemoral or femorofemoral crossover graft. Both anastomoses were performed end-to-side. The aortic anastomosis was performed, using a Statinsky clamp as shown in Plate 165 C. The distal anastomosis was end-to-side to the distal end of the common femoral artery since both profunda femoris and superficial femoral arteries were patent. It is believed this is a more satisfactory procedure and will give better long-term patency than an axillofemoral bypass if the patient's condition warrants this more major procedure. It is possible to do it through an extraperitoneal approach, but for a short operative procedure such as this the transperitoneal facilitates the construction of the proximal anastomosis.

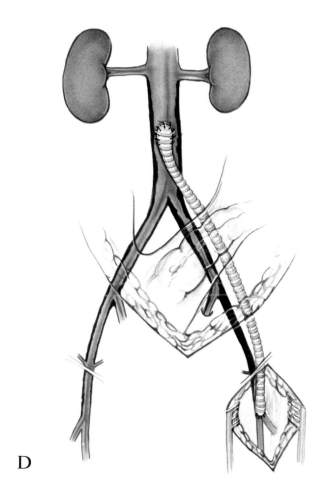

D

Plate 168

ILIOFEMORAL BYPASS
DACRON GRAFT,
RETROPERITONEAL METHOD

A. This demonstrates atherosclerotic occlusive disease in the right common iliac and external iliac arteries with complete occlusion of the latter; this is not suitable for endarterectomy because of the flimsy structure of the common femoral and external iliac arteries. The bypass graft was implanted from the proximal end of the common iliac artery to the distal end of the common femoral artery because the latter anastomosis is much more readily accomplished by making a relatively long end-to-side type of anastomosis; this, at the same time, increases the caliber of the common femoral artery, often an advantage when there is a large posterior plaque that it is best not to remove.

B. This demonstrates the location of the incisions: the abdominal one is a right pararectus extended obliquely proximally toward the costal arch; the lower one is the routine incision used for exposure of femoral vessels.

C. This demonstrates the double exposure. Through the pararectus incision the fascia of the external oblique, internal oblique and transversalis muscles is divided. The rectus muscle is retracted medialward. The nerve supply to the very distal portion is usually divided, but the other nerves are preserved. The peritoneum is stripped out of the right iliac fossa and is carefully separated from the transversalis fascia, which is divided and then retracted medially with the intestines. This gives very good exposure of the right external iliac, hypogastric and common iliac arteries. The femoral arteries are exposed in the routine manner in the femoral triangle. A tourniquet clamp is placed around the proximal end of the right common iliac artery; bulldog clamps are placed on the hypogastric and external iliac arteries. The ureter can be seen crossing over the external iliac artery and vein between the two bulldog clamps. A longitudinal arteriotomy has been made in the common iliac artery where it is essentially normal. Bulldog clamps are shown on the right common femoral, superficial femoral and profunda femoris arteries but are not placed there until after the proximal anastomosis of the graft to the common iliac arteries has been made.

D. This demonstrates the 8-mm., knitted, single velour Dacron graft that has been implanted end-to-side to the common iliac artery and the common femoral artery at its bifurcation. The graft is usually preclotted before performing the anastomoses, which are done according to the technique described in Plates 135 to 137. The groin incision is closed in layers with fine interrupted linen sutures. The abdominal incision is also closed in layers, using interrupted mattress sutures of linen or cotton to the fascia of the transversalis, internal oblique and external oblique. Stay sutures of nylon are also used. The skin is closed with interrupted mattress sutures of silk. The retroperitoneal area is drained for 24 hours with Penrose drains brought out through a stab incision in the flank. The ureter can be seen crossing over the graft just distal to the hypogastric artery. It is usual to place the graft behind it, but as yet no trouble has been encountered if the graft has been placed over it. If for some reason reoperation is necessary in the late follow-up period, there are advantages in having the ureter posterior to the graft since there is much less danger of injuring it under these conditions. In most instances, however, it seems preferable to place it anterior just in case it might become obstructed. Actually, it seems to make little difference in which location the ureter is placed.

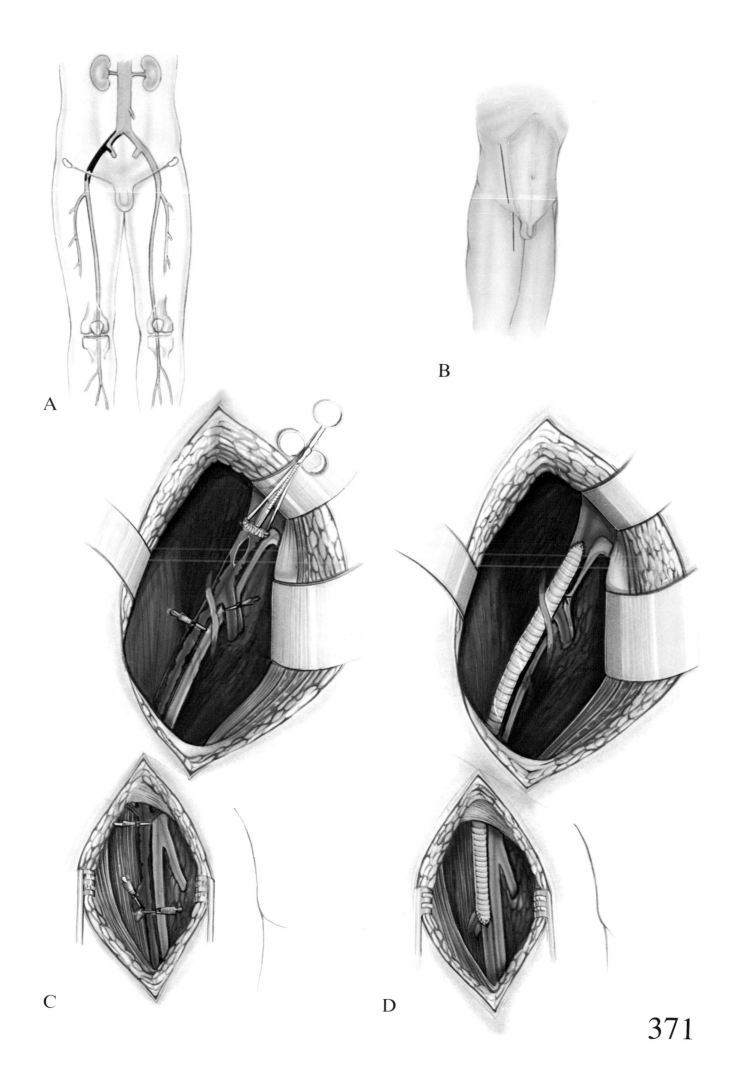

A

B

C

D

371

Plate 169

TECHNIQUE OF ANASTOMOSIS
OF KNITTED DACRON
GRAFT TO PROFUNDA
FEMORIS ARTERY

A. There are many instances when the only outflow tract to the lower limb from the femoral artery is the profunda femoris artery, so it is important to understand the various methods of constructing the anastomosis between the knitted Dacron graft and the relatively small profunda femoris artery. This illustration demonstrates one very satisfactory method of performing it by interrupting the superficial femoral artery close to its origin. The distal end is usually ligated and the anastomosis is then constructed to the distal end of the common femoral artery, utilizing the small cuff of superficial femoral artery so as not to encroach on the lumen of the profunda femoris. This gives a satisfactory streamlined anastomosis.

B. This is a similar procedure without division of the superficial femoral artery and still making the anastomosis essentially to the very terminal cuff of the common femoral artery and a very small part of the proximal end of the superficial femoral artery. The proximal ligature eliminates any cul-de-sac in which a thrombus might form and then propagate into the anastomotic site. One advantage of this method over the one shown in *A* is that the superficial femoral artery is left in continuity, which lends stability to the anastomosis as there is less danger of the prosthesis tending to twist the profunda femoris artery. The decision of which method to use will depend on the condition of the terminal part of the common femoral artery.

C. This demonstrates a more distal anastomosis to the proximal end of the profunda femoris artery, yet still using a portion of the cuff of the distal end of the common femoral artery. This, of necessity, requires division of the superficial femoral artery to permit the anastomosis to be made streamlined and carried distally on the profunda femoris after endarterectomizing the proximal end of it. It is thought that this gives better long-term patency than applying a patch graft to the profunda femoris and implanting the Dacron prosthesis to the common femoral artery.

D. This demonstrates extensive occlusive atherosclerotic disease involving the external iliac artery with complete occlusion of the common femoral and superficial femoral arteries and of the proximal portion of the profunda femoris artery down to its bifurcation. Under these conditions it is found more advantageous to implant the prosthesis more distally in the profunda femoris artery rather than to endarterectomize so much of the proximal end of it and place the anastomosis at the bifurcation of the profunda femoris. Not infrequently with serious disease in the proximal profunda femoris the artery is found to have soft pliable walls and a good lumen, so that a satisfactory end-to-side anastomosis, as shown, can be constructed between the prosthesis and the mid portion of the profunda femoris artery. In a few instances it has been necessary to implant the graft to the distal end of the lateral circumflex branch of the profunda femoris for salvage of an extremity. It is remarkable what satisfactory results can be accomplished with revascularization of the profunda femoris artery and its branches, so when necessary these procedures should be performed.

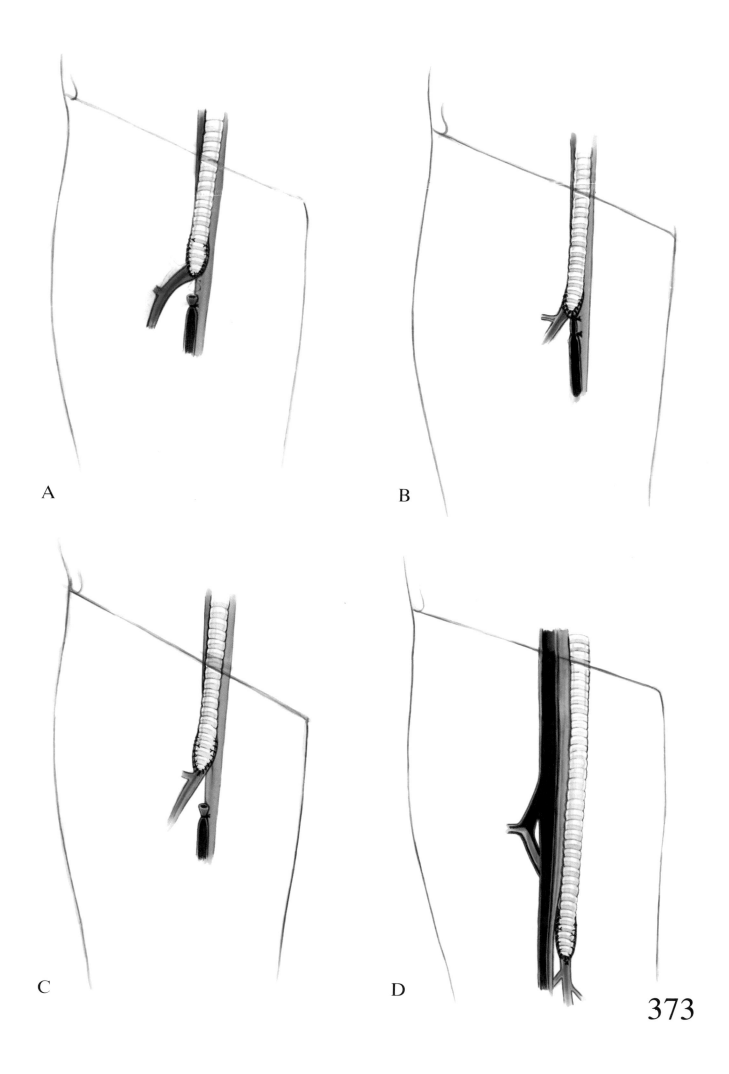

A

B

C

D

373

Plate 170

AORTIC BILATERAL FEMORAL KNITTED DACRON GRAFT AND SAPHENOUS VEIN BYPASS AUTOGRAFT FROM LEFT ILIAC LIMB OF GRAFT TO DISTAL POPLITEAL ARTERY

A. This demonstrates complete occlusion of the abdominal aorta secondary to atherosclerosis with proximal thrombus formation, occlusion of the common iliac arteries and severe atherosclerotic disease of the external iliac and common femoral arteries. There is also complete occlusion of the left superficial femoral artery and severe disease of the left profunda femoris artery. The distal popliteal artery and the outflow arteries are patent.

B. An endarterectomy and a thrombectomy of the proximal abdominal aorta have been performed. The distal abdominal aorta has been resected, the common iliac arteries ligated, and an aortic bifurcation knitted Dacron prosthesis implanted, using interrupted mattress sutures. The distal anastomoses were end-to-side to both common femoral arteries. On the left side, because of complete occlusion of the superficial femoral artery and advanced atherosclerotic changes in the profunda femoris, it was necessary to implant a saphenous vein bypass autograft from the iliac limb of the Dacron prosthesis in the groin to the distal popliteal artery by the end-to-side technique, which is one of the easiest anastomoses to construct.

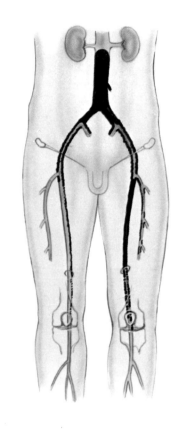

A

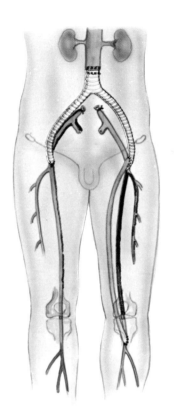

B

375

Plate 170 (Continued)

AORTIC BILATERAL ILIAC KNITTED DACRON GRAFT WITH BILATERAL KNITTED DACRON TUBULAR GRAFTS TO RENAL ARTERIES

C. This demonstrates atherosclerotic disease of the abdominal aorta and the origins of the renal arteries with resulting secondary hypertension. The exposure is obtained with the usual long paramedian or midline abdominal incision, exposing the aorta, the renal arteries and the inferior vena cava through an incision in the posterior peritoneum. The exposure of the right renal artery can be facilitated by freeing up the right colon and then retracting it and the small intestine cephalad. Another approach is to reflect the spleen, the pancreas and the left colon to the right and expose the aorta and the renal arteries retroperitoneally. The illustration shows a tourniquet clamp on the aorta placed above the renal arteries. In this patient the left renal vein passed posterior to the aorta, which facilitated the exposure. Even with the left renal vein anterior to the aorta, a tourniquet clamp can be placed proximal to the renal arteries and distal to the superior mesenteric artery in most patients. Bulldog clamps have been placed on the proximal end of the common iliac arteries to permit collateral blood flow through the hypogastrics into the external iliac and femoral arteries.

D. This demonstrates the completed aortic and renal artery reconstructive grafting procedure. In this case, a bifurcation graft was used. Some surgeons may prefer a tubular aortic graft, but with disease in the iliac arteries the bifurcation graft was the best for this patient. Six-millimeter, knitted Dacron tubular grafts are anastomosed to the aortic graft; they are all preclotted before inserting the grafts. The renal arteries are divided. Ten cubic centimeters of dilute heparin saline solution are injected into the renal arteries distally, then bulldog clamps placed on them. One usually has at least an hour or longer before renal damage will occur after occluding the renal arteries, and it may be even longer. After the aortic and renal artery anastomoses have been completed and the aorta flushed out, a clamp is placed on the prosthesis distal to the renal grafts to allow blood to flow to the kidneys. It is then a simple procedure to complete the distal anastomoses as shown in the illustration.

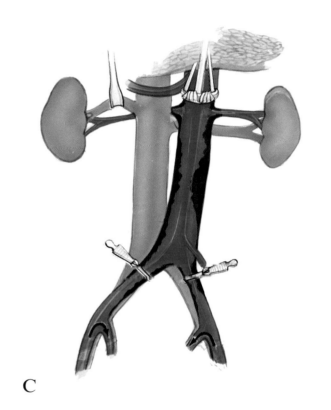

C

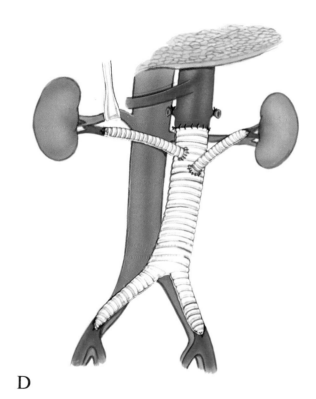

D

377

Plate 171

INNOMINATE ARTERY
ENDARTERECTOMY

A. This demonstrates the location of the supraclavicular sternum-splitting type of incision that gives the best exposure of the innominate artery at its origin from the arch of the aorta to its bifurcation into the common carotid and the subclavian arteries.

B. The cervical portion of the incision is carried through the sternocleidomastoid, the sternohyoid and sternothyroid muscles near their insertion into the manubrium. The sternum is split, and the dissection in the right upper mediastinum demonstrates the arch of the aorta (a), the left innominate (b) and the right innominate (c) veins, which join together to form the superior vena cava. The innominate artery (d) is partially hidden by the left innominate vein, but its bifurcation into the right common carotid (e) and right subclavian arteries (f) is visible. The right vagus nerve is seen crossing the subclavian artery, and circling around behind it is seen the right recurrent laryngeal nerve.

C. The left innominate vein has been doubly ligated and divided, allowing the distal end to retract, which exposes the innominate artery to much better advantage, especially its origin; just beyond it is seen the left common carotid artery.

D. Fifteen minutes after 4000 units of heparin have been given intravenously to completely heparinize the patient, arterial control of the innominate artery is obtained with a curved clamp with narrow blades and multiple fine teeth. This is placed on the aorta proximal to the innominate artery because the atheromatous plaque protrudes in some cases into the aortic lumen. Distal control is obtained with bulldog clamps on the right common carotid and right subclavian arteries.

E. The large atheromatous plaque that almost completely occludes the innominate artery is demonstrated. It has a thin, clear-cut distal edge at the origin of the subclavian and common carotid arteries. The main part of the plaque is elevated with a Penfield dura elevator. In some cases the atheromatous plaques extend distally into the origin of the common carotid and subclavian arteries. It is important to clear out the former especially, making sure that no free intimal flap is left at the distal end of the endarterectomy.

F. This demonstrates the lumen of the innominate artery after completion of the endarterectomy. All the atheromatous plaques and most of the media have been removed. Note that the intima distal to its bifurcation has thinned out and is firmly adherent to the arterial wall, so that it is not necessary to suture it down.

G. This demonstrates the completed operation, with the arteriotomy closed by use of a running over-and-over type of suture; all the occluding clamps have been removed and the arterial blood flow re-established through it and the subclavian and common carotid arteries. The clamps on the aortic arch and the subclavian artery are removed first to permit blood to flow down the arm before releasing the clamp on the common carotid artery; this will assure that no clot or air emboli are carried into the cerebral circulation. The sternum incision is closed with stainless steel wire sutures. The muscles at the base of the neck are sutured back to their points of insertion with linen or cotton sutures, and the skin is closed with mattress sutures of silk or synthetic material. In some instances it may be advisable to drain the mediastinum for 24 hours; if the pleura has been opened inadvertently, the pleural space should be drained.

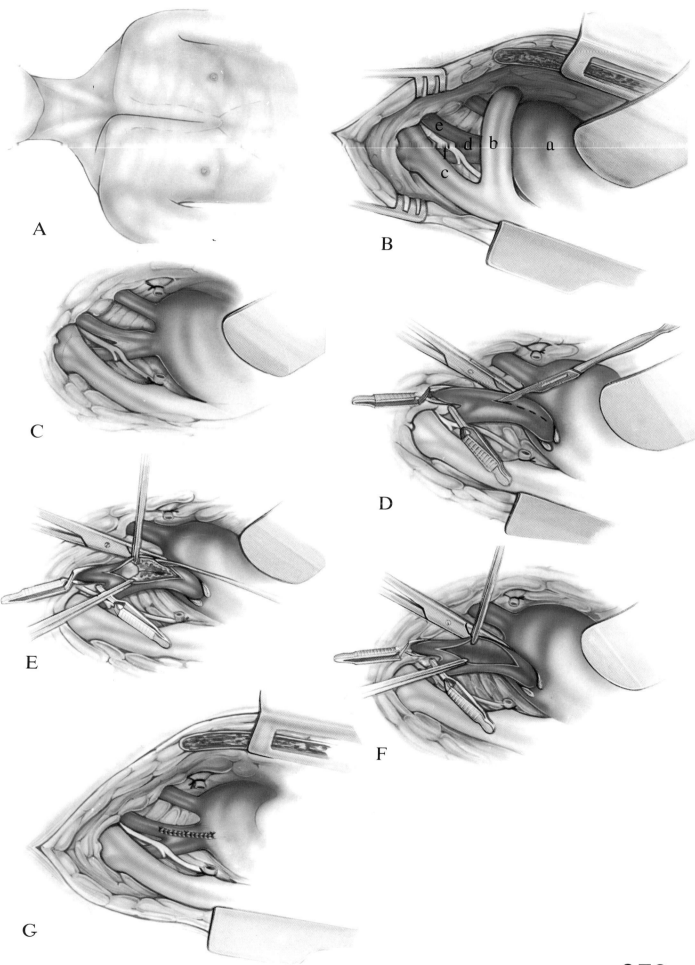

A

B

e
f d b a
c

C

D

E

F

G

379

Plate 172

ENDARTERECTOMY OF THE RIGHT COMMON, INTERNAL AND EXTERNAL CAROTID ARTERIES

A. The carotid arteries are best exposed through an incision at the anterior border of the sternocleidomastoid muscle placed about a centimeter posterior to the angle of the jaw to avoid injury to the mandibular branch of the facial nerve.

B. The external jugular vein is ligated and divided and the dissection is carried down to the common carotid artery and the internal jugular vein. The facial vein is ligated and divided, then the artery and vein are separated. The ansahypoglossal nerve (a) is retracted laterally. The bifurcation of the common carotid artery is localized. The dissection is carried distally to expose the hypoglossal nerve (b), seen coursing obliquely over the internal and external carotid arteries. This nerve varies somewhat in position and is shown more distally on the arteries than it is usually encountered. As it is a motor nerve to the tongue, it should be dissected free and trauma to it carefully avoided. The superior thyroid artery (c) is freed up, and also the lingual artery, the next branch of the external carotid. The dissection is carried between the internal and external carotid arteries after injection of 1 per cent lidocaine solution in this area to anesthetize the carotid body. There may be a small artery arising from the bifurcation of the common carotid that needs to be controlled. Three thousand units of heparin are injected into the internal jugular vein.

C. After 15 minutes arterial control is obtained with a large bulldog clamp on the common carotid artery and two smaller ones on the internal and external carotid arteries. The superior thyroid and the lingual arteries are controlled with small silver clips, which are removed after suture of the arteriotomy.

D. A longitudinal arteriotomy is performed in the common carotid and the internal carotid artery beyond the upper edge of the atheromatous plaque. Note the ulcerated nature of the plaque in the common carotid and the origin of the internal carotid. At the apex of the arteriotomy, however, in the internal carotid artery the intima is very smooth, thin and normal in appearance.

E. The bulldog clamp on the internal carotid artery has been temporarily released. This demonstrates a brisk backflow of arterial blood, a positive Henle-Coenen sign. It is unnecessary to use a bypass graft when such an excellent backflow is observed since it indicates an adequate collateral blood supply. If the blood merely dribbles out of the internal carotid artery, a bypass graft should be used.

F. If a bypass graft is not used, it is very important to inject 10 cc. of dilute heparin saline solution (20 units per 1 cc.) into the distal end of the internal carotid artery, using a fine polyvinyl catheter. This is additional insurance against a blood clot forming in the extracranial portion of the internal carotid artery. If a clot were present when the circulation is restored, it would embolize the intracranial arterial system with resulting hemiplegia. It is also important to make sure that there is no air in the polyvinyl tubing or syringe, since an air embolus will result in serious brain damage.

G. The endarterectomy has been commenced on the near side of the arteriotomy, freeing up the thick atheromatous plaque with a Penfield dura elevator (a).

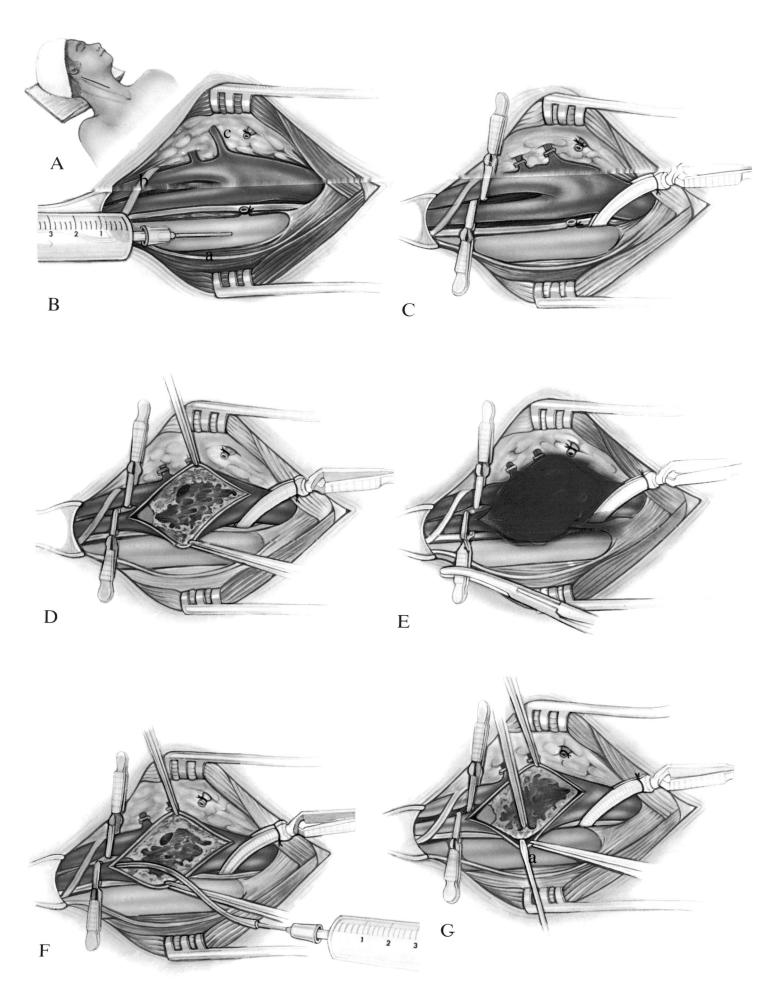

A

B

C

D

E

F

G

381

Plate 173

ENDARTERECTOMY OF THE RIGHT COMMON, INTERNAL AND EXTERNAL CAROTID ARTERIES *(Continued)*

A.   The atheromatous plaque is elevated with a small, right-angled clamp.

B.   The thin normal media and intima are carefully divided at the distal end of the thick atheromatous plaque, using fine-pointed, curved scissors. This is a very important step and should be done carefully so as not to leave any loose intimal flaps that might be a nidus for a thrombus to develop. If done with care using fine scissors, the distal edge of the media and intima will remain firmly attached to the adventitia and so will not need suturing. After completing this it is a simple matter to remove the large plaque to the proximal end of the arteriotomy, again making certain that no loose intima plaque edges are left at the proximal end of the endarterectomy.

C.   Any loose intimal fragments are carefully cut away with fine curved scissors as shown. These are most apt to occur near the orifice of the external iliac artery.

D.   It should be noted the arteriotomy was carried distally only in the internal carotid artery since this is the most important artery to endarterectomize perfectly. However, there is frequently a thick plaque involving the orifice and a short distance distally of the external carotid artery; this can be cleared out as shown with a curved Schnitt type of clamp. The end point of the endarterectomy, of course, cannot be seen, but many times the patency of the artery can be re-established.

E.   The endarterectomy has been completed. This shows the small triangle of normal intima on the posterior wall of the proximal end of the internal carotid and the distal end of the common carotid arteries. The cleaned out proximal lumen of the external carotid artery is also shown. Note that the intima of the internal carotid and the common carotid arteries have not been sutured down, as the large plaque was removed without leaving any loose flaps at either end of the endarterectomy.

F.   A short segment of a polyvinyl catheter that fits the lumen of the internal carotid artery snugly, but not too tightly, has been inserted. This is used as a stent for the closure of the internal carotid arteriotomy. One stay suture is being placed approximately a third of the distance down the arteriotomy and another one will be placed an equal distance farther proximally to hold the stent in place.

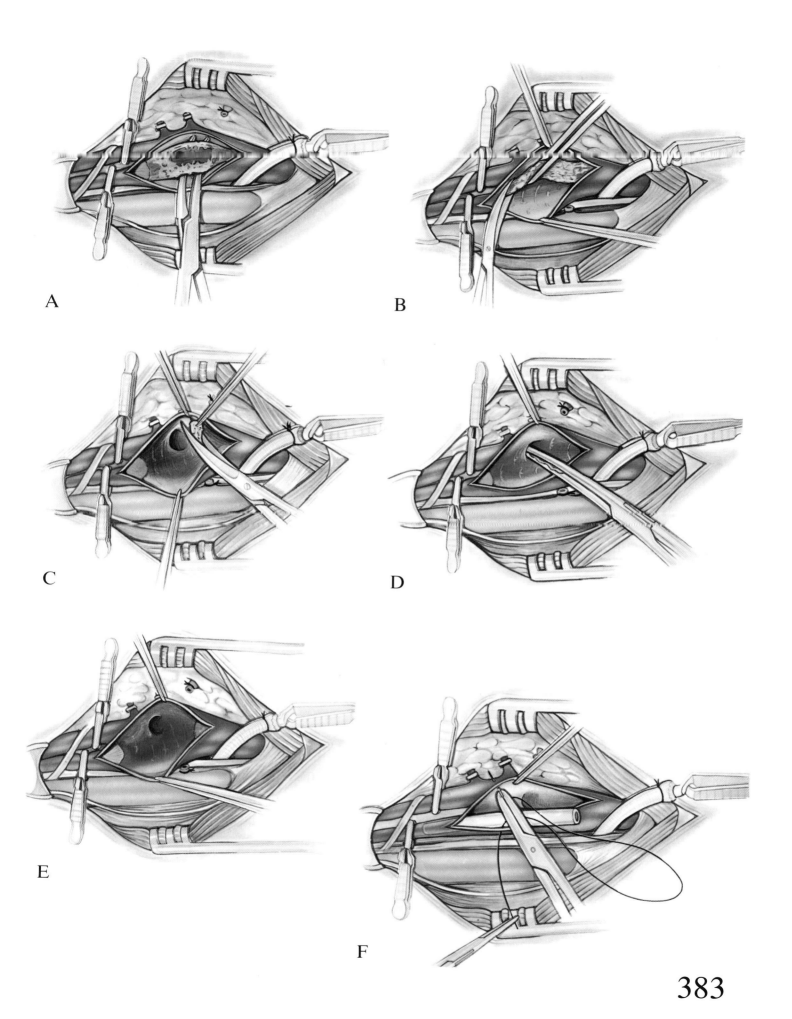

A

B

C

D

E

F

383

Plate 174

ENDARTERECTOMY OF THE RIGHT COMMON, INTERNAL AND EXTERNAL CAROTID ARTERIES *(Continued)*

A. This demonstrates the stent in place and the over-and-over suture of the internal carotid artery portion of the arteriotomy. It is customary to use a 6-0 monofilament synthetic or a Teflon-coated Dacron suture. The great advantage of the stent is that it obviates the necessity of using a patch graft to close the arteriotomy because, with the fine needle and suture, it is possible to take very small bites of tissue that produce a smooth, streamlined, evenly closed arteriotomy. The suturing is then continued proximally to the stay suture to which it is tied. The stent is removed after the common carotid artery portion of the arteriotomy has been reached. The common carotid artery is so large that a stent is not necessary, but great care should be taken nevertheless to obtain a smooth, neat closure of it.

B. This demonstrates the completed suturing of the arteriotomy. The bulldog clamps are still in place. Dilute heparin saline solution is being injected into the common carotid artery to determine if there are any leaks in the suture line which can be closed with individual stitches, if present, instead of struggling with them after the blood flow has been re-established.

C. Sometimes there is some leakage from the suture line that does not require individual stitches. This can be controlled very quickly by placing a piece of rubber sheeting (a) over the arteriotomy; then a rolled up gauze sponge (b) is placed over the sheeting and pressure is exerted against it and the artery.

D. The self-retaining retractor has been removed. The skin edges of the neck incision are brought together and held with towel clips. This produces moderate pressure against the gauze roll and rubber sheeting. This is a quick and satisfactory method of controlling this type of bleeding because the rubber is very thrombogenic, and when it is removed it does not pull the blood clot away with it, as so often occurs if only the gauze sponges are used.

E. This demonstrates the completed endarterectomy with all the bulldog clamps and the silver clips removed. The hypoglossal and the vagus nerves are intact. The incision is closed with one layer of interrupted fine linen or cotton sutures in the deep fascia, and interrupted synthetic mattress sutures to the skin. In some cases, because of continued oozing, probably the result of heparin administration, a small Penrose tubing is used for drainage; it is removed in 24 hours. It has never been necessary to neutralize the effect of the heparin.

F. It is customary at all operations to have a shunt ready to use if necessary. These can be made readily out of a polyvinyl pediatric feeding tube, size 8 French. Approximately 15 cm. of the end of the tube is selected for the shunt. The smooth end is the one inserted into the internal carotid artery and the cut end, in which another opening has been made, is placed in the common carotid artery. Four-0 silk sutures arc wrapped around the graft and tied. These are used to suture the shunt to the edge of the arteriotomy at each end and to prevent the graft from slipping out during the endarterectomy procedure.

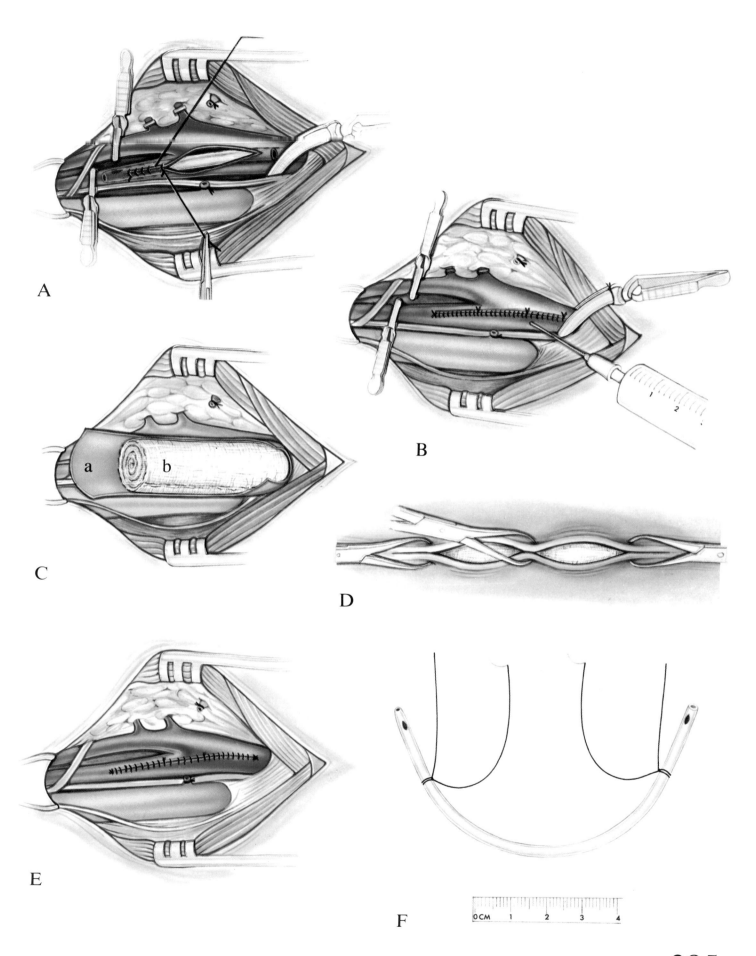

A

B

C

a   b

D

E

F

385

Plate 175

INTERNAL CAROTID BYPASS GRAFT

A. The plastic bypass graft has been inserted and the stay sutures holding it in place have been tied. It is very important in inserting this graft that no air be allowed to escape distally to embolize the intracranial arterial circulation, so it is best to insert the proximal end first, allowing blood to flow out through it to evacuate all the air in it before inserting the other end into the common carotid artery. The common carotid and internal carotid arteries are controlled with a double loop of 0 silk sutures around each that is held snugly with a small hemostat. The long bypass graft permits an easy access to the arterial plaques to perform the endarterectomy, whereas a short one within the arteriotomy tends to handicap the procedure.

B. After completion of the endarterectomy the plastic graft is used in the internal carotid artery as a stent. It is also left in place while closing the proximal end of the common carotid section of the arteriotomy. Both these arteries are then controlled with bulldog clamps as the graft is removed so that the arteriotomy closure can be completed.

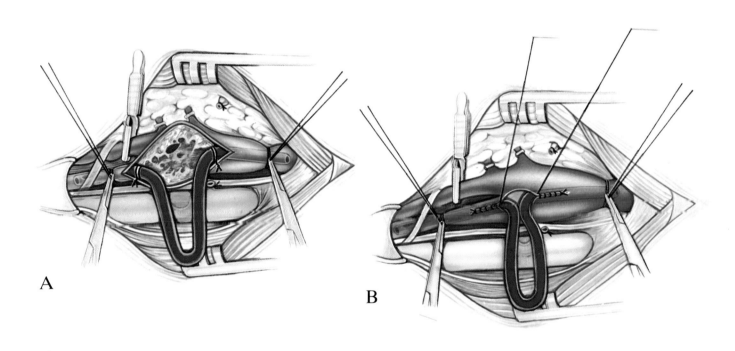

A

B

387

Plate 175 (Continued)

EXCISION OF CAROTID BODY TUMOR

C. This demonstrates a large carotid body tumor, which can be seen bulging out through the left side of the neck. The line of the incision used to excise it is shown. These tumors are pulsatile and have a loud bruit over them, so occasionally surgeons operate on them with the mistaken diagnosis of a carotid arterial aneurysm. If there is any doubt as to the diagnosis, a preliminary angiogram should be obtained. They are extremely vascular, so it is important to stay outside their ill defined capsule, thus enabling the resection to be carried out without too much bleeding, since hemorrhage here is difficult to control.

D. The carotid body tumor is demonstrated lying between and posterior to the internal carotid artery (a) and the external carotid artery (b). The hypoglossal nerve (c) is shown coursing over the distal end of the tumor. The internal jugular vein has been displaced laterally and posteriorly. The vagus nerve (d) can be seen proximal to the tumor and lying posterior to it. Numerous small blood vessels, that are the blood supply of the tumor, can be seen arising from the internal and external carotid arteries.

E. It is seldom necessary to resect the internal carotid artery and implant a graft to restore arterial continuity because it is possible by very careful dissection to isolate the small arteries arising from the internal and external carotid arteries and ligate them with fine, nonabsorbable ligatures, thus preserving the arteries intact as shown. The hypoglossal nerve and the vagus nerve can also be preserved in the great majority of cases.

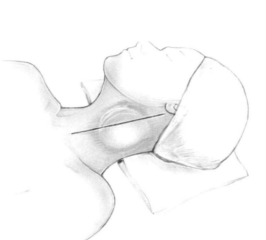

C

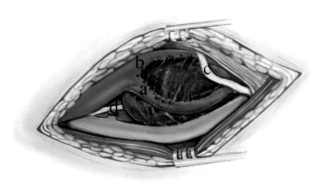

D

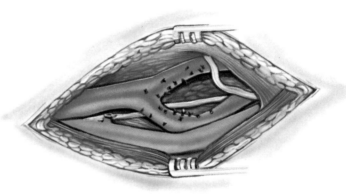

E

Plate 176

RECONSTRUCTIVE ARTERIAL PROCEDURE FOR THROMBOSED COMMON FEMORAL ANEURYSM WITH OCCLUSION OF SUPERFICIAL FEMORAL AND PROFUNDA FEMORIS ARTERIES

A. An oblique longitudinal incision is made from 5 to 8 cm. above the inguinal ligament to 5 or 6 cm. distal to the aneurysm. The procedure is done under general inhalation or catheter epidural anesthesia.

B. The distal end of the external iliac artery proximal to the aneurysm and the superficial femoral and profunda femoris arteries distal to it are isolated. The common femoral artery is carefully dissected free proximal to the aneurysm. The inguinal ligament is divided if necessary to obtain more adequate proximal control. A bulldog clamp is placed proximal to the aneurysm; distal control at this stage is unnecessary because the outflow arteries are occluded. The aneurysm is opened through a long arteriotomy. The patient is given 4000 units of heparin intravenously during this exploratory part of the operation.

C. The intrasaccular thrombus has been removed from the aneurysm. The common femoral artery has been divided proximal to it and a longitudinal arteriotomy performed in the anterior wall to facilitate the implantation of the graft. The major portion of the aneurysmal sac has been resected. A thrombus that had been propagated into the profunda femoris was removed with a curved Schnitt clamp, a bulldog clamp having been placed distal to the thrombus to control the backbleeding after the thrombectomy. It was released after clearing out the proximal portion of the artery, which demonstrated an excellent backflow from the profunda femoris artery. The lateral circumflex branch is also demonstrated arising from the profunda femoris.

D. A short 8-mm., knitted Dacron graft is then sutured end-to-end by the end-to-side technique with Teflon-coated 4- or 5-0 Dacron sutures. A longer end-to-side anastomosis is then made, with the distal end of the graft between the posterior wall of the aneurysmal sac proximal and distal to the origin of the profunda femoris artery. The posterior wall of the distal part of the graft has been cut away obliquely to facilitate the construction of a long anastomosis. The proximal end of the anastomosis is commenced with the double needle suture (a) of 4-0 Teflon-coated Dacron. After tying the mattress stitch it is used to commence the anastomotic suture line. The needle of suture (a) first passes through the graft and the cuff of the aneurysmal sac as shown, which constitutes an over-and-over type of stitch.

E. Suture (a) is then brought back, passing it through only the cuff of the aneurysm and thus making a mattress stitch; then it continues on, alternating the same type of stitch as is shown in *D.* After it is carried to the midpoint of the anastomosis, it is tied to a stay suture. The proximal half of the other side of the anastomosis is then completed in a similar manner, using the other needle end of suture (a). After completing one half of the anastomosis with suture (a), each end is tied to a stay suture, then the distal half of the anastomosis is completed by mattress suture (b), using the same method of stitching.

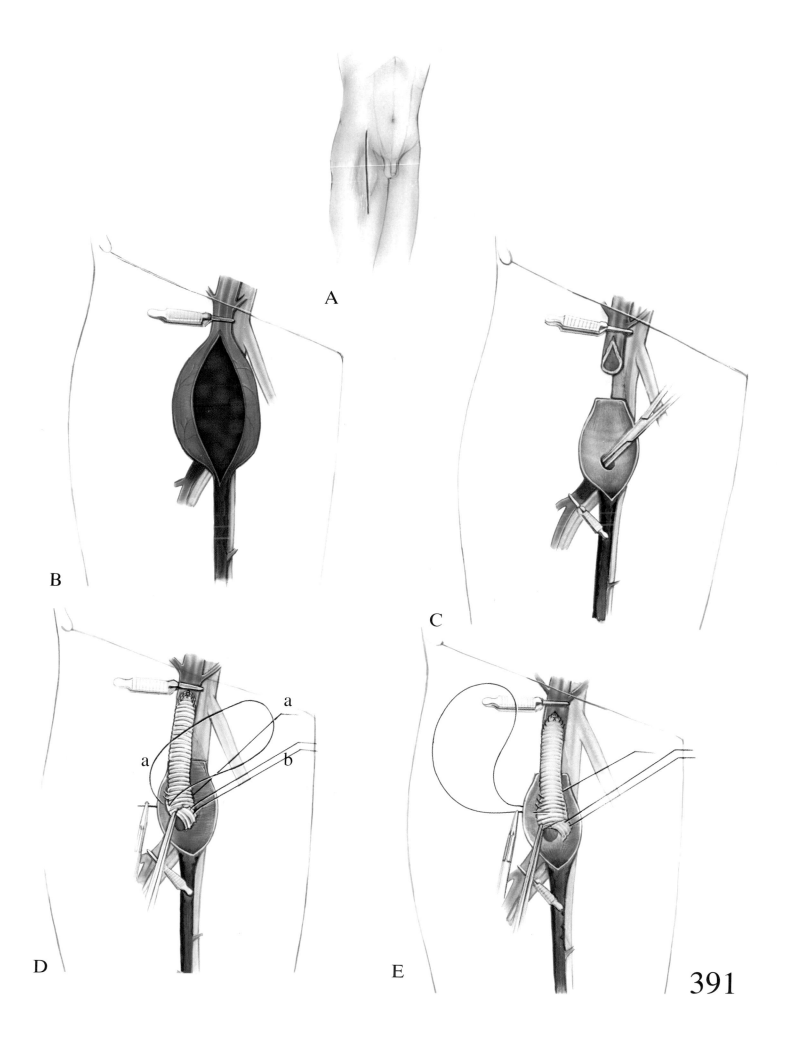

A

B

C

D

a
a
a
b

E

391

Plate 177

RECONSTRUCTIVE ARTERIAL PROCEDURE FOR THROMBOSED COMMON FEMORAL ANEURYSM AND FOR PULSATILE COMMON FEMORAL ANEURYSM

A. The implantation of the graft is completed, with the proximal anastomosis to the proximal common femoral artery and the distal one to the posterior portion of the aneurysmal sac that includes the origin of the profunda femoris artery. The superficial femoral artery has been ligated. In some instances the extra free edges of the sac can be excised so that the suture line of the anastomosis is performed with a continuous over-and-over type of stitch.

B. Sometimes, however, because the edges are so thin-walled, reinforcement of the suture line is recommended. This is accomplished by suturing the free edges of the aneurysmal sac across the distal end of the prosthesis, which will control suture line bleeding. This cuff must not be too tight, as it will narrow the anastomotic lumen. It is important not to use too much of the posterior aneurysmal sac at the site of anastomosis because this will result in another aneurysm. The lumen at the site of the anastomosis should be reconstructed so that it is the same caliber as the prosthesis.

C. This demonstrates a longer incision for a more extensive reconstructive procedure because, in addition to a thrombosed femoral aneurysm, the external iliac artery is occluded and the profunda femoris artery badly diseased. The proximal part of the superficial femoral artery was occluded, but it was patent from the mid thigh distally and satisfactory for the implantation of a graft.

D. The operative procedure consists of implanting a knitted Dacron aortic bifurcation prosthesis, with the left iliac to the left common femoral artery and the right one to the cuff of the femoral aneurysm, as demonstrated in Plate 176. An additional knitted Dacron tubular graft 6 mm. in diameter is then implanted end-to-side to the right iliac limb of the aortic graft and end-to-side to the superficial femoral artery 20 cm. beyond the origin of the profunda femoris artery. If the superficial femoral artery is not suitable for implanting the graft, a long saphenous vein bypass autograft, or if that is not long enough, a composite graft (consisting of a tubular proximal Dacron graft and a distal short segment of saphenous vein autograft to cross the knee joint area) is anastomosed to the iliac limb and carried down to the distal popliteal artery. (See Plates 202, 203, and 204.)

E. This demonstrates an excellent method of reconstructing the femoral arteries after excising a femoral aneurysm, using a graft of the long saphenous vein anastomosed end-to-end by the end-to-side technique to the proximal common femoral artery and distally to the proximal end of the superficial femoral artery. The proximal portion of the profunda femoris artery had to be removed, so another section of the saphenous vein was anastomosed end-to-side to the main saphenous vein graft and then end-to-end by the end-to-side technique to the profunda femoris artery. If the saphenous vein is not of sufficient caliber, a knitted Dacron prosthesis is implanted by the same technique. The continuity of the profunda femoris artery should always be restored if possible in case the superficial femoral artery becomes occluded as the result of an advance in the atherosclerotic disease in it; this would result in occlusion of the saphenous vein graft, and without a functioning profunda femoris artery the extremity might be lost.

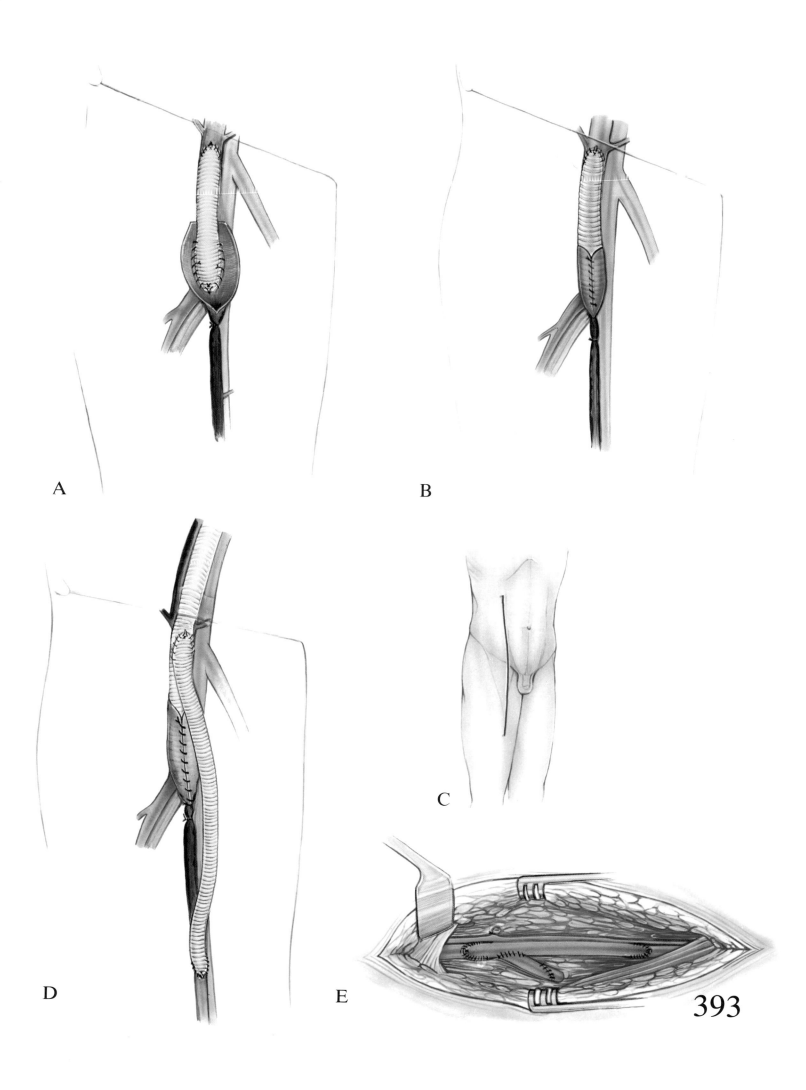

A

B

C

D

E

393

SAPHENOUS VEIN
BYPASS GRAFT

Introduction

The restoration of arterial continuity in atherosclerotic obliterative disease of the lower extremity during the last two decades has been performed by reverse saphenous vein bypass autografts, arterial bypass homografts, synthetic prosthetic bypass grafts and endarterectomy of the occluded arteries. Reverse saphenous vein bypass autografts have given such excellent results compared to the other methods that the latter have been abandoned, and so will not be described in this book. The bypass venous autograft procedure has resulted in the restoration of a patient's walking ability, with complete relief of intermittent claudication in the majority. It has also saved many limbs that, before this new field in vascular surgery was developed, would have required major amputations. The best method to accomplish these good results is to excise the long saphenous vein carefully, then implant it in the reverse direction as an autograft to bypass the arterial blood stream, from the common femoral artery proximal to the occluded superficial femoral artery, down to the popliteal artery, preferably distal to the knee joint. This can be accomplished in the majority of patients, and in some with occluded popliteal arteries the graft can be anastomosed more distal to the anterior tibial, peroneal or posterior tibial artery in the lower leg. The end-to-side type of anastomosis is the best method of implanting the vein graft, as first described by the French surgeon Kunlin, in 1949. It is recommended that the distal anastomosis should be constructed first, as it is the more difficult to construct and is made more so if it is done after the proximal one, and since for long-term patency it is of such vital importance to accomplish a flawless anastomosis.

The success of this operative procedure depends on the following ten requirements.

1. Accurate arteriograms of the arteries proximal and distal to the occluded artery should be obtained, preferably a day or two prior to the operation so that they can be carefully evaluated in order that the best type of procedure for each case can be determined.

2. An autogenous long saphenous vein must be available with an adequate outside diameter (4.0 to 6.0 mm.) and long enough to reach from the common femoral artery to the distal popliteal artery, usually 45 to 50 cm. in length. It must be dissected with extreme care to avoid trauma to it and each tributary must be carefully ligated. The vein is implanted in reversed direction to permit the blood to flow through it in the normal direction so that it is not necessary to remove or destroy the venous bicuspid valves.

3. An adequate inflow of blood into the graft from the proximal

arteries is an absolute essential. A femoropopliteal graft should never be implanted if there is aortoiliac obliterative disease with a poor outflow from the external iliac artery.

4. Adequate outflow arteries distal to the graft are necessary, but it is not necessary that all three arteries of the trifurcation of the popliteal artery should be patent, so that normal or near normal outflow arteries are not as essential as the patency of the inflow arteries. It is important, however, that the distal popliteal artery must be of good texture and not calcified at the site for the distal anastomosis so that a flawless anastomosis can be accomplished. Many successful results have been obtained when the distal anastomosis has been made to an isolated segment of the popliteal artery with only collateral vessels arising from it.

5. Aseptic technique is essential in order to isolate the skin from possible sources of infection. Self-adhering thin transparent plastic sheets should be used to cover the skin after it has been prepared with an alcohol solution of hexachlorophene. The skin is then dried thoroughly with ether, as it is essential that the plastic remain adherent to the skin at the edges of the incision throughout the operation. In addition, pre- and postoperative prophylactic antibiotics are administered by intramuscular injections of 500,000 units of penicillin and 250 mg. of streptomycin to help prevent postoperative infections. The preoperative injection is given as the patient leaves for the operating room. This is because it is of utmost importance to have the antibiotics circulating in the blood and lymph during the operative procedure; in this way they are more effective as prophylactic measures than if administered after the operation is completed or after evidence of postoperative infection develops. Following the operation the antibiotics are administered four times daily for approximately five days. These measures are of especial importance in all types of reconstructive arterial surgery because infection in an anastomotic suture line may mean loss of the graft and sometimes the extremity, or even the life of the patient. It is necessary also, of course, to maintain all the other usual aseptic precautions without eliminating any of them.

6. It is extremely important to prevent thrombosis in the arteries proximal and distal to the occluding clamps that are placed on them during the reconstructive arterial procedures. This is accomplished by complete anticoagulation of the patient's blood by giving 3,000 to 5,000 units of heparin intravenously after the surgical dissection has been nearly completed and 15 minutes before the arteries are to be occluded, to give it ample time to be well disseminated. This amount of heparin gives satisfactory anticoagulation for 3 to 4 hours and does not require neutralization. This step is of sufficient importance that the surgeon should perform the injection himself, into the largest vein available in the operative field, to make sure that it gets into the blood stream. It is not necessary to continue anticoagulation in the postoperative period. It is believed that postoperative anticoagulation will not keep a poorly constructed anastomosis patent, and it is not necessary for a well constructed one, so that it is best to eliminate it to prevent problems from postoperative bleeding.

7. Multiple transfusions must be available for this type of surgery. Many times only one or two will be necessary but, even with the greatest of care and attention to hemostasis, five to ten may occasionally be required in the more extensive and prolonged operative procedures.

8. An anesthetic should be selected that will not result in a fall in blood pressure, as it is important to maintain the patient's blood pressure at its normal level in order to insure an adequate flow of blood into and

through the graft. It is a mistake to start using vasopressor drugs to keep the patient's blood pressure normotensive. Induction with Pentothal Sodium and maintenance with a muscle relaxant, supplemented with gas oxygen administered through an endotracheal tube, has been found to be a satisfactory method; sometimes it is supplemented with a little ether for relaxation.

9. Meticulous careful gentle technique in the exposure and isolation of the arteries for the implantation of the graft and also in the excision of the long saphenous vein graft is essential for success. Stripping of the vein is so traumatic to the walls and the valves that this method of removal makes it unsuitable for grafting procedures. The end-to-side type of anastomosis gives the best results. Technical errors in the construction of the anastomoses are the most common cause of the vast majority of early postoperative graft failures and also most of those that fail within a year after their implantation; for success, therefore, the construction of the anastomoses must be flawless and, preferably, performed as demonstrated in the following plates. A five year failure rate of 20 per cent or less for long 45 to 50 cm. reversed autogenous saphenous vein bypass grafts in the lower extremity is considered evidence of the skill of the vascular surgeon in selecting the optimum places for the proximal and distal anastomoses and his ability to construct them with flawless technique. It is emphasized also that these techniques which are described are basic for all types of autogenous venous bypass grafts elsewhere in the body.

10. Adequate time and patience are essential to carry out these meticulous procedures to obtain the optimum results. The surgeon never should be in a hurry or be a "clock watcher"; otherwise the incidence of his technical errors will increase enormously. Early graft failures that require immediate re-operation have a very high percentage of secondary failure, and such failures usually are permanent. Everything must be done, therefore, to make sure that the primary operative procedure to implant the venous autograft is flawless, so that it will function for many years in its new role as an artery.

The long saphenous vein in some patients unfortunately may be a single trunk of optimal caliber only in the proximal thigh. Then it splits into a double trunk in the middle and distal thigh and the proximal lower leg, each with a caliber of 3.0 to 3.5 mm., which is too small to be used singly for a long graft. Under these conditions both the single and the double trunks should be excised intact distal to the knee, to be used as a long reverse saphenous vein bifid autograft. The distal double trunks become the proximal end of the graft and the proximal single trunk is the distal part of the graft. The distal popliteal anastomosis is constructed in the usual manner with the single trunk. An angioplasty is performed to the open ends of the two trunks by incising them each for 1.0 to 1.5 cm. The anterior adjacent two cut edges are sewn together with a running suture of 6-0 Teflon-coated Dacron. This makes a large venous cuff to use to construct the proximal anastomosis. (See Plate 199.)

Another method of utilizing the bifid portion of these saphenous veins is to perform a long angioplasty by incising the entire length of the double trunks. The adjacent two edges of each are sewn together with running sutures of 5-0 or 6-0 synthetic over a catheter stent of the correct size. This long angioplasty produces a single-lumen venous graft. Some of these have done well but the failure rate within a year has been too high, and the ones that remain patent become dilated and aneurysmal after a few years, so for these reasons this method has been abandoned, and also because

396

the other method of preserving and utilizing the two trunks as a bifid graft has given such good results and is a much less tedious procedure to perform.

In other patients only the proximal 15 to 20 cm. of the long saphenous vein will be of sufficient caliber to use as a graft, because the distal trunks are too small to use as a bifid graft. Under these conditions a composite graft may be constructed by anastomosing the portion of the saphenous vein with a good caliber to a 6.0 or 8.0 mm. knitted Dacron standard type prosthesis, in order to increase the graft length so that it will reach from the common femoral artery to the distal popliteal artery. For success the end-to-end anastomosis of the vein to the prosthesis must be a long tapered one so that it will be well streamlined. (See Plate 202.) It is best first to preclot the Dacron graft, then to construct the anastomosis either before or after the venous portion of the graft has been anastomosed to the popliteal artery. The Dacron prosthesis anastomosis to the common femoral artery is always the last to be constructed. In some patients who do not have a saphenous vein because it is diseased or has been removed, or in those in whom it is not large enough, the cephalic vein in the upper extremity has been used to construct this type of composite graft, providing it is of sufficient caliber. (See Plate 203.) The portion of this vein in the upper arm has been found to be the most satisfactory part of it to utilize for this type of composite graft.

Other methods of restoring the arterial continuity of the lower limb have been tried. Thromboendarterectomy, or, as the English surgeons term it, the Disobliteration Operation of the superficial femoral artery and sometimes the popliteal artery, antedates the utilization of the saphenous vein as a bypass graft in the lower extremity. This procedure, however, has been found to be totally inadequate except when a very short segment of the superficial femoral or popliteal artery is involved. Late patency rates have been extremely disappointing when the major portion of the artery must be endarterectomized, whether it is performed by the open, closed or the gas endarterectomy method. In my own experience the only ones that have remained patent for more than three years include a few limbs in which short segments of the superficial femoral or popliteal arteries have been endarterectomized. A few others have also remained patent following secondary operative procedures two to three years after the endarterectomies were performed on stenotic areas that developed in the endarterectomized segments. The normal lumen in these is restored by longitudinal arteriotomies and closure with autogenous venous patch grafts. A five-year follow-up, however, of 78 limbs with long thromboendarterectomies of the superficial femoral artery revealed 55 failures, a 71 per cent failure rate. For this reason I have discontinued this procedure except for the rare case with a very short segment that can be endarterectomized. Synthetic prostheses were implanted in 31 limbs as femoropopliteal bypass grafts and at the end of five years there were 25 failures, an 81 per cent failure rate. Frozen irradiated arterial homografts were implanted in 190 limbs, with 115 failures in five years, a 61 per cent failure rate. In contradistinction to these poor results there were 295 limbs in which saphenous vein bypass grafts were implanted and there were only 58 failures at the end of five years, a 20 per cent failure rate. From these results it is obvious why, in my opinion, the autogenous reverse saphenous vein bypass autograft is the procedure of choice for the treatment of patients with femoropopliteal atherosclerotic occlusive disease.

Plate 178

TECHNIQUE OF ILIOFEMORAL AND FEMOROPOPLITEAL ARTERIOGRAMS

A. Every surgeon who does reconstructive femoropopliteal arterial procedures should know how to perform iliofemoral and femoropopliteal arteriograms. The following method has proved to be the most satisfactory in obtaining excellent angiograms and reducing the incidence of complications to 0.001 per cent or less. As a rule, bilateral angiograms are obtained at the same time. The necessary equipment consists of (a) two 70-cm. pieces of 16-gauge transparent plastic tubing with a male and female Luerlok type of end piece. The purpose of these is to allow the surgeon and assistant to keep their hands away from the x-radiation during the injections. Each is attached to a large 50-cc. plastic syringe (b) at one end, and at the other end to an 18-gauge spinal needle (c). The metal basin (d) is for 60 per cent Renografin solution. Bilateral iliofemoral and femoropopliteal arteriograms require approximately 200 cc. of this solution. One of the 12-cc. syringes (e) is used first to draw up 7 cc. of 2 per cent lidocaine solution with the 16-gauge needle (f). This is mixed with the Renografin solution to lessen the pain of the dye injection. The smaller needles (g), gauge 22, are used to inject 1 per cent lidocaine solution in each groin for local anesthesia. The curved Kelly clamps are placed on the polyvinyl plastic tubing a short distance from the 50-cc. syringes to keep the Renografin solution in the tubing and the syringe until the time of injection.

B. This demonstrates the location of the spinal needles after their insertion into the common femoral arteries just distal to the inguinal crease. They should be directed toward the umbilicus as they are advanced gently. This permits threading them well up into the external iliac arteries. The large syringes with 50 cc. of 60 per cent Renografin are connected to them by means of the plastic tubing.

C. This demonstrates the patient lying on the operating table with a portable x-ray machine in place. A 14 by 17 inch x-ray film in an 8-1 grid type of cassette is placed under the extremity from the mid lower leg to the mid thigh. The feet are held together with a thin towel or bandage to aid in obtaining a better view of the outflow vessels between the tibia and fibula of both legs. For patients with superficial femoral artery occlusions the angiograms are obtained by injecting 50 cc. of 60 per cent Renografin over a 15-second period. This will always give an excellent angiogram unless the outflow tract is more seriously involved, in which case it may require a 20- to 25-second injection period. For patients with occlusive femoral atherosclerotic disease it is important to use a large amount of solution and to inject it over this long period of time, and also to use a long x-ray exposure of 1.5 seconds at 15 MA with K.V. of 67 to 74, the latter depending on the size of the extremity. A second film is taken with the plate placed under the upper thigh and buttocks to show the proximal femoral and the iliac arteries. This injection is made as rapidly as possible with 30 cc. of 60 per cent Renografin while the patient does a Valsalva maneuver. This x-ray exposure is at 300 MA with K.V. of 67 to 74 for 0.5 to 0.3 second, depending on the girth of the patient. The dye refluxes well up into the iliac arteries, demonstrating the external iliac, and down the common femoral, profunda femoris and superficial femoral arteries. The films are viewed and, if they are satisfactory, the needles are withdrawn; if not, the angiograms may be repeated. The patient remains flat in bed for two hours and then may be ambulatory. The advantage of this method of angiography is that excellent angiograms are routinely obtained, complications are essentially zero, and the surgeon can immediately determine what reconstructive arterial procedure should be performed. Angiograms of the aorta and its major branches should be done by radiologists with the aid of fluoroscopy and rapid film changing equipment.

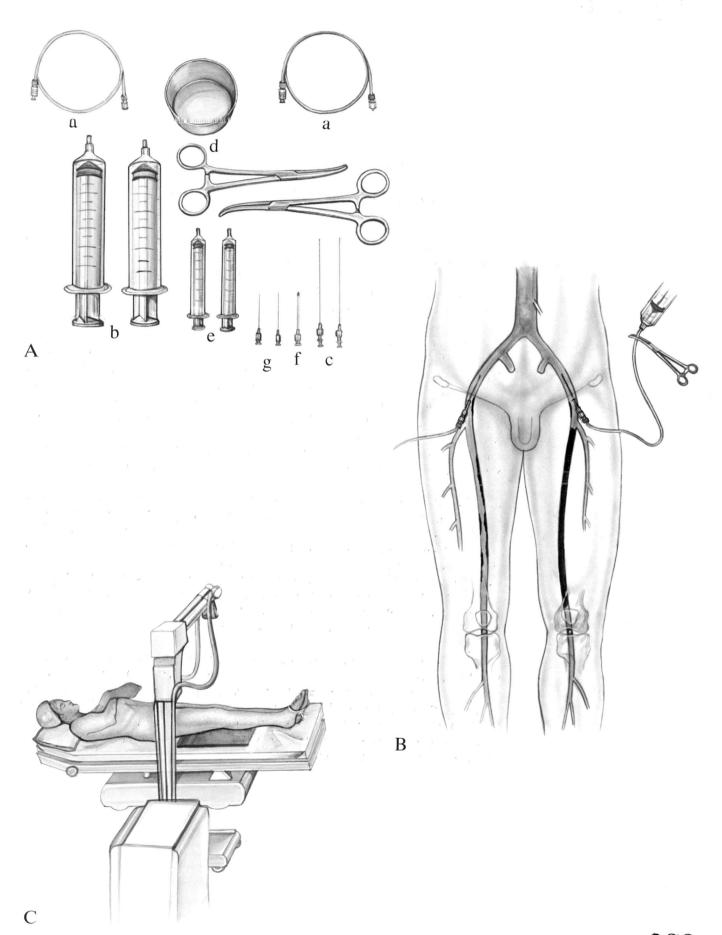

A

B

C

399

Plate 179

PROCUREMENT OF THE SAPHENOUS VEIN AUTOGRAFT

A. The long saphenous vein is sometimes difficult to isolate, especially at the level of the knee. It is important not to lacerate it accidentally while making the incision to obtain it because it may be difficult to repair satisfactorily. For this reason it is a great help to mark its course with an indelible skin pencil the day before the operation while the patient is standing, as shown.

B. This shows the position of the patient on the operating table, with the hip slightly flexed, externally rotated and abducted, and the knee flexed approximately 15 degrees. This position is maintained by placing a folded towel around the dorsum of the foot, then fastening both ends of it to the sterile sheet beneath the foot with a Kocher clamp. The skin of the lower abdomen, both groins, the legs and the feet is prepared with an alcoholic solution of hexachlorophene, then covered with a self-adhering, thin, transparent synthetic sheet to completely isolate the skin after drying it with ether and a towel. The operative area from the lower abdomen to the toes is then draped with sterile towels and sheets.

C. This shows the single long incision which is most commonly used to remove the long saphenous vein, extending from above the groin crease to a short distance distal to the knee. The lower part of the incision is made close to the skin mark that has been placed, but not directly over it, to prevent injury to the vein. This incision gives the best exposure of the saphenous vein and reduces the possibilities of injuring it, which is of vital importance for a successful result. In addition, it gives adequate exposure for isolating the common femoral, profunda femoris and popliteal arteries. When it is closed correctly at the end of the operation, necrosis of the skin edges of the incision rarely if ever occurs.

D. This shows the multiple incisions that can be used if the surgeon prefers. It usually works out very well if one is fortunate enough to find a single trunk saphenous vein without too many tributaries. In my experience, too often the latter arise behind the skin bridges, so that there is danger of injuring the main vein trunk during the ligation of the branches; while I have favored the single incision, I do use both. Also, it is impossible with the multiple incisions to remove a saphenous vein with bifid trunks.

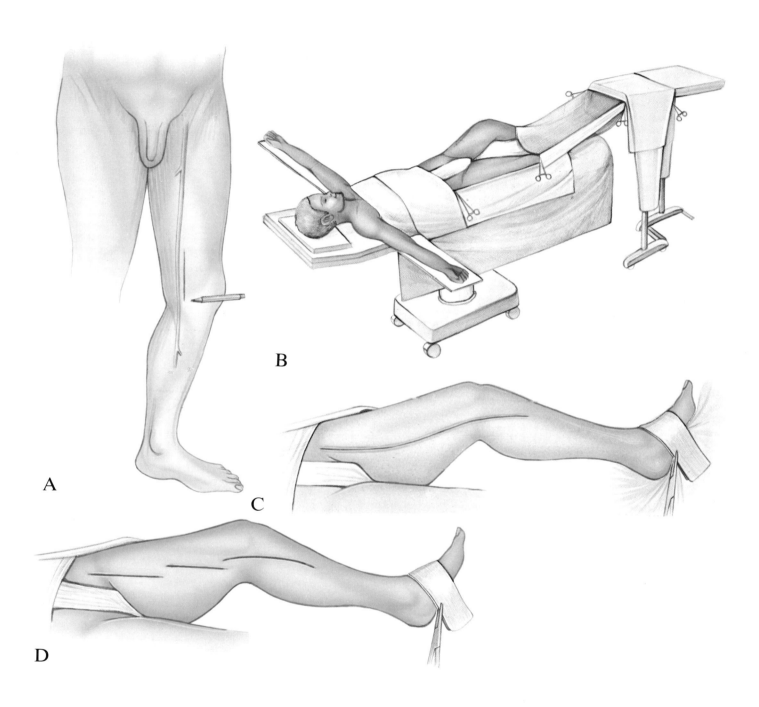

A

B

C

D

401

Plate 179 (Continued)

EXPOSURE OF THE DISTAL POPLITEAL ARTERY

E. This shows the exposure of the distal portion of the popliteal artery in most patients for the distal anastomosis. This portion has fewer branches and atheromatous plaques than the proximal and middle sections so that, technically, a better anastomosis can be constructed. It is not always possible to determine from the femoropopliteal arteriogram whether the popliteal artery is suitable for implanting a graft, although many times it is; in questionable situations it is good practice to expose the distal popliteal artery distal to the knee joint before proceeding further with the operation in case the artery is so atherosclerotic that a graft cannot be implanted. Care must be taken not to injure the long saphenous vein. The insertion of the sartorius muscle is severed, then the deep fascia is incised posterior to the tibia. The medial head of the gastrocnemius muscle (a) is easily retracted posteriorly to expose the popliteal artery (b) and vein (c), and the posterior tibial nerve (d). The popliteus muscle (e) is seen beyond the artery and vein.

F. This shows the exposure of the proximal and distal portions of the popliteal artery to determine the best site for the distal anastomosis. The sartorius muscle (a) is displaced posteriorly after dividing the distal tendinous portion of it to expose the proximal popliteal artery. If this section of the artery is too atherosclerotic for the distal anastomosis, the distal portion of it is often more readily accomplished by dividing the tendons of the semitendinosus (b) and gracilis (c) muscles. The proximal ends of these are marked with 0 black ligatures to facilitate finding them when closing the incision. The exposure is further facilitated by incising the tendinous portions of the medial head of the gastrocnemius muscle (d).

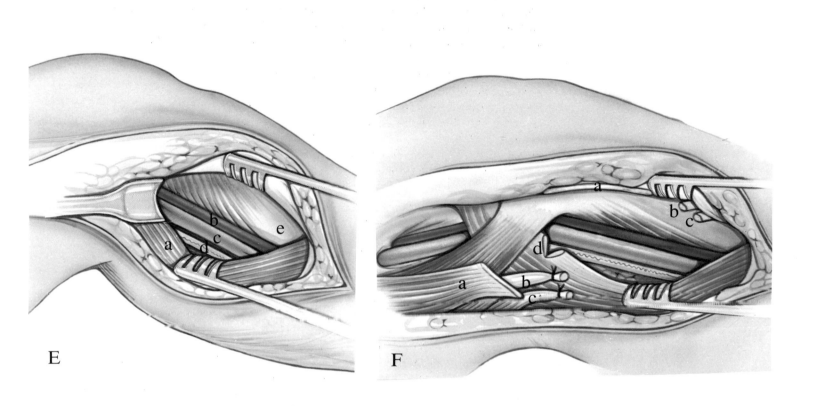

E

F

403

Plate 180

EXPOSURE OF DISTAL
POPLITEAL ARTERY *(Continued)*

A. The popliteal vein lies in front of the artery so it must be separated carefully by retracting the two vessels apart and cutting the areolar tissue between them by sharp scissor dissection. A second popliteal vein is frequently found on the other side of the artery and this must also be separated carefully. Venous bleeding from the vein can be very troublesome to control and may jeopardize the construction of a good anastomosis, so laceration of the popliteal veins must be avoided.

B. After isolation of the artery for a centimeter, a small right-angle retractor is passed beneath it. Further dissection of the artery is greatly facilitated by traction with this instrument. It is recommended that at least 3 cm. of the artery be isolated so that a satisfactory anastomosis can be constructed. Occasionally a tributary arises from the far side of the artery; this should be doubly ligated and divided before it is torn, since if this occurs it may result in serious injury to the popliteal artery before the proximal end is secured. The retractor is also helpful in determining the texture of the arterial wall by palpation of the vessel against it to select the thinnest and softest part of its wall where the anastomosis can be accomplished most satisfactorily.

C. This shows the exposure of the distal popliteal artery with its bifurcation into the posterior tibial (a) and the anterior tibial (b) arteries. It is necessary to partially divide the medial head of the gastrocnemius and the tibial origin of the soleus muscles to obtain this exposure. More distal exposure of the posterior tibial artery can be obtained by continuing the dissection in this same plane, which occasionally may be desirable. The anterior tibial artery cannot be isolated further through this approach because of its right angle turn to pass through the interosseous membrane. The anterior tibial vein must be doubly ligated and divided, as shown, in order to expose the arteries sufficiently to obtain distal control of them. This more extensive exposure is necessary when the distal anastomosis must be made to the popliteal at or near its bifurcation, or even more distally.

D. As a result of the trauma from isolating the popliteal artery, it often becomes markedly vasoconstricted. This is a good sign because it means that the artery has a soft pliable wall and will be satisfactory for the implantation of a graft. This section of the artery is isolated between two bulldog clamps and distended by injecting it with a solution of weak heparin in normal saline, using a 2-cc. syringe with a 26-gauge needle. Great care must be taken to make sure the needle is in the arterial lumen during the injection to avoid separating the media and intima. This simple maneuver relieves the vasospasm and has been found to be far superior to any other method; done carefully, it results in no damage to the artery.

E. This shows the section of the artery that was dilated. Fortunately this dilated state persists for hours. As a result, the construction of a perfect distal anastomosis is greatly facilitated, which is very important as it is the outflow tract from the graft.

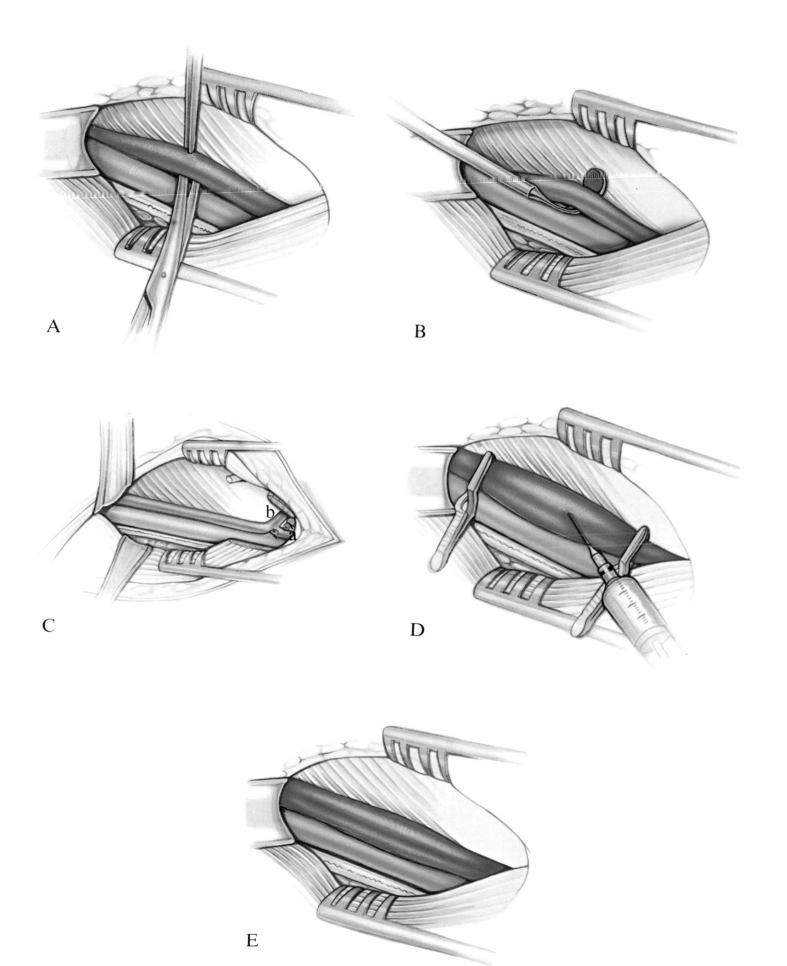

A

B

C

D

E

405

Plate 181

EXPOSURE OF COMMON
FEMORAL ARTERY

A. This shows the next step, which is to isolate the common (a), the superficial (b) and the profunda femoris (c) arteries and the proximal end of the long saphenous vein (d) in the groin through a slightly oblique longitudinal incision extending above the groin crease. The surgeon should watch for a small constant tributary (e) of the femoral vein that comes out behind the superficial femoral artery and crosses the profunda femoris artery. It frequently is best to doubly ligate and divide this, as there is danger of injury to the profunda femoris artery in obtaining control of it if it is torn or lacerated. It is recommended that the proximal anastomosis should, with very few exceptions, be made to the common femoral artery in order to attain an adequate proximal arterial inflow into the graft, which is so necessary for long-term patency of the graft. The results have not been nearly so good if the graft is anastomosed to the superficial femoral artery because of the smaller volume flow in it as a result of the marked narrowing of its origin and proximal portion from atheromatous plaques, so frequently observed.

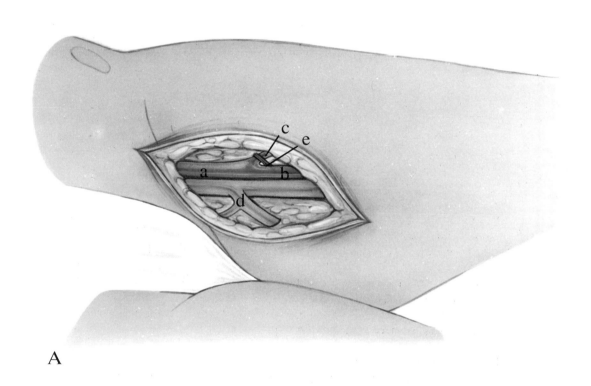

A

Plate 181 (Continued)

PROCUREMENT OF THE
SAPHENOUS VEIN AUTOGRAFT

B. This shows the next step, which is the excision of the long saphenous vein through a single incision. The dissection is begun distal to the knee and should be carried distalward to where the single trunk of the vein becomes bifid. It is extremely important to develop a technique that will run the least danger of accidentally lacerating the saphenous vein trunk, since if this occurs it reduces the success rate of the grafting procedure because of the difficulty in obtaining a satisfactory repair. It has been found that by upward retraction of the skin and subcutaneous tissues with tooth forceps the dissection of the saphenous vein can best be performed with scissors, keeping the blades parallel to the vein trunk. Finger dissection between it and the skin before incising it is also useful. The majority of the tributaries are doubly ligated and divided. Others that may be missed are ligated during the final preparation of the graft after it is excised. The dissection of the vein, especially a small one, can best be performed from the groin distally.

C. The distal bifid trunks are ligated and divided 2 cm. beyond their junction. These short sections are removed with the main trunk so that it will be possible to perform an angioplastic procedure to make a larger vein cuff for the proximal anastomosis if the common femoral artery is thick-walled or the main trunk of the vein graft is only 3.5 to 4.0 mm. in diameter. An acorn-tipped Mark's needle is inserted into one of the short venous trunks or the main trunk if a bifid one is not used. This type of needle is recommended because it will not slip out or cause injury to the vein as a sharp pointed one tends to do.

D. This shows the needle securely ligated in place with a 0 silk ligature. It is used to inject a weak heparin in normal saline solution during the dissection of the vein to prevent blood clots from forming in it and later to dilate it after it has been removed. It also acts as a label on the distal end of the vein, which is to become the proximal end of the graft, so that there is no chance that the graft will be implanted in the wrong direction.

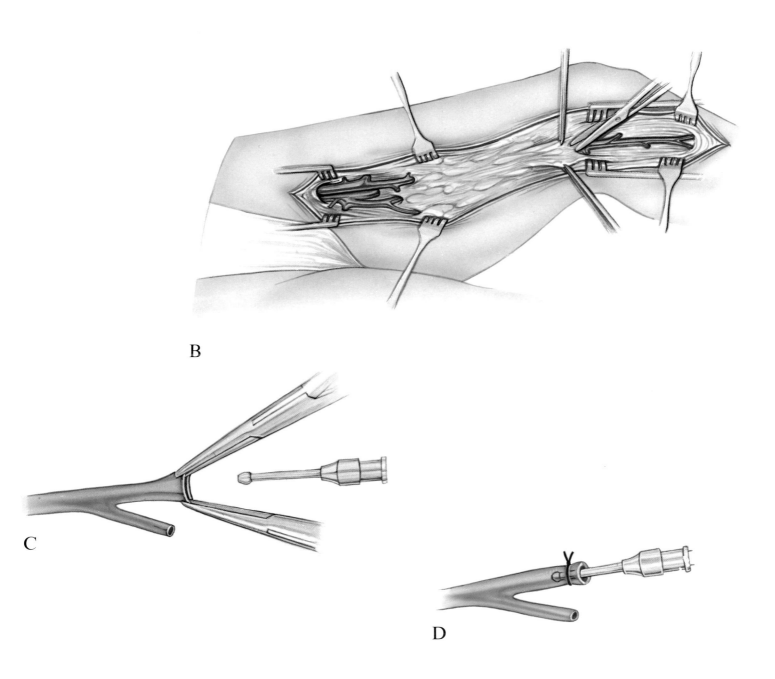

B

C

D

409

Plate 182

PROCUREMENT OF THE
SAPHENOUS VEIN AUTOGRAFT
(Continued)

A. This shows the long saphenous vein almost completely freed up through a single long incision. Dilute heparin in normal saline solution is being injected through the distal end. This method of obtaining the vein graft is most satisfactory, as the exposure of it is so complete and simple.

B. This shows the method of removing the long saphenous vein when multiple incisions are utilized. Strong retraction is necessary at the skin bridges between the incisions in order to secure tributaries which seem to arise beneath them so frequently. The only advantage of this method is that the shorter incisions may heal more satisfactorily with less danger of skin necrosis. This, in my opinion, does not outweigh the difficulty encountered in removing the vein, with the danger of injuring it under the skin bridges. In addition, if the single incision is closed with interrupted sutures to the deep fascia where it has been incised, and interrupted mattress silk sutures to the skin *without any sutures in the subcutaneous fat,* primary healing will always take place without skin sloughs.

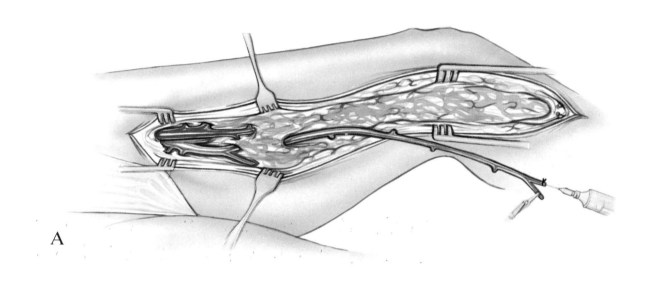

A

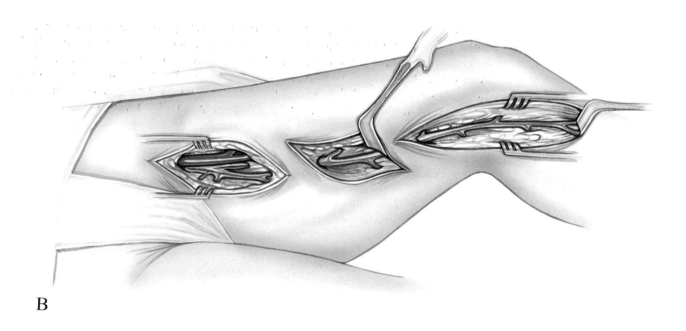

B

411

Plate 183

MAKING THE TUNNEL FOR THE SAPHENOUS VEIN AUTOGRAFT

A. This demonstrates the method of making a tunnel in the popliteal space behind the medial head of the gastrocnemius, with the index fingers of both hands. There is less danger of injuring the popliteal vein by this technique than if an instrument is used; furthermore, crossing bands of tissue in the tunnel can be cleared or avoided by use of the fingers. It also gives an adequate-sized tunnel.

B. This shows that a large Penrose tube has been passed through the tunnel to mark it and to help in placing the graft. Another tunnel is being made in a similar manner over the adductor longus tendon and Hunter's canal, and beneath the sartorius muscle. After completion of the tunnel, it is cleared by finger dissection of any crossing strands of tissue that might interfere with the graft, and another large Penrose tubing is threaded through it to facilitate placing the graft later.

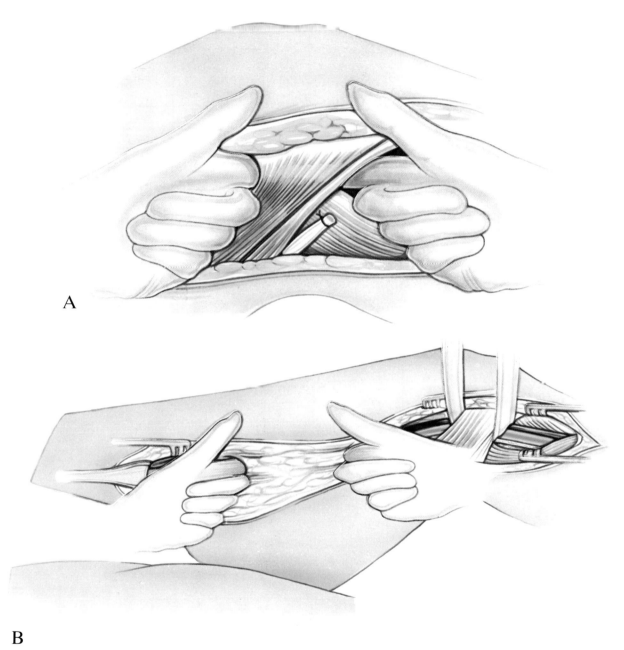

A

B

413

Plate 183 (Continued)

HEPARINIZATION OF
THE PATIENT

C. This shows that the long saphenous vein has been removed. The ligated proximal end of it at its junction with the femoral vein is near the tip of the needle, which has been inserted into the common femoral vein for the injection of 40 mg. of heparin for general heparinization. The anticoagulant effect of this amount lasts for approximately four hours, which is usually sufficiently long for a femoropopliteal saphenous vein bypass procedure. It gives good protection against intra-arterial thrombosis of the arteries that have been dissected out for the anastomotic sites and later during the time they are occluded to implant the graft. The vein graft is thoroughly flushed out with heparin in normal saline solution. It is then stored in a basin containing this solution.

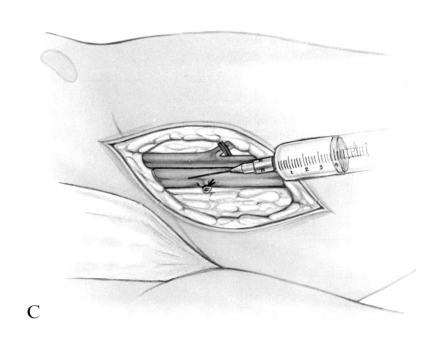

C

Plate 184

PREPARATION OF THE AUTOGENOUS SAPHENOUS VEIN GRAFT

A. This shows the saphenous vein graft that was excised and placed in the basin with dilute heparin-saline solution, leaving it at room temperature.

B. This demonstrates the proper way to ligate the tributaries of the vein graft. The assistant holds the vessel firmly with the second and third fingers of the left hand against an improvised table made of folded sheets and a moist towel. He grasps the end of the tributary with a fine hemostat, and with traction the vein is tented upward. A fine silk ligature is then used to ligate the tributary at a point a millimeter or two distal to its junction with the main trunk.

C and D. These demonstrate a tributary ligated correctly so that the ligature has not caught the adventitia of the main trunk. As shown, it is much better to leave a small portion of the tributary proximal to the ligature.

E and F. These demonstrate an improperly ligated tributary. The ligature was placed at its junction with the main trunk, so that in the process of ligating it some of the adventitia of the main vessel wall was caught in the ligature to produce a narrowing of its lumen. This is a serious mistake to make, especially if a number of tributaries are ligated in this manner, because it results in narrowed areas that cause turbulence, thrombosis and occlusion of the graft.

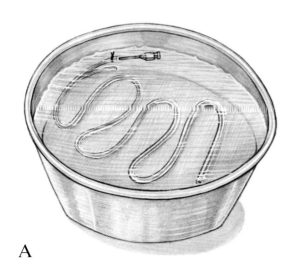

A

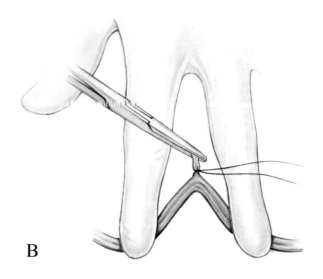

B

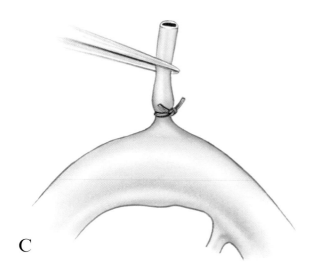

C

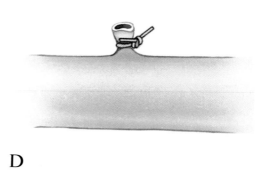

D

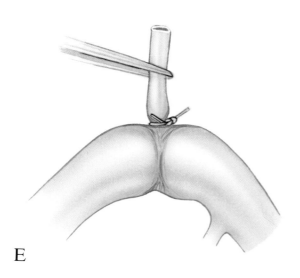

E

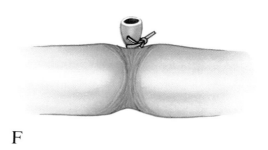

F

417

Plate 185

PREPARATION OF THE AUTOGENOUS SAPHENOUS VEIN GRAFT *(Continued)*

A. This demonstrates how to eliminate the point of constriction caused by a poorly placed ligature. It is necessary to use a fine pair of scissors with rounded points. With the vein distended with heparin-saline solution it is possible to pass the tip of one blade of the scissors under the constricting adventitial band and divide it. Extreme care must be taken not to incise the vein wall, which is the reason for using the blunt-tipped scissors.

B. This demonstrates that these constricting bands can be eliminated by this maneuver. It is better, however, to avoid making them, as it is time consuming to correct them. In addition, the vein wall may inadvertently be damaged with the scissors, which means that it must be repaired. This may be difficult to accomplish satisfactorily with a thin-walled venous graft.

C. Venous grafts always go into a state of vasoconstriction during the process of removal and frequently look too narrow to be suitable for a bypass graft. One must remember, however, that the normal size when first exposed can be re-established by gentle hydraulic pressure, using heparin-saline solution injected through the Mark's needle, with a bulldog clamp occluding the graft as shown in the illustration. It is always gratifying to see the vein restored to its normal size. The illustration demonstrates the distal vasoconstricted portion and the portion between the large bulldog clamp and the syringe restored back to its normal state. It is usual to find additional tributaries that have been divided but not ligated during this maneuver, so the dilatation is done in segments, ligating each tributary as it is discovered. Occasionally the tributary may have been divided so close to the main trunk that it cannot be ligated; under these conditions it is best secured with a mattress suture of 5-0 silk. The advantage of the silk is that it is thrombogenic and is usually slipperier, especially if coated with bone wax, so that it does not pick up too much adventitia and cause a constriction at the point of repair.

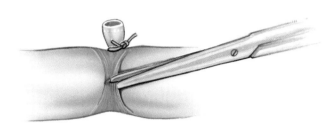

A

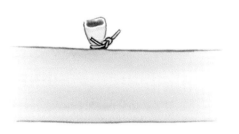

B

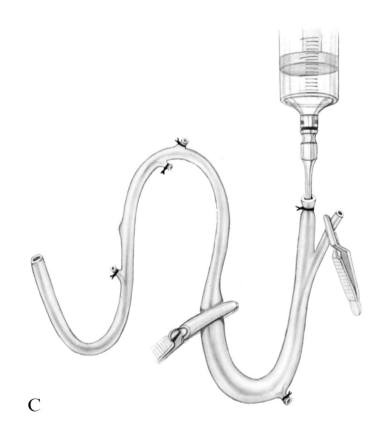

C

Plate 186

PREPARATION OF THE AUTOGENOUS SAPHENOUS VEIN GRAFT *(Continued)*

A. This shows the graft completely distended throughout its full length. It is fortunate that once the vein is distended by this method it never returns to the state of vasoconstriction, so it is not necessary to repeat the dilatation, even after several hours.

B. This shows the vein hanging freely without touching the table, with a bulldog clamp (a) on the end. It is again distended under moderate pressure to make the vein graft straighten out similar to the way it will lie when it is implanted. A second bulldog clamp (b) is then applied at the proximal end of the graft, as shown. This should be placed exactly parallel to the one at the other end of the graft. These two bulldogs then act as markers so that when the vein is laid down exactly as it was hanging one can be absolutely sure that, by keeping the bulldog clamps in the same positions, it will not be twisted.

C. This shows the placing of a fine silk suture from one end of the graft to the other, after laying it down on the operating field with the two bulldog clamps, (a) and (b), still in place. Very small bites of adventitia are taken, so that the suture does not enter the lumen of the vein. The placing of the suture is greatly facilitated by having the first assistant keep tension on the graft, as shown, with his forefinger. Neither end of the suture is tied because it should be removed after the vein graft is implanted; this is readily accomplished by gently pulling it out. After the suture has been placed the bulldog clamps are removed and the graft is placed back in the basin of heparin-saline solution. The black thread serves as a marker on the vein to help to prevent any twist in it as it is implanted. If this should occur, failure of the graft is almost certain to occur. Without a marker it is more difficult to be sure that it has been implanted untwisted, so it is absolutely essential to have some method such as this to prevent such a serious technical error.

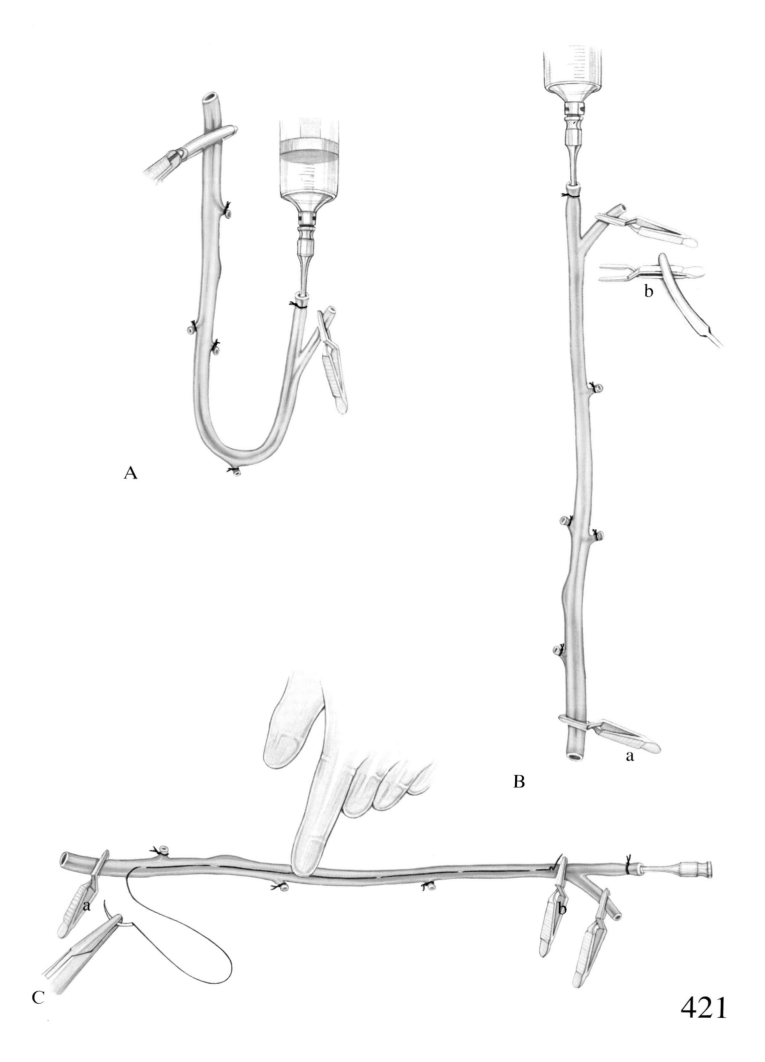

A

B

a

b

C

a

b

421

Plate 187

PREPARATION OF THE
AUTOGENOUS SAPHENOUS
VEIN GRAFT *(Continued)*

A.   This demonstrates a saccular type of aneurysm that is occasionally encountered in a saphenous vein autograft with extremely thin walls. It is best to repair these for fear they may grow larger, or even rupture.

B.   This short type of aneurysm can be closed successfully in a transverse manner without narrowing of the lumen of the graft. This is done with a running everting mattress suture which is started in the midline of the vein, working toward both sides.

C.   The suture is then pulled taut, which approximates the base of the aneurysm transversely. Each suture then comes back as a running over-and-over stitch to reinforce the mattress suture line. It is placed outside the latter and they are tied together in the middle where the suturing was commenced.

D.   This shows a linear type of aneurysm which cannot be closed transversely without producing too much kinking of the graft, so it is closed in a longitudinal manner. This type usually has a narrow base from side to side and the main trunk is a little dilated, so it is much more suitable for the linear type of aneurysmorrhaphy.

E and F.   The same method of suturing is shown as for the other type, except it is done in the longitudinal direction, as shown in these illustrations.

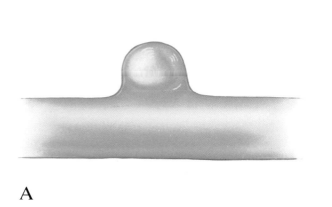

A

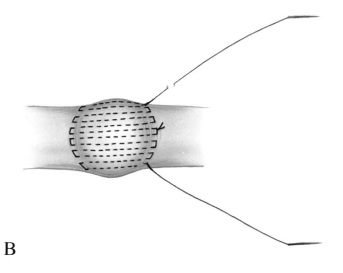

B

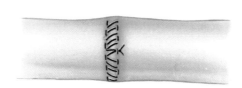

C

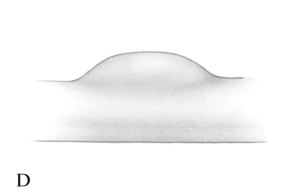

D

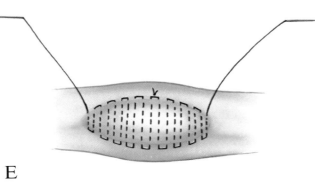

E

F

423

Plate 188

CONSTRUCTION OF THE POPLITEAL ANASTOMOSIS

A. This illustration demonstrates exposure of the popliteal artery from the adductor hiatus to the distal part of the popliteal space, exposing the proximal and distal thirds of the artery. The proximal portion of the artery in this case was unsuitable for the construction of an anastomosis, so the distal section was selected because it was soft and pliable. Saphenous vein autografts function very satisfactorily even though they cross the knee joint, so it is much better to select the best portion of the artery for the distal anastomosis with this type of graft rather than use a more sclerotic proximal section of the popliteal artery.

B. A self-retaining retractor is used to keep the incision open, and the gastrocnemius muscle is retracted with the additional help of a Richardson retractor at the proximal end of the incision. Two bulldog clamps are then placed 3 cm. apart on the distal part of the popliteal artery that had been previously isolated and dilated. It is of utmost importance to prevent blood from entering this isolated portion of the artery during the implantation of the graft because, if it does, a thrombus may form after completion of the popliteal anastomosis, which will embolize the outflow arteries when the graft is opened. In order to keep the anastomotic field dry the surgeon should make certain that the bulldog clamps prevent blood from entering this section of the artery and that there are no overlooked tributaries entering it. This is done by forcing the blood out of it, then watching to see if it fills with the clamps still in place. If it does, the source of the blood is searched for until found and then controlled.

Blood is then allowed to fill this section of the artery again by loosening one of the bulldog clamps, making it much easier to open the artery. This is done by making a longitudinal incision with a small-bladed, sharp knife, with the blood vessel being held with small tissue forceps on each side. After the lumen is opened a short distance the arteriotomy is then enlarged longitudinally with a fine pair of angled Pott's scissors. It should be made at least twice as long as the width of the vessel and sometimes a little longer to facilitate the making of a more perfect anastomosis.

C. The arteriotomy is spread open, which reveals a relatively thin arterial wall that is very suitable for the implantation of a graft. There is a small plaque visible on the posterior wall, which is left undisturbed.

D. In order to prevent thrombosis developing in the distal arterial tree, which is unlikely to occur because of the previous heparinization, it is an additional safeguard to inject 10 to 15 cc. of the dilute heparin in normal saline solution through a small-calibered plastic tube inserted beyond the distal bulldog clamp. The same amount is injected proximal to the proximal bulldog clamp, although this is not so necessary as the distal injection.

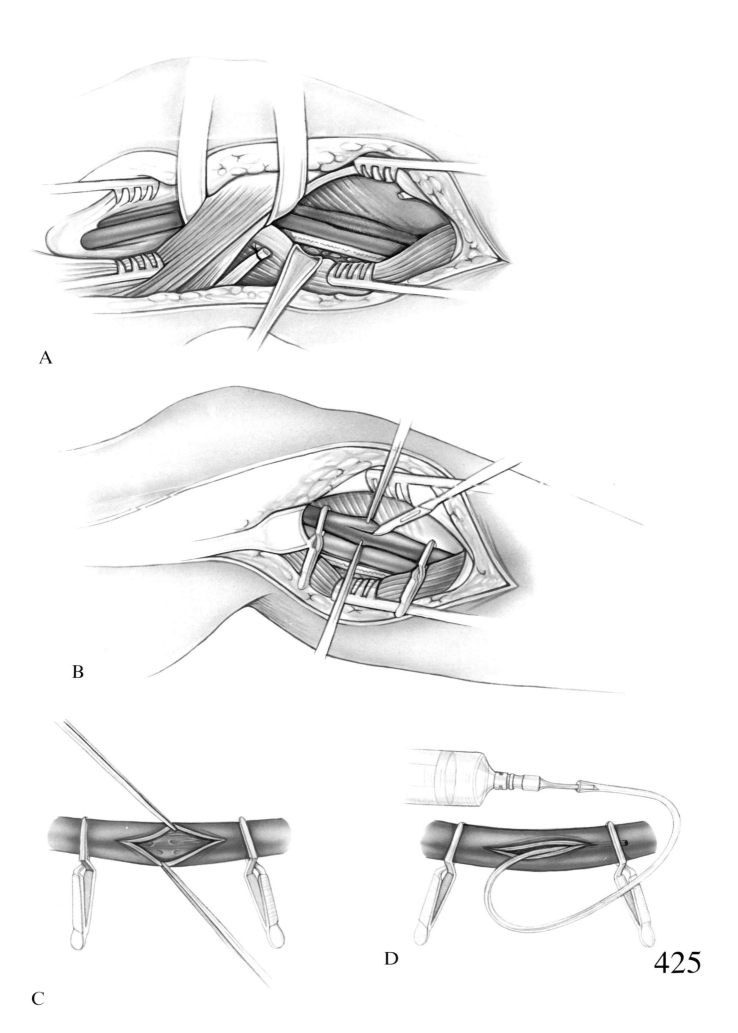

A

B

C

D

425

Plate 189

THE MAKING OF A DOUBLE-NEEDLED SUTURE

The illustrations in this plate demonstrate a method of making a double-needled suture by tying two single-needled ones together. There are certain advantages in this since one can make them as long or as short as desired, depending on the depth the blood vessel lies in the incision that has to be sutured, which is helpful for any location. The knot that is formed by tying the two sutures together also acts as a buttress, so that when two very thin-walled vessels are being sutured together, the suture is much less apt to tear through the vessel walls. In addition, the knot also lets the surgeon know when he has reached the mid point of the suture as he is placing it. Teflon-coated Dacron 5-0 sutures with a straight taper cutting point needle are used routinely to construct most saphenous vein to artery anastomoses. It helps to rub the sutures with bone wax to make them slide through the tissues and to prevent them from dragging the adventitia with each stitch. Sometimes 6-0 is preferred for constructing small anastomoses. Some of the new monofilament synthetic sutures are preferred for the small anastomoses for this reason.

A.   The first step is to tie a single overhand knot with the ends of the two sutures over an instrument held by the first assistant. The knot is placed so that the double-needled suture will be the optimum length for the particular suturing that is to be performed. Thus, when one is working on shallowly placed blood vessels, short sutures are much more satisfactory, whereas in a deep wound it is necessary to have much longer ones.

B.   The knot is snugged up tightly, which makes it an extremely secure knot except in the case of synthetic sutures.

C.   This shows two additional throws that are made with synthetic sutures. This is done by using the long ends of the sutures with the needles. The figure shows only one of the extra throws, but experience has shown that two make it much safer, so that even with the slipperiest materials it is a very secure knot.

D.   This shows the completed double-needled suture.

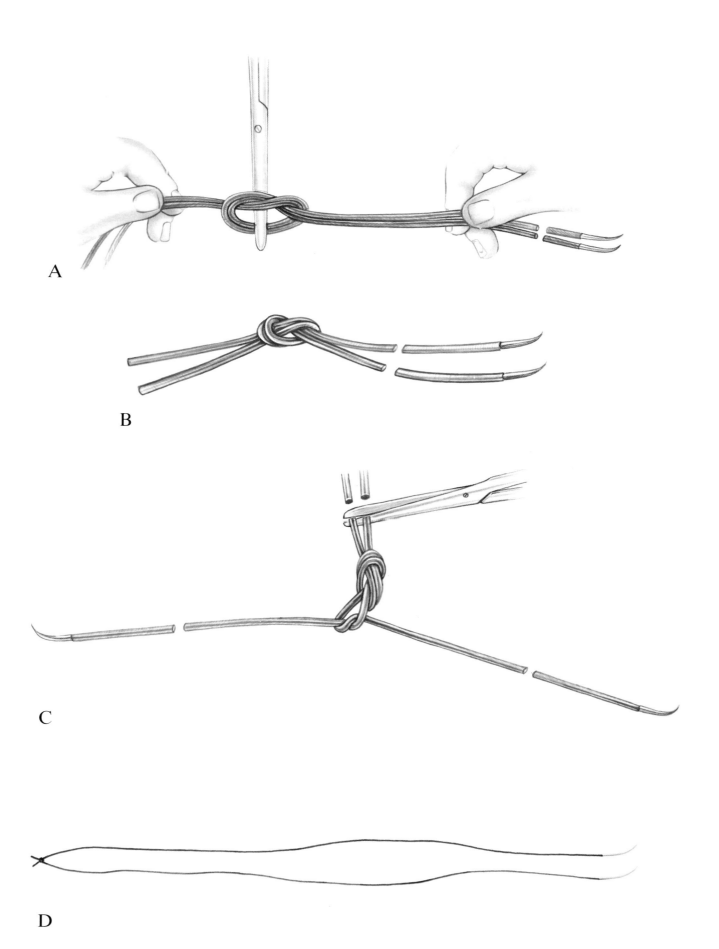

A

B

C

D

427

Plate 190

THE CONSTRUCTION OF THE POPLITEAL ANASTOMOSIS

A.   This demonstrates the incision made in the distal end of the saphenous vein autograft, which was the proximal end of the vein, since the graft will be implanted in the reversed manner from which it lay in the extremity. This is because the bicuspid venous valves allow blood to flow only from the distal end of the vein to the proximal end of it. The incision is made on the side of the graft opposite the black silk marker suture so that it can be visualized readily, as the graft is implanted, to aid in keeping it from becoming twisted. This incision should be approximately between 10 and 12 mm. in length, or about two to three times as long as the diameter of the popliteal artery.

B.   Small sections of the corners of the graft cuff are removed. It is important not to make it pointed on the end, but to leave a small transverse section of the vein graft because this facilitates making a more perfect anastomosis.

C.   The double-needled suture that has been prepared is then placed in the graft as shown, the needles going from the outside to the inside of the vessel. A small pair of straight scissors or a hemostat is placed in the lumen of the vein, which helps in placing these sutures by gently stabilizing the end of the graft.

D.   As the sutures are pulled through it is very important that the adventitia be grasped with fine forceps to prevent it from being caught in the suture, which if it occurs tends to kink and narrow the proximal part of the anastomosis. This is a serious technical error in the construction of the anastomosis. It should be avoided, as it will surely result in early failure of the graft because of the localized narrowing, which causes turbulence of the blood stream with thrombus formation.

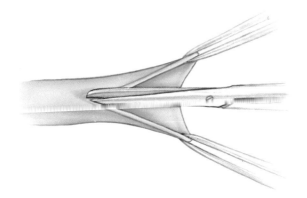

A

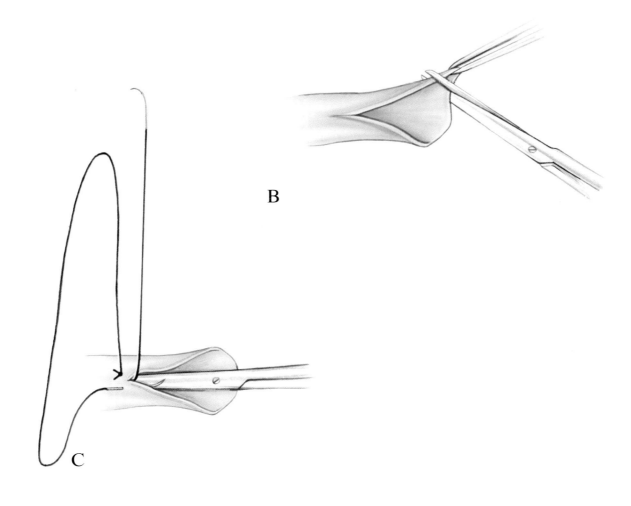

B

C

D

Plate 191

THE CONSTRUCTION OF THE POPLITEAL ANASTOMOSIS
(Continued)

A. This shows the distal end of the vein graft with the mattress suture in place. The popliteal artery is controlled by two bulldog clamps, with the arteriotomy between them. The double-needled suture is now passed from the inside of the artery to the outside so that it will result in an intima-to-intima approximation of the vein graft to the artery. There is an additional advantage to passing the needles in this direction through the artery, as it greatly reduces the chance of separating the media or an intimal plaque from the arterial wall, a serious fault if it occurs in the construction of the anastomosis that may result in the thrombosis of it.

B. The first assistant then grasps the vein graft in his right hand and the top of the cuff of the distal end of the vein graft with fine forceps, bringing them over to the site of the arteriotomy. The vein graft is held up perpendicularly so that in tying the suture the adventitia of the vein graft is not caught, which would produce constriction of it at this point. Note that the silk marker suture is plainly visible on the front of the graft.

C. The next step is to insert a similar double-needled suture first through the end of the graft and then through the distal end of the arteriotomy, as shown. It is important that the cuff of the graft be on slight tension rather than leaving it a little loose, which will result in its wrinkling and producing turbulence of the blood flow that will often cause thrombosis. (See Plate 207.)

D. The distal mattress suture has been ligated and the proximal part of the suture line commenced. Note that the suturing is from the outside to the inside of the vein and through the arterial wall from the inside to the outside. This is to give a better intima-to-intima approximation and to prevent loosening of the media or intimal plaques. Tension is kept on the vein graft with the forceps (a) to prevent the suture from pulling adventitial strands along with it, which tends to produce points of constriction and irregularity in the anastomosis. Forceps (b) is placed behind the suture loop as it is pulled through, as shown, to prevent it from falling backward, which it will always do if this precaution is not taken; this often results in suture line leaks because of poor approximation of the vessel edges. Forceps (c) holds the edge of the artery to facilitate placing each stitch.

E. This shows another method of controlling the loop of the running suture as it is pulled taut; the first assistant places his forefinger behind it, leaving the points that the stitch passes through the vessel visible so that it will fall true. The finger should not push the suture too far forward because this will also result in a faulty suture line. Again note the forceps (a) maintaining tension on the vein graft.

F The suturing is continued as a running stitch to the midpoint of this side of the anastomosis. Note that the sewing is done by the surgeon using a straight needle and pushing it away from him. This method greatly facilitates the suturing, especially if a straight needle is used or one with a slight curve to the tip. (See Plate 14.) I personally prefer the straight one with a cutting point for this type of anastomosis. If necessary, a slight curve can be put on it when it is difficult to use the straight needle, such as at the corners; it is then readily straightened out again. The great advantage of the straight needle is that with each stitch it can be picked up with the needle holder without having to use the other hand or an instrument to do this. In addition, a straight needle will pass more easily through tough atheromatous plaques and scar tissue than a curved needle.

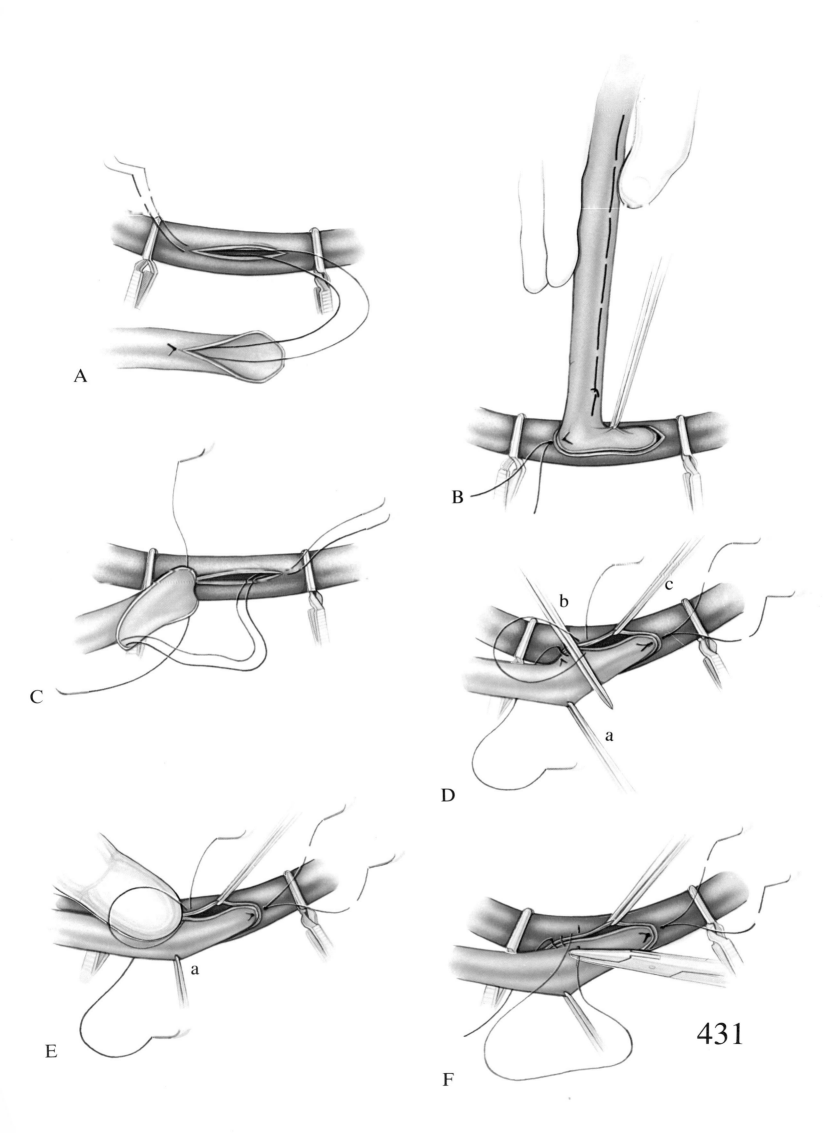

A

B

C

D

E

F

431

Plate 192

THE CONSTRUCTION OF THE POPLITEAL ANASTOMOSIS
(Continued)

A.   The far side of the anastomosis is then completed, using one of the sutures at the distal end of it that has been placed and tied already as a mattress suture. In order to obtain a better intima-to-intima approximation, two or three additional mattress sutures may be used at the beginning of this portion of the suture line to obtain good eversion of the vessel edges. Since this is the lumen to the proximal end of the outflow tract, it is essential that this part of the anastomosis be constructed with extreme care.

B.   The suturing is then continued with a running over-and-over stitch to the mid point where the other one had stopped. The two ends are then ligated together, which completes the far side of the anastomosis.

C.   The edges of the vein graft and the artery on the unsutured side are then opened to examine how accurately the intimas of the two vessels have been approximated. Sometimes there are rough edges due to plaques that can be trimmed, but usually it is very pleasing to see how neatly the intima surfaces have come together without any raw areas. This maneuver can be performed more readily if the proximal half of this side of the anastomosis has not already been completed.

D.   This demonstrates the over-and-over suturing of the proximal half of the anastomosis on the near side. Again, great care must be taken not to kink the graft at the start of this suture line, so again the adventitia of the vein must be firmly retracted with fine forceps, by the assistant, as shown.

E.   This shows another method useful for difficult anastomoses in which the proximal half of both sides of the anastomosis are first completed after placing the proximal and distal mattress sutures. Each suture has been anchored at the halfway point by ligating it to a stay suture placed at these points.

F.   The remainder of the anastomosis is completed by beginning at the distal end of the anastomosis with a few mattress sutures and then an over-and-over type of suture to join the other suture at the midway point, where the two are ligated together. When the arterial wall is soft and pliable without atheromatous plaques the suturing may be performed as shown, with the needle passing first from the outside to the inside of the artery, and then from the inside to the outside of the vein. This avoids the adventitia of the latter being caught in the sutures with resulting irregularities in the anastomotic cuff. On the contrary, if plaques are encountered in the artery the suturing must be done in the reverse direction, to prevent dislodging the plaques, so that with each stitch the needle first passes from the outside to the inside of the vein and then from the inside to the outside of the artery, as shown in *D*. It should be emphasized again that the construction of these anastomoses, beginning at each end and working toward the middle, is much better than if the suturing is started at one end and then carried all the way to the other end, because this makes it much more difficult to do the perfect anastomosis that is so essential to success.

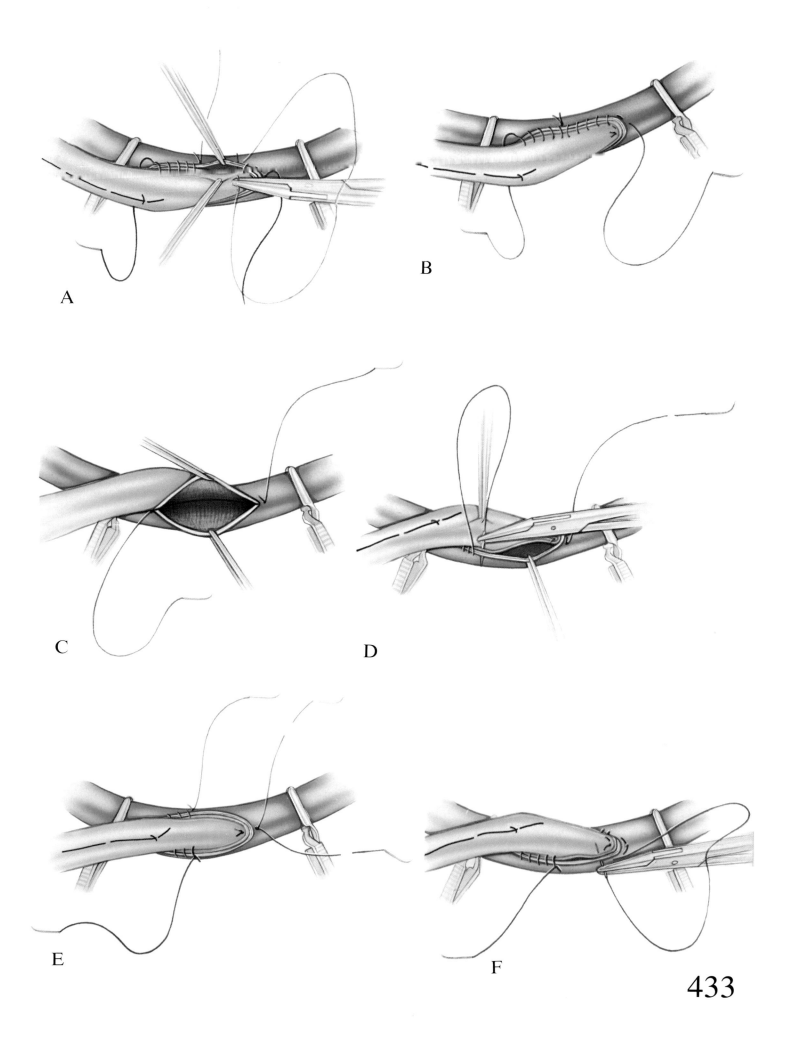

A

B

C

D

E

F

433

Plate 193

COMPLETION OF THE
POPLITEAL ANASTOMOSIS

A. This illustration shows the entire femoropopliteal saphenous bypass graft with the silk marker in its wall and the completed anastomosis to the popliteal artery, with the bulldog clamps still occluding this vessel. Dilute heparin in normal saline solution is injected into the graft to determine if there are any significant leaks in the suture line. As can be seen, after it has been fully dilated and is under pressure, there is one at the very distal end ncar one of the mattress sutures at point (a). This is an important maneuver to perform before allowing blood to flow through the graft, because it is much easier to find and correct using the heparin-saline solution than to be troubled with blood leaking out after opening the graft which would tend to obscure the field and make it difficult to obtain a neat closure without interfering with the contour of the anastomosis. As a rule, all that is necessary is a single simple suture, as is shown being placed. Occasionally there may be a tear in a thin-walled vein graft which necessitates the use of a mattress suture.

B.   After the leaks are controlled, or if the anastomosis is tight after completion, 20 cm. of dilute heparin in normal saline solution is injected through the proximal end of the graft and the distal anastomosis into the arterial outflow tract by opening the blades of the distal bulldog clamp on the popliteal artery with an instrument, as shown. The clamp is closed again quickly before blood regurgitates into the anastomotic area. The same procedure is then performed into the proximal outflow tract by temporarily releasing the proximal bulldog clamp.

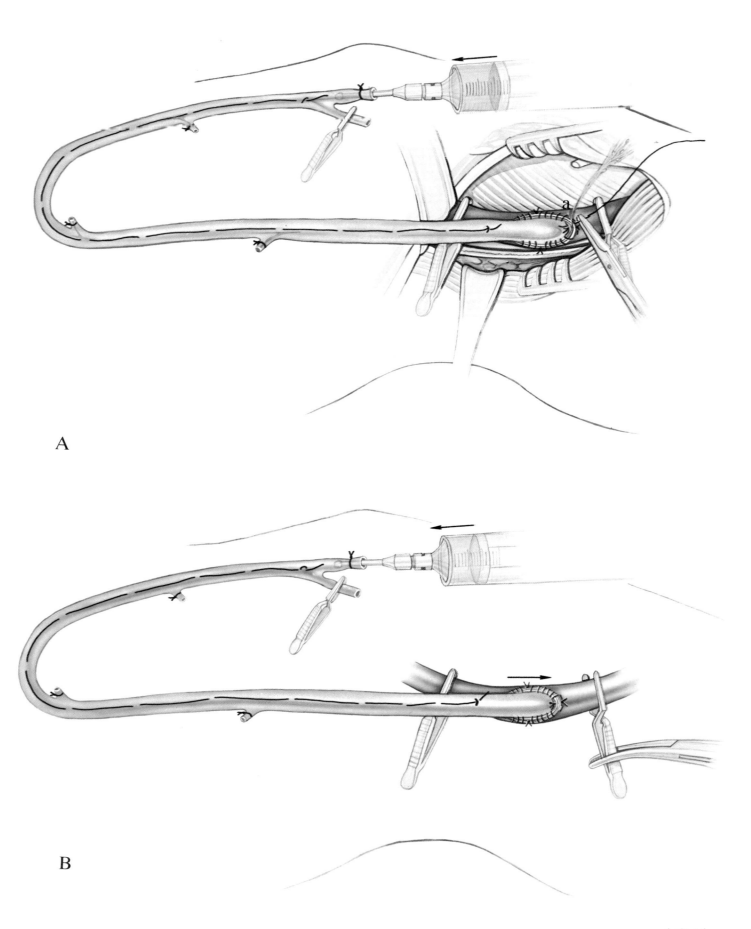

A

B

435

Plate 194

THE CONSTRUCTION OF THE COMMON FEMORAL ANASTOMOSIS

A. This demonstrates the method of pulling the saphenous vein graft proximally through the two tunnels that have been made previously. A large right-angle clamp is used for the distal tunnel behind the gastrocnemius muscle and a long slightly curved one for the longer proximal tunnel beneath the sartorius muscle. It is during this maneuver that the black silk marker thread on the vein graft proves invaluable, because with it one can be absolutely sure that there is no twist in the graft. The knee should be straightened so that the correct length of vein graft will be used, not too short and not too long. If the 15-degree flexion of the knee joint is maintained during this measurement, it will be found after constructing the proximal anastomosis that the graft will be under too much tension when the knee is straightened, and this will narrow the anastomotic lumen. It is better to have the graft a little too long than too short, but it should not be loose enough to bend or buckle. The vein graft should be pulled proximally so that it is quite snug and then allowed to slacken off about 2 cm., which will leave it at the right degree of tension. It should be the proper length so that after an angioplasty to the bifid distal trunks the larger vein cuff so constructed can be used for the proximal anastomosis. This maneuver is especially helpful when the main trunk of the saphenous vein is relatively small, so that it would be difficult to make a satisfactory anastomosis, especially to a thick-walled common femoral artery. See Plate 195 for the details of this angioplastic technique.

B. This shows the grafting procedure completed. Note that the silk marker suture on the vein graft has been removed. The proximal anastomosis with the angioplasty to the proximal end of the graft was made to the common femoral artery, using the same technique as for the distal anastomosis. Before allowing blood to flow through the graft it is tested for leaks by distending it with dilute heparin-saline solution injected into the proximal end of the vein graft, with a bulldog clamp applied distal to the point of injection, using a 10-cc. syringe and a 22-gauge needle. If leaks are found, these are controlled with individual sutures. The bulldog clamps on the popliteal, superficial femoral and profunda femoris arteries are then removed to allow blood to flow from the latter one down through the graft. This is another check on whether there are any bleeding sources that should be controlled; if not, the occluding clamp on the common femoral artery is removed. If bleeding continues as an ooze from the proximal anastomosis, this is best controlled by placing a piece of thin rubber sheeting over the anastomosis. Gentle pressure with a few rolled sponges is applied over the rubber by clipping the skin edges together with towel clips for a few minutes. The rubber produces rapid clotting of blood and when it is removed it does not pull the clots away with it as gauze will do.

C. The incision is closed, first suturing the tendons of the semitendinosus, gracilis and sartorius muscles if they were divided, using linen sutures. They are also sutured to the medial part of the knee joint capsule. The groin incision is closed carefully in two layers to obliterate the dead space over the graft with interrupted sutures of fine linen or cotton. A second layer is placed in the deep fascia where it was opened. It is of utmost importance *that no additional sutures* be placed in the subcutaneous tissues because if used this will invariably result in necrosis of the skin edges, whereas without them necrosis seldom, if ever, occurs. The skin edges should be approximated with interrupted vertical mattress sutures of silk. Drainage of the proximal and distal portions of the incision with Penrose tubing may occasionally be necessary if there is troublesome oozing. The drain should be removed after 24 hours.

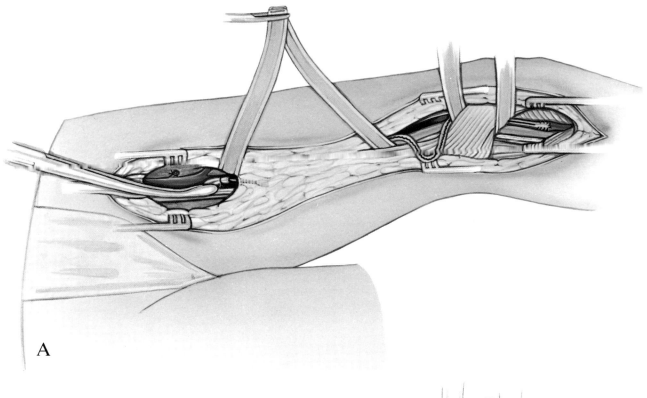

A

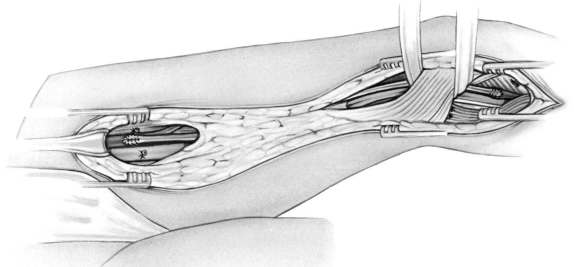

B

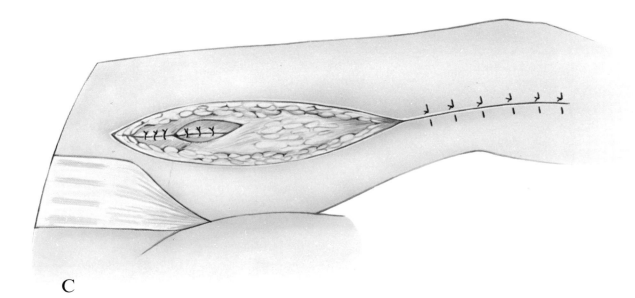

C

437

Plate 195

ANGIOPLASTIC PROCEDURE
TO PROXIMAL END OF
SAPHENOUS VEIN
BYPASS GRAFT

A.   This shows the proximal end of the long saphenous vein graft removed from below the knee with the short segments of the two distal trunks to demonstrate the angioplastic procedure that is carried out to make a larger venous cuff for the proximal anastomosis.

B.   This shows the ends of the two distal trunks stretched out straight. The adjacent sides are incised with scissors, as shown.

C.   This shows that the two trunks have been opened, leaving the main trunk intact.

D.   The vessel is now turned end for end, as this part of the vein graft will be used for the proximal anastomosis. The two edges (a) and (b) are sutured together with a running over-and-over suture of 6-0 Teflon-coated Dacron, using a taper-pointed needle to avoid tearing the thin vein wall, which may happen if a cutting point needle is used.

E.   This demonstrates the completed proximal anastomosis to the common femoral artery of a saphenous vein graft in which the angioplastic procedure has been performed to the branches at the proximal end. Note that it makes a wider cuff, which helps to make a better anastomosis if a thick-walled femoral artery is encountered. This type of artery is encountered frequently; it has a thick media and intima which interfere with the construction of a satisfactory anastomosis, especially when the venous cuff of the main trunk of saphenous vein is small. This angioplastic procedure permits the use of much larger bites of the vein cuff with each stitch, thus obtaining a better intima-to-intima approximation between the venous graft and the artery.

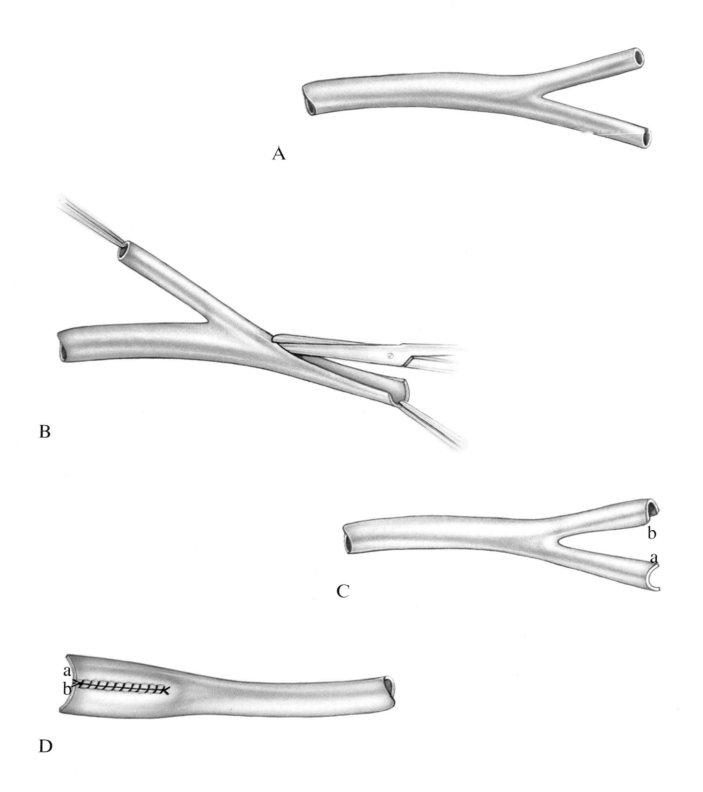

A

B

C

D

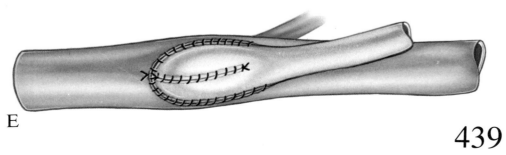

E

439

Plate 196

EXPOSURE OF THE
ENTIRE POPLITEAL ARTERY

A. This shows exposure of the entire popliteal artery through the medial approach. This necessitates dividing the tendons of the gracilis (a), semitendinosus (b), sartorius (c), and the semimembranosus (d) muscles; in addition, the medial head of the gastrocnemius muscle (e) must also be severed. The reason for this more adequate exposure of the popliteal artery is that occasionally the most suitable place to implant a saphenous vein bypass autograft will be directly behind these structures, so that it is necessary to divide them in order to be able to construct a satisfactory distal anastomosis. In the case illustrated here the proximal part of the popliteal artery is occluded; the distal part was so calcified that it would have been impossible to have anastomosed a graft to either of these sections of it. Sometimes there is a soft pliable area in the middle portion of the popliteal artery, as there fortuitously was in this case, and a graft was implanted to it satisfactorily.

B. This shows that the saphenous vein autograft has been anastomosed to the popliteal artery (a). So that it could be shown after the suturing of the muscles, the illustration shows it to be a little more distal than it was actually placed at the operation, but even in this location it would have been very difficult to construct a good anastomosis without severing all the tendons and muscular structures on the medial side of the knee joint. The medial heads of the gastrocnemius and the semimembranosus tendons have been reconstituted, using interrupted mattress sutures of No. 60 linen or No. 20 cotton. The sartorius, semitendinosus and gracilis tendons will be sutured back into place in the same manner. In addition to the mattress suture, interrupted single sutures are placed longitudinally between the capsule of the knee and the tendons of the semimembranosus, semitendinosus and the gracilis. These tendons are also sutured to each other with interrupted stitches. It is important that the sutures be of nonabsorbable material, because catgut ligatures will not hold. With this type of repair no weakness or difficulty with the knee joint has been encountered following the numerous procedures that have been performed. Additional operative time for this type of closure is required, but in order to construct a perfect anastomosis and end up with a stable knee joint it is well worth the effort and extra time.

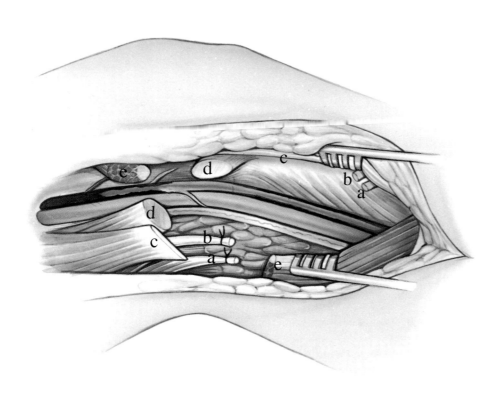

A

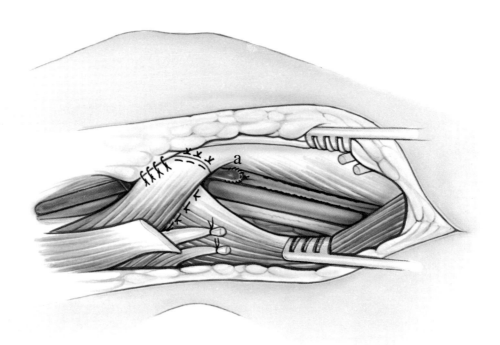

B

441

Plate 197

PROXIMAL ANASTOMOSIS WITH AN AUTOGENOUS VEIN PATCH GRAFT TO THE COMMON FEMORAL AND SUPERFICIAL FEMORAL ARTERIES

A. This shows an arteriotomy incision made in the distal end of the common femoral and the proximal end of the superficial femoral arteries. In the mid portion is seen a narrow take-off of the profunda femoris artery. Note the very thick wall of the common femoral artery to which it would be very difficult to construct a satisfactory saphenous vein anastomosis. For that reason it is worthwhile to do a limited excision of the thick media and intima of the arteriotomy incision and remove the plaque that is encroaching on the orifice of the profunda femoris artery.

B. This shows these vessels after the excision has been accomplished. The edges of the arteriotomy incision are still quite ragged and, although the arterial wall is thinner, it would still be difficult to obtain a good streamlined anastomosis.

C. This shows that a vein patch graft has been implanted, using a running over-and-over stitch with a 5-0 Teflon-coated Dacron suture on a straight cutting point needle. Note that there is a portion of a polyvinyl catheter within the artery as a stent. This is very important, because the diameter of the artery with the vein graft should be maintained the same diameter as the patient's femoral artery in order to prevent an aneurysmal dilatation at the site of the patch graft and the anastomosis. Note that large bites of the arterial wall are used with the arterial suture and small ones in the vein patch in order to save the thinner, better textured venous graft for the anastomosis. The incision in the venous graft has been made with a knife with the stent still in place, which makes it much easier to accomplish.

D. This demonstrates the removal of the stent through the incision in the vein graft.

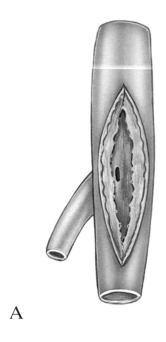

A

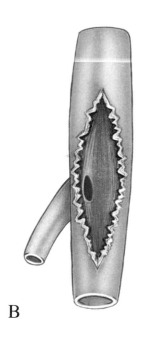

B

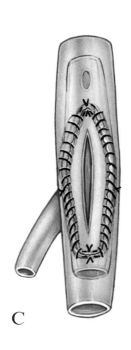

C

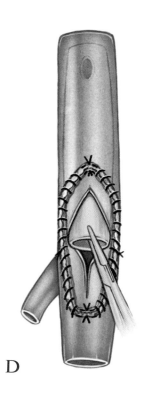

D

Plate 198

PROXIMAL ANASTOMOSIS WITH AN AUTOGENOUS VEIN PATCH GRAFT TO THE COMMON FEMORAL AND SUPERFICIAL FEMORAL ARTERIES *(Continued)*

A. This demonstrates one of the advantages of implanting the vein graft to the patch graft in these thick-walled arteries: it is possible after removing the stent to examine both sides of the suture line and cut away any projecting raw edges that sometimes protrude into the vessel lumen between the stitches. If the anastomosis is made directly to the artery, this is possible on only one side of the anastomosis.

B. This demonstrates the completed anastomosis of an autogenous vein graft to autogenous vein patch graft. It is well streamlined and there is very little widening of the artery as the result of the vein graft and the veno-venous anastomosis.

C and D. This demonstrates what is sometimes necessary if the proximal end of the vein graft is very small. The proximal graft cuff can be enlarged so that a better proximal anastomosis can be made by doing an angioplasty to the bifid end of the graft. This results in a more adequate anastomotic lumen and at the same time maintains good streamlining. (See Plate 195.)

E. This demonstrates the long femoropopliteal saphenous vein bypass graft implanted in this manner. The distal anastomosis was made directly to the popliteal artery. In some cases, however, because of the thickness of the popliteal arterial wall, it has been found advantageous to use this same vein patch graft anastomotic technique for the distal anastomosis, but it is not necessary nearly so often as for the femoral anastomosis.

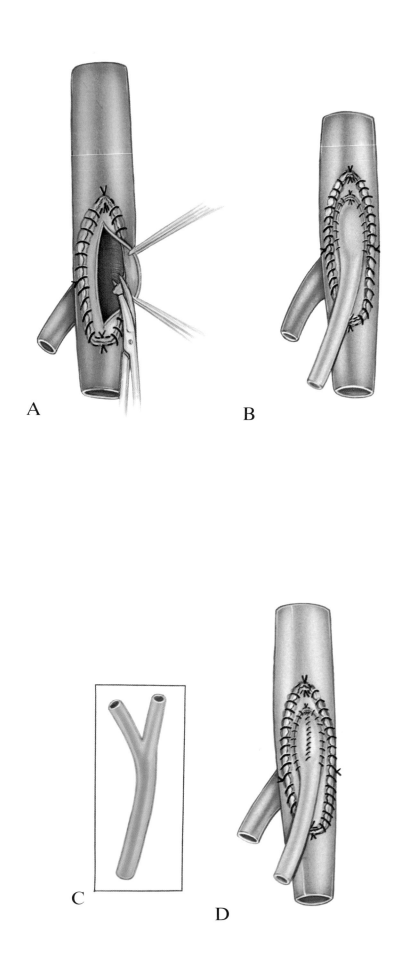

A

B

C

D

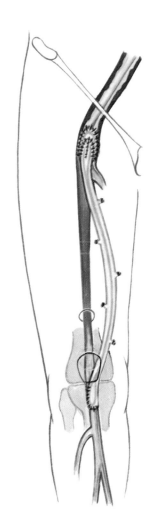

E

445

Plate 199

BIFID REVERSED
FEMOROPOPLITEAL
SAPHENOUS VEIN GRAFTS

A. As the dissection of the saphenous vein is carried distalward from the groin, it is not uncommon to find that it divides into two trunks at the mid thigh or a little distal to this level. Under these conditions it is advisable in most cases to continue the excision of both trunks distal to the knee joint. In some cases the two trunks rejoin at or just distal to the knee joint so that under these conditions it makes an ideal type of graft; more frequently, however, they do not. The removal of this type of vein is made easier by dissecting it out from the groin distalward in the extremity; almost of necessity a single long incision is required. The completely excised bifid vein with the single and double lumen portion is shown with all the tributaries ligated.

B. This shows the bifid vein implanted in the reverse manner. The distal anastomosis has been made to the popliteal artery distal to the knee joint in a patient with a complete occlusion of the superficial femoral and most of the popliteal artery. The proximal anastomosis has been made to the common femoral artery. This has been accomplished after selecting the correct lengths of graft to use by straightening the knee joint and discarding the extra length of each graft limb. It is important to always excise a longer section of saphenous vein than is thought to be necessary. The end of each graft limb over a distance of 12 to 15 mm. is incised with scissors and the top edges sewn together with a 6-0 suture with a running over-and-over type of stitch; this can be readily anastomosed to the common femoral artery, permitting a two-channel outflow tract.

C. This demonstrates the inside of this proximal cuff made from the distal ends of the bifid portion of the graft. Note what a satisfactory venous cuff has been constructed by this technique, which makes it readily possible to construct a very satisfactory proximal anastomosis even to a thick-walled femoral artery, which would not be possible if only one of the small trunks were used.

D. This demonstrates an unusual configuration of one of these bifid saphenous vein grafts in which the two trunks would not lie parallel to each other as shown in *B.* This intertwining of the two limbs was discovered as the vein graft was being dilated under pressure with dilute heparin in normal saline solution. It was necessary therefore to construct the proximal cuff of the graft as shown, so that the intertwining of the two limbs was maintained instead of trying to make them lie parallel with each other. The graft has functioned well since it was implanted. Both these cases demonstrate how the surgeon can improvise with saphenous vein autografts to make satisfactory long femoropopliteal grafts that will function by preserving the bifid portion of the graft instead of utilizing only one trunk, which would jeopardize the patency of it because of the impossibility of making a satisfactory proximal anastomosis with the narrow single venous trunk to the femoral artery. It is also considered a better procedure than incising the entire length of both of the limbs and sewing them together to make a single tube graft. This method has been used, but the section with the long angioplasty in it tends to become aneurysmal. If the bifid portion is in the middle of the graft, both trunks should be left intact and utilized.

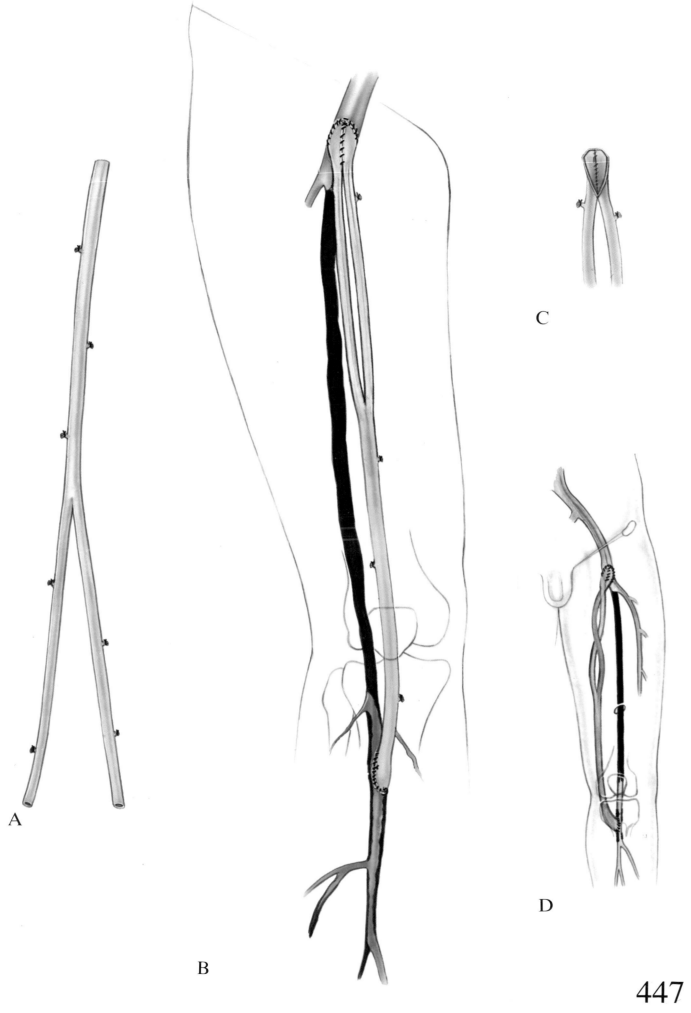

A

B

C

D

447

Plate 200

FEMORAL, POSTERIOR TIBIAL
SAPHENOUS VEIN
BYPASS GRAFTS

It is necessary in some patients, because of complete occlusion of the popliteal and the proximal sections of the outflow arteries from it, to carry a grafting procedure to one of the latter in the mid lower leg or more distally. These are usually desperation procedures, as they are done to save a limb and are not performed only for the treatment of intermittent claudication. The percentage of late patency is not so good as in the femoropopliteal grafting procedures, but it is certainly worth performing if a satisfactory saphenous vein graft is available and one of the outflow vessels has a satisfactory lumen in it. It is possible also if the saphenous vein is not long enough to utilize a composite type of graft consisting of a proximal section of a Dacron prosthesis and a distal portion of the saphenous vein autograft across the knee joint and in the lower leg. (See Plates 202 and 203.)

A.   The outflow artery for these procedures should be exposed first to make sure that it will be possible to anastomose the vein graft to it. The location of the distal anastomosis will vary, depending on where the angiograms demonstrate the widest caliber of the artery. The posterior tibial artery is exposed on the inner side of the mid lower leg. It may be necessary to go more distally in some patients, but the more proximal the anastomosis is placed the better the patency rate. The incision is 6 to 8 cm. long and about 1 cm. behind the posterior edge of the tibia.

B.   The dissection is carried down the intermuscular septum, separating the flexor digitorum longus muscle (a) from the soleus muscle (b), to the neurovascular bundle (c).

C.   This shows the end-to-side anastomosis of the saphenous vein autograft (c) to the posterior tibial artery (d) constructed with 6-0 synthetic sutures, lying between the flexor digitorum longus (a) and the soleus (b) muscles. The posterior tibial nerve (e) is identified and carefully preserved. The graft is brought proximally through a tunnel along the neurovascular bundle and through the popliteal space behind the medial head of the gastrocnemius muscle, then along Hunter's canal beneath the sartorius muscle to the incision in the femoral triangle, where it is anastomosed end-to-side to the common femoral artery.

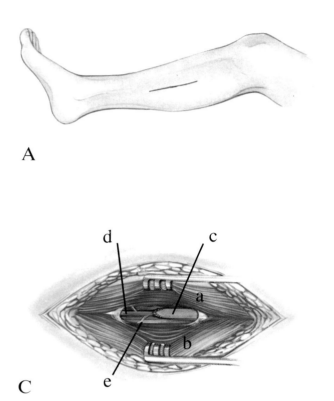

A

C

d   c

                     a

          b

e

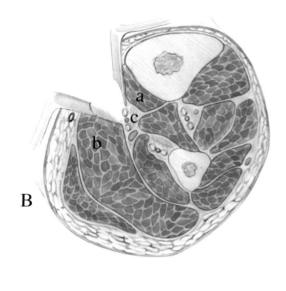

B

449

Plate 200 (Continued)

FEMORAL, ANTERIOR TIBIAL
SAPHENOUS VEIN
BYPASS GRAFTS

D.   The anterior tibial artery may be the best one to use in some patients. It is exposed through an anterior incision lateral to the tibia about 6 to 8 cm. long and usually at the mid lower leg.

E.   The dissection is carried down between the tibialis anticus (a), the extensor digitorum longus (b) and the extensor hallucis longus (c) muscles to the neurovascular bundle (d).

F.   This demonstrates the distal anastomosis of the saphenous vein autograft (d) to the anterior tibial artery (e) lying between the tibialis anticus (a) and the extensor digitorum longus (b) and extensor hallucis longus (c) muscles. It is constructed with 6-0 monofilament synthetic sutures. The deep peroneal nerve (f) is seen and should be carefully preserved. As this anastomosis lies anterior to the interosseous membrane, it is necessary to make an opening through it and a tunnel through the calf muscles to the popliteal space through which the vein graft is brought proximally, passing behind the medial head of the gastrocnemius muscle, then anteriorly to Hunter's canal underneath the sartorius muscle to the incision in the femoral triangle, where it is anastomosed end-to-side to the common femoral artery. In a few patients the superficial femoral artery may be of sufficient caliber so that it can be used for the proximal anastomosis, especially when the saphenous vein is not long enough to reach the common femoral artery.

D

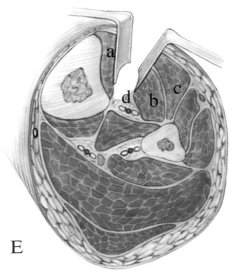

E

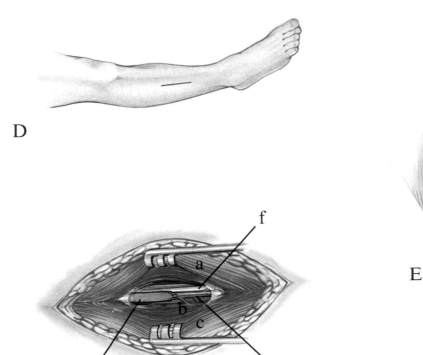

F

451

Plate 201

A FEMORAL PERONEAL SAPHENOUS VEIN BYPASS AUTOGRAFT

A. This demonstrates the patient lying prone for a postlateral exposure of the peroneal artery that is carried out posterior to the fibula in the mid lower leg. The artery should first be exposed through this small incision to determine if it is suitable for the implantation of a saphenous vein autograft before proceeding with the rest of the operation.

B. This cross-section of the mid lower leg shows the exposure obtained by following the lateral interosseous fascial septum. The soleus (a) and the flexor hallucis longus (c) muscles are retracted forward and the peroneal longus muscle (b) is retracted downward. The dissection is carried to the medial edge of the fibula, where the peroneal artery and veins (d) are found. After it has been determined that the peroneal artery will accept a vein graft, the patient is turned supine and the extremity redraped. The long saphenous vein is removed by careful excision through a long incision (or multiple incisions) from the saphenofemoral junction distalward beyond the level of the exploratory incision for the peroneal artery. At the same time it can be determined if the femoral artery is satisfactory for the proximal anastomosis. A tunnel is made from the groin under the sartorius muscle through the popliteal space behind the medial head of the gastrocnemius to the distal end of the popliteal space, then through the muscles along the neurovascular bundle to the exploratory incision for the peroneal artery.

C. The patient is then turned prone again and redraped. The lower leg incision is opened. This shows the peroneal longus muscle (c) and the fibula (d) in the upper part of the illustration; the flexor hallucis longus muscle (e) that was dissected from the fibula, and the soleus muscle (f) are seen in the lower portion. The distal anastomosis is constructed between the saphenous vein graft (a) and the peroneal artery (b), which has previously been dilated with dilute heparin-saline solution, to aid in the construction of a flawless end-to-side anastomosis, using 6-0 monofilament synthetic sutures. After it is constructed it is tested with dilute heparin-saline solution, then the patient is turned supine again. The graft is brought out through the tunnel that had been previously made to the groin incision, making sure there is no twist in the graft, and constructing an end-to-side anastomosis between the graft and the common femoral artery. The incisions are closed without drainage, using a few fascial sutures and interrupted silk sutures to the skin.

D. This demonstrates a 62 cm. by 5 mm. reversed saphenous vein autograft implanted in the left leg of a patient 69 years of age with severe occlusive atherosclerotic disease involving the superficial femoral, popliteal and proximal outflow arteries and with ischemic gangrene of several toes of his left foot. This graft was implanted five years ago and it still continues to function, with salvage of the extremity and the healing of the ischemic lesions of the toes of the foot.

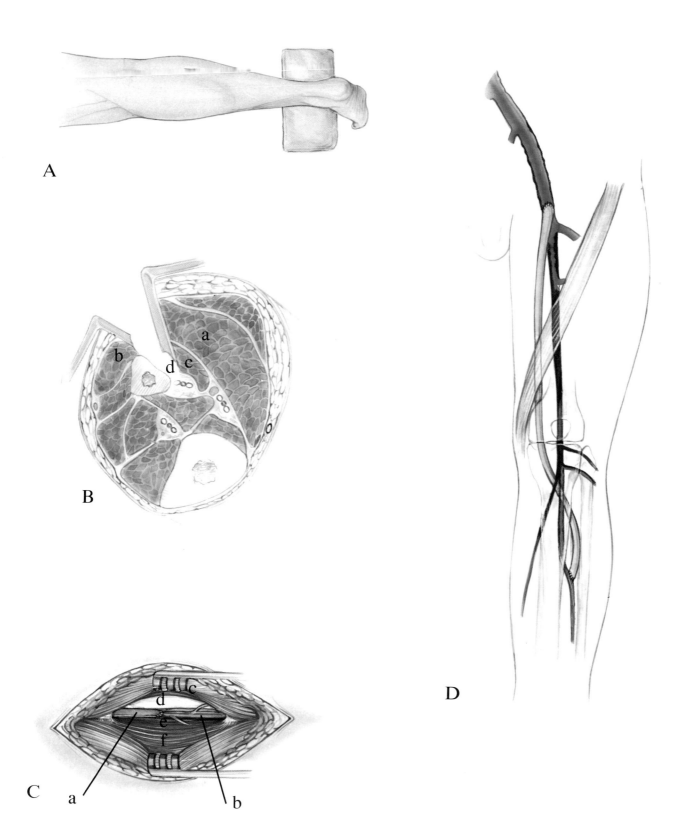

A

B

a
b
d c

C

d c
e
f
a b

D

453

Plate 202

FEMOROPOPLITEAL COMPOSITE DACRON AND AUTOGENOUS SAPHENOUS VEIN BYPASS GRAFT

Femoropopliteal saphenous vein bypass autografts from the common femoral artery to the popliteal artery distal to the knee joint have a five-year patency rate of 80 per cent compared to 19 per cent for synthetic prostheses and 29 per cent for femoral endarterectomy. Unfortunately the long saphenous vein in some patients is not of sufficient caliber, except for the proximal 15 to 20 cm., to utilize as a saphenous bypass graft. For this reason a composite graft has been used successfully and consists of a 6- or 8 mm. knitted Dacron prosthesis for the proximal portion, and for the distal portion that crosses the knee joint, a segment of saphenous vein autograft. This method has the additional advantage that the proximal anastomosis, or take-off of the Dacron prosthesis, may be made to the common or external iliac arteries if the common femoral artery does not have a satisfactory lumen. The following methods of constructing a composite graft of this type have been utilized with encouraging success rates. As there is a great disparity between the size of the Dacron and the venous portions of the graft, a special technique is necessary to create a streamlined type of anastomosis between them.

A. The construction is by a long end-to-end type of anastomosis utilizing the end-to-side type of suture technique. A 6- or 8-mm. standard type knitted Dacron prosthesis is selected and first preclotted, then a large wedge-shaped section of it is cut away with straight scissors, as shown, leaving a long tapered end to the graft which should equal the length of the planned anastomosis.

B. The ideal saphenous vein graft should be 5 to 6 mm. in diameter, although 4.0 to 4.5 mm. ones can be used. If it is smaller than this, the method of anastomosis shown in Plate 203*B* should be used. If possible the venotomy is carried through a small venous branch, as shown; this facilitates the construction of the anastomosis. The length of the anastomosis in most instances should be approximately 2.0 to 2.5 cm. The smaller the vein diameter, the longer the anastomosis should be.

C. Two double-needled mattress sutures are placed first at each end of the anastomosis using 5-0 Teflon-coated Dacron sutures with straight needles. These are tied to approximate the grafts.

D. A polyvinyl catheter of the same diameter as the venous autograft is used as a stent. The suturing is continued with the same sutures always sewing by passing the needle first through the wall of the Dacron graft, then the venous graft, thus avoiding the suture dragging the adventitia of the vein with resulting irregularities in the contour of the venous portion of the anastomosis. It is best to carry the suturing from each end of the anastomosis, ligating the first suture to a stay stitch at the mid point of the anastomosis; then the second suture is tied to the first one. The graft is then turned end-for-end so that the suturing can be placed through the grafts in the same manner on the opposite side. This has the additional advantage that it avoids a tendency for the graft to twist at the site of the long anastomosis, which occurs if both sides are sutured in the same direction.

E. This demonstrates the completed streamlined type of tapering anastomosis that can be constructed between a 6- or 8-mm. Dacron graft and a 5-mm. venous graft.

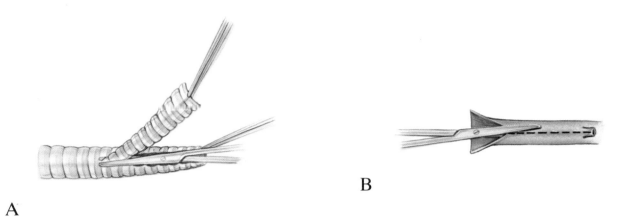

A

B

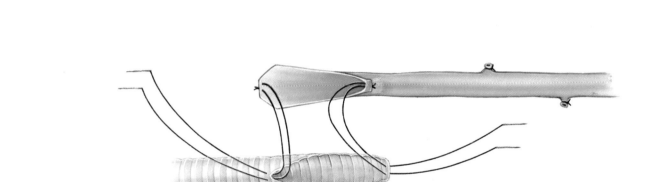

C

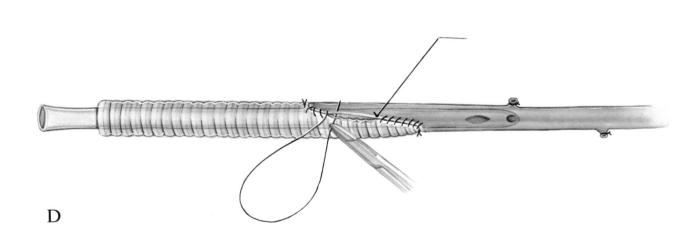

D

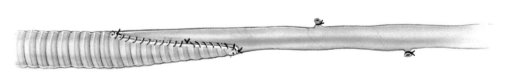

E

455

Plate 203

TYPE I. FEMOROPOPLITEAL COMPOSITE DACRON AND AUTOGENOUS SAPHENOUS VEIN BYPASS GRAFT

A. This illustration shows a femoropopliteal composite bypass graft in the left lower extremity, consisting of a 27 cm. by 6 mm. knitted Dacron prosthesis and a 20 cm. by 5 mm. saphenous vein autograft. The Dacron prosthesis is first preclotted, then the long streamlined anastomosis is made between it and the saphenous vein autograft. The anastomosis (a) to the distal popliteal artery is made next. The graft is drawn through the tunnel behind the medial head of the gastrocnemius and sartorius muscles. After straightening the knee, an end-to-side anastomosis (b) is made between the Dacron end and the common femoral artery with a slight amount of tension on it. The correct amount of tension is important, otherwise it will tend to bend and buckle when the knee is flexed. The anastomosis (c) between the prosthesis and the saphenous vein may leak at the suture line, so it is recommended that it be visualized in order to suture any bleeding points that may be present. The incisions are then closed in the routine manner.

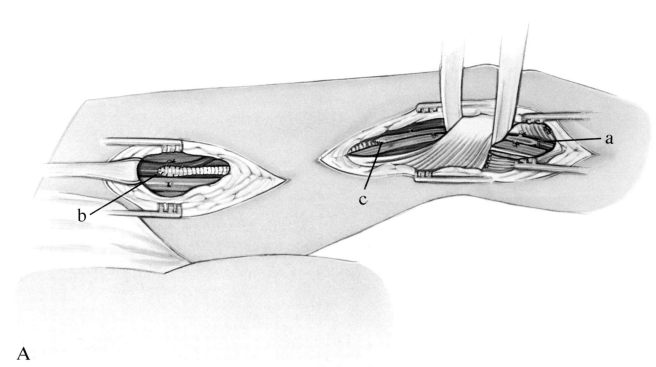

A

Plate 203 (Continued)

TYPE II. FEMOROPOPLITEAL COMPOSITE KNITTED DACRON AND SAPHENOUS VEIN BYPASS AUTOGRAFT

B. One of the easiest end-to-side anastomoses to construct is between a Dacron prosthesis and a saphenous vein autograft, even of small size. If the vein graft portion is 3.0 to 3.5 mm. in diameter, it is considered too small to make a satisfactory long end-to-end anastomosis as described in Plate 202. For this reason another method of constructing the composite graft has been utilized: after preclotting the Dacron tube, the proximal anastomosis is made to the common femoral artery. The graft is occluded with a bulldog clamp at the site of anastomosis to restore the blood supply through the profunda femoris during the remainder of the grafting procedure. The graft is brought distally beneath the sartorius muscle and sutured to the tendinous attachment of the adductor longus muscle (a) with the proper amount of tension on it. A small ellipse of the anterior wall of the distal portion of the prosthesis (b) is removed for the site of the Dacron-venous anastomosis.

C. This is constructed in the routine method, using either 6-0 or 5-0 synthetic sutures and keeping the knee in extension to get the correct tension on the venous graft. This can be accomplished because the distal end of the Dacron prosthesis has been fixed to the adductor longus tendon. After completion of the anastomosis the proximal end of the vein graft is occluded with a bulldog clamp and the Dacron prosthesis is flushed out through its distal end, which has not been hemostatically sealed. A ligature of 2-0 Dacron is then placed around it just distal to the anastomosis.

D. This demonstrates the exposure for the removal of the cephalic vein in the arm if a saphenous vein is not available. Sometimes the full length of this vein may be used, but frequently it is not long enough, so either the portion in the forearm or that in the upper arm may be used successfully in the construction of a femoropopliteal bypass composite Dacron-venous type of graft.

E. This demonstrates a long femoropopliteal composite graft of this type that permits the use of a smaller calibered saphenous or cephalic vein. It also enables the surgeon to obtain the optimum tension on the two portions of the graft, especially the Dacron portion, and at the same time to suture it to a fixed stricture (a) so that it will not twist the more tender venous graft after completion of the anastomosis. In addition, with either the Type I or Type II procedure the Dacron graft does not become kinked on genuflexion.

458

A

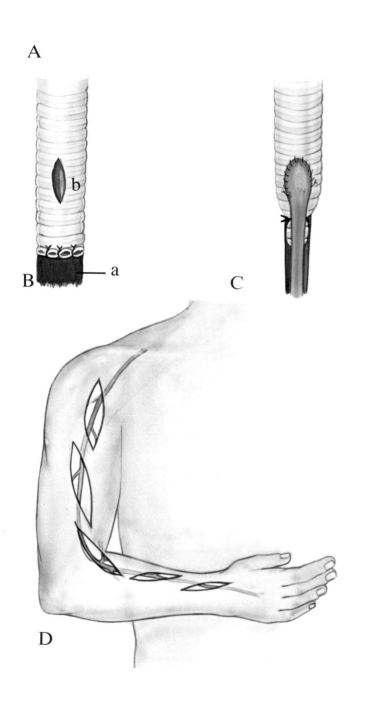

B b

a

C

D

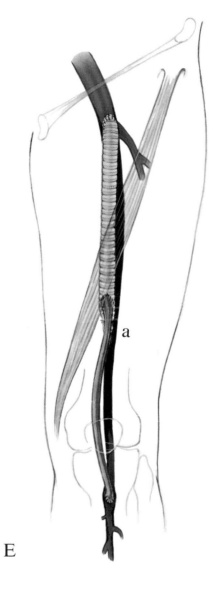

E

a

459

Plate 204

COMPOSITE DACRON
SAPHENOUS VEIN BYPASS
ILIOPOPLITEAL GRAFT

A.   This demonstrates the angiographic findings in a patient with bilateral severe iliofemoral obliterative arterial disease. The patient, a man aged 61 years, had a large ischemic ulcer 5 cm. in diameter over his right heel. The collateral blood supply on the left through his hypogastric artery and distal profunda femoral and popliteal arteries was sufficient so that this extremity was giving him no symptoms. On the right side a satisfactory common iliac artery, a distal popliteal artery and outflow arteries are shown.

B.   This shows a long composite graft that was implanted from the distal right common iliac artery to the distal popliteal artery. In addition, the common femoral and proximal portion of the profunda femoris artery were endarterectomized, and a side-to-side anastomosis was constructed between the prosthesis and the segment of the common femoral artery from which the profunda femoris arose, after ligating it proximal to the anastomosis and the superficial femoral artery distal to it. The Dacron prosthesis was 48 cm. by 8 mm. and the saphenous vein autograft was 16 cm. by 4 mm., which was all the length that was available. The latter was just sufficiently long to satisfactorily cross the knee joint area. It is felt that, without any question, the utilization of the distal venous segment across the knee joint is an important factor in the long patency rate of this type of reconstructive procedure. Following this procedure in this patient there was an excellent return of arterial pulses in the extremity and the foot. The heel ulceration developed deep red granulation, so that it was possible to cover it with a split-thickness skin graft with a complete take. The composite graft has remained patent and still continues to function five years postoperative, with salvage of the limb and no recurrence of the ulceration, an excellent result that could not have been obtained by any other method.

C.   This demonstrates the utilization of this composite Dacron saphenous vein grafting procedure to restore the circulation to the lower leg by utilizing a long saphenous vein bypass graft from the femoral limb of an aortic Dacron bifurcation prosthesis that has been implanted into the common femoral artery. In this case the venous graft was only 4 mm. in diameter, but it was possible to implant it into the Dacron graft by performing the angioplastic technique between the two distal trunks of the graft to make a wider cuff for the proximal anastomosis. (See Plate 195.)

D.   This demonstrates another variation of this technique in which a composite Dacron-venous bypass graft of the lower extremity has been anastomosed to the femoral limb of an aortic bifurcation graft because the venous graft was not sufficiently long to reach from the common femoral artery to the distal popliteal artery. It is recommended that this method be used if a femoropopliteal bypass graft is performed months or years after an aortofemoral graft was implanted. This is because of the thick fibrous scar that forms in the groin after these secondary procedures, which almost surely will cause a vein graft to occlude but is much less likely to do so if the proximal portion of the graft is Dacron, as it is in these composite grafts.

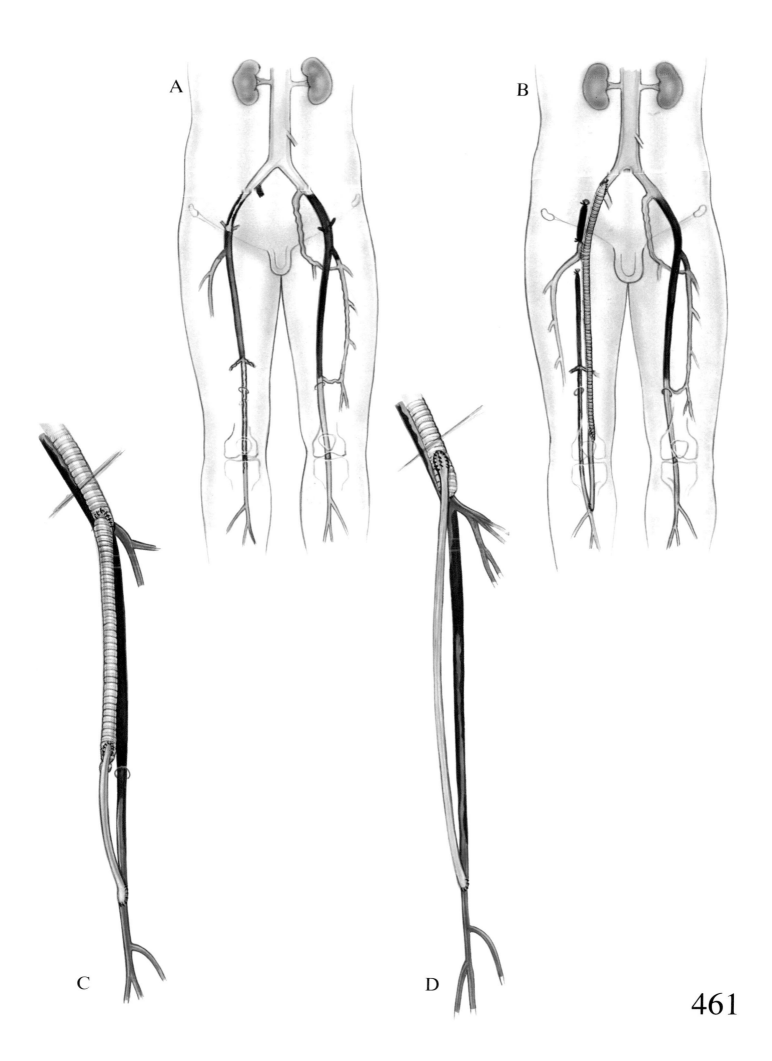

Plate 205

COMPOSITE FEMORAL ENDARTERECTOMY AND DISTAL AUTOGENOUS SAPHENOUS VEIN BYPASS GRAFT

These procedures were developed with the hope that since they were performed entirely with autogenous tissues they would give better and longer patency rates than were obtained with prosthetic grafts. But except for *B* this was not true.

A. This demonstrates one method of a composite procedure, including an endarterectomy of the femoral artery and saphenous vein bypass graft, a long vein patch extending the entire length of the common femoral artery and a portion of the distal end of the external iliac artery. The proximal end of the saphenous vein graft is anastomosed to the distal end of the patch graft. The results have proved disappointing for long-term patency because of aneurysmal dilatation of the common femoral artery, so this method has been discontinued.

B. This demonstrates the most satisfactory method of performing the composite endarterectomy and the saphenous vein bypass autograft by combining it with a local endarterectomy of the common femoral artery, then anastomosing the saphenous vein bypass graft to a venous patch on the common femoral artery (Plates 197 and 198). The results with this technique proved satisfactory with the limited endarterectomy.

C This shows another variant in which the patch graft to the common femoral artery is in continuity with the vein graft. It is difficult to obtain a satisfactory result with this technique although it looks simpler to perform in the drawing than the others. It is believed that the reason for this is the difficulty of obtaining good streamlining of the patch graft and the anastomotic lumen.

D. This shows another composite method of femoropopliteal reconstruction by performing a closed type of endarterectomy of the common femoral and the proximal half of the superficial femoral arteries. The arteriotomies are closed with autogenous vein patch grafts. A short segment of the saphenous vein is used as a bypass graft from the distal end of the endarterectomized femoral artery to the distal popliteal artery. They all failed, unfortunately, because of stenosis of the endarterectomized segment of the superficial femoral artery, requiring replacement of the latter with a Dacron tubular graft, with salvage of the vein graft.

E. This demonstrates a similar procedure, performed by the open method and the long arteriotomy was closed with a long vein patch graft in continuity with a short saphenous vein bypass graft. Again it was disappointing because of poor long patency rates.

F. A further attempt was made in a few patients by implanting a separate long patch graft to close the endarterectomized superficial femoral artery, and the vein bypass graft was anastomosed to the distal end of it and to the distal popliteal artery. The results with this procedure were better than in *D* or *E*, but still were not sufficiently good to warrant continuing this type of procedure.

It became obvious that the failures always occurred in the endarterectomized femoral artery. Because of the poor results in these patients, all these methods except the one in *B* have been discontinued and are no longer performed.

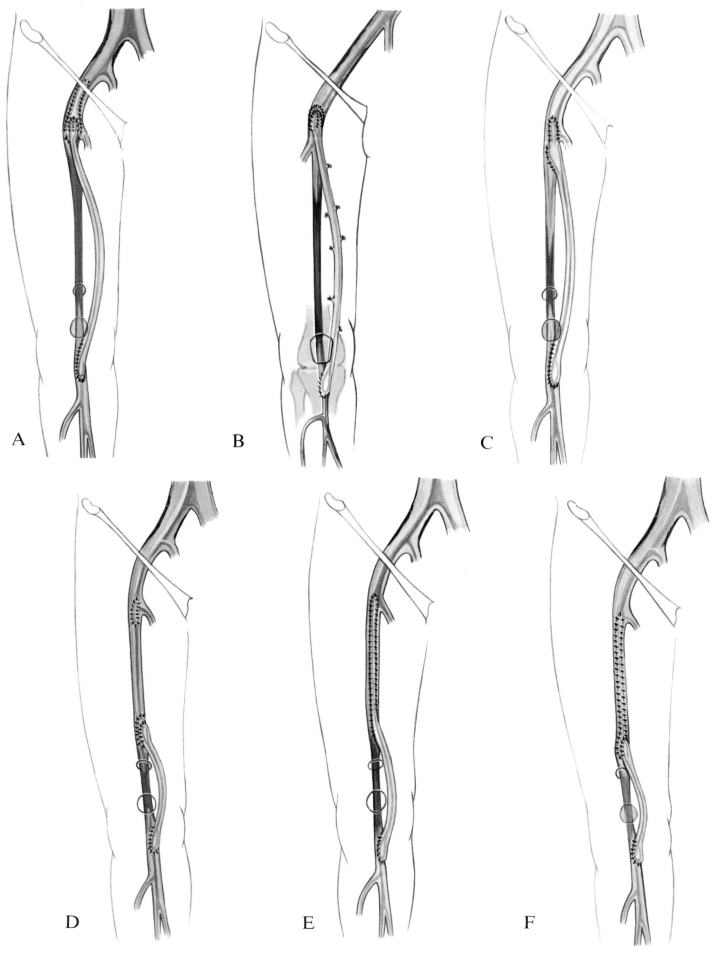

A

B

C

D

E

F

463

Plate 206

THE CORRECT METHOD OF CONSTRUCTING AN END-TO-SIDE VENOUS ARTERIAL ANASTOMOSIS

A. This demonstrates the end of the vein used for the venous arterial anastomosis. It is incised longitudinally equal to the length of the anastomosis that is planned.

B. This demonstrates the cuff of the vein with the corners trimmed. Two mattress sutures (a and b) are placed from outside in on the vein at the end of the venous incision and the cuff, and then passed through the artery from inside out. The one at the acute angle of the venotomy is placed first and ligated. Then the other one at the end of the venous cuff is tied. A ski-shaped needle, as shown, is the preferred type to use.

C. In order to construct a streamlined end-to-side anastomosis the vein cuff, after the tying of the two mattress sutures at each end, should be on a slight amount of tension so that there is no wrinkling of the venous cuff. It should not be too short either, as this will cause buckling of the artery, with poor streamlining of the anastomosis. The suturing is commenced and carried from each end to the middle of the anastomosis. The two sutures are tied there after tying the first one (a) to a stay suture that is placed at that point. This procedure is carried out on each side of the anastomosis.

D. This demonstrates the completed anastomosis and shows a little ballooning of the vein cuff, suggesting the head of a cobra snake. It produces some turbulence but does not seem to cause thrombosis to interfere with patency. For further details see Plates 190, 191, 192 and 193.

E. This demonstrates a modification of the end-to-side venous arterial anastomosis, described by Kunlin, a French surgeon. The venotomy in the venous autograft is made longitudinally, carrying the incision to and through the side of a small branch of the vein at the proximal end of the venotomy, when it is present.

F. The small tab of vein which is produced in this manner facilitates the construction of the anastomosis at the acute angle. Since this is the most difficult part of the anastomosis to construct, especially with small-calibered grafts, it is recommended that this method be used if this small venous branch is found.

G. This demonstrates the completed anastomosis utilizing this technique. It is again of utmost importance that the cuff be sutured under a slight degree of tension to prevent it from wrinkling.

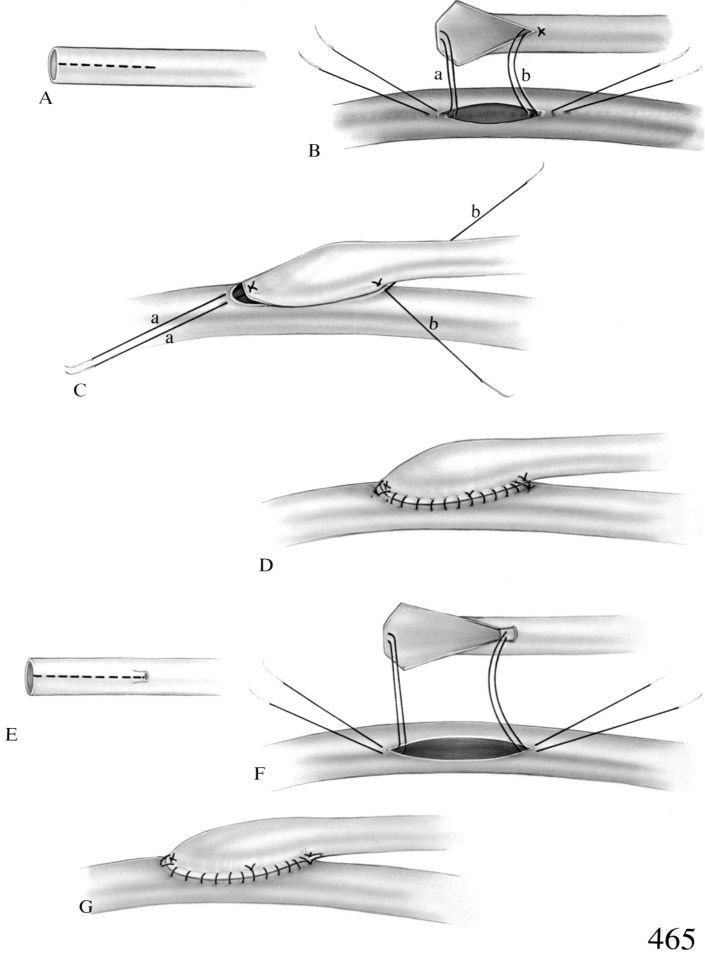

A

B

C

D

E

F

G

465

Plate 207

TECHNICAL ERRORS IN CONSTRUCTING END-TO-SIDE VENOUS-ARTERIAL ANASTOMOSES

Most failures in the treatment of femoral atherosclerotic occlusive disease with femoropopliteal saphenous vein bypass autografts are due to technical errors in the construction of the venous-arterial anastomoses. The flawless technique of constructing these anastomoses is of utmost importance in obtaining long-term successful results. The following errors are the ones most commonly seen, and all of them can be prevented if flawless technique is adhered to.

A. One of the commonest technical errors is to have too long a venous cuff. This illustration demonstrates the two primary mattress sutures in place at each end of the anastomosis, which resulted in wrinkling of the venous cuff. It is essential that the vein cuff should be on a slight amount of tension to eliminate this wrinkling.

B. This demonstrates the completed anastomosis with a cuff that is too long, resulting in transverse creases which produce turbulence and favor thrombosis.

C. This shows a very common error at the beginning of the anastomosis that occurs if the suture material adheres to the adventitia. It is therefore of utmost importance to use a suture that is slippery and slides through the tissues without dragging them. This error may also result from taking too long a stitch in the venous cuff and a short one in the arterial wall. It may also occur if the adventitia of the vein wall is caught when tying the mattress suture. With careful technique and the use of monofilament synthetic sutures this error can be avoided.

D. This demonstrates more irregularity in the contour of the vein cuff near its proximal end, again because the suture drags the adventitia with it as it is pulled taut. This error can be avoided by grasping the adventitia very firmly and holding it with a fine forceps as each stitch of the suture is pulled through.

E. Again the same effect may occur in the distal part of the anastomosis if care is not taken to avoid the same complication as seen in the preceding illustration.

F. This demonstrates the narrowing of the arterial lumen at the site of the anastomosis because the suturing has been carried from outside in on the artery, then through the venous wall so that the adventitia of the artery is caught in the suture, resulting in narrowing of the arterial lumen. All these errors can be avoided by sticking to the rules for performing a flawless venous-arterial anastomosis. Even use of a monofilament suture will not always obviate these types of errors unless special precautions are taken to prevent them.

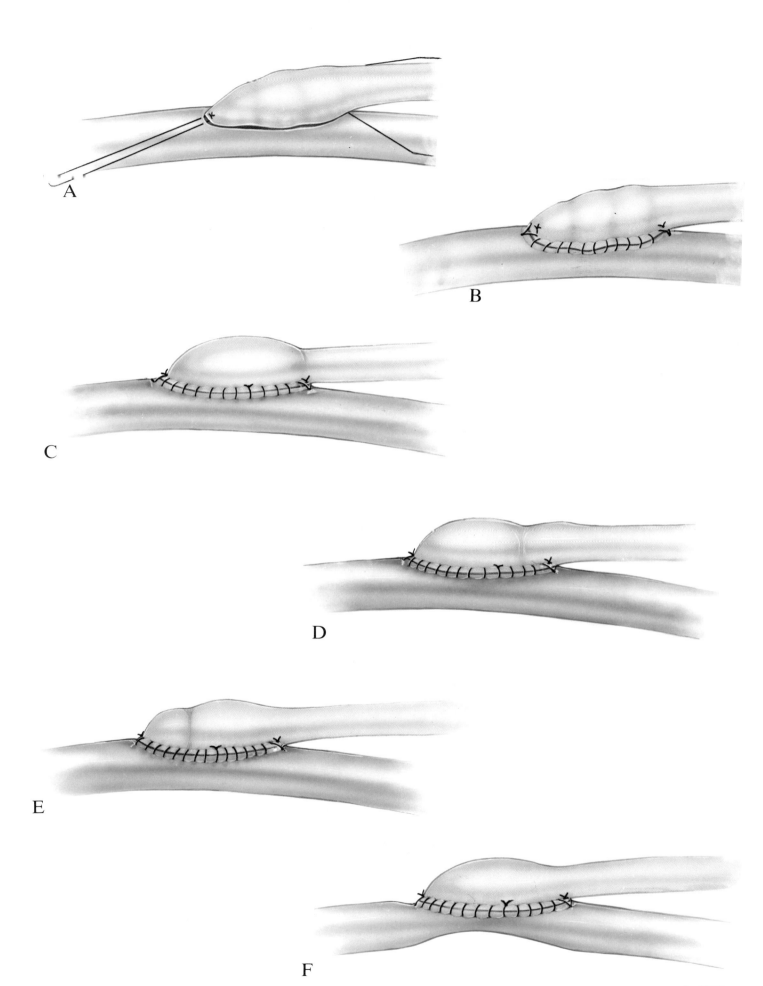

A

B

C

D

E

F

467

OTHER VASCULAR PROCEDURES

Plate 208

END-TO-END BLOOD VESSEL ANASTOMOSES BY THE END-TO-SIDE TECHNIQUE

A.   An end-to-end anastomosis between the two ends of a divided vein or artery is usually accomplished by suturing the ends together in three segments, using a running type of stitch and a fine synthetic suture, after cutting each end of the blood vessel cleanly straight across. This technique frequently results in varying degrees of stenosis at the site of the suture line, depending on the thickness and structure of the blood vessel that is being anastomosed. The one great advantage of this method is that it is possible to bring the two ends together more readily without tension. It has also been found a very useful method of suturing two synthetic prostheses together, although if they are of different sizes the following method demonstrates a satisfactory method of end-to-end anastomosis by what I have termed the end-to-side technique to suture two vein grafts together, two arteries together or a plastic prosthesis and artery together. The two ends are incised for a distance equal in length to or a little greater than the diameter of the blood vessel to be sutured. The incisions are longitudinal and are made on the opposite sides of the two ends.

B.   The corners of both ends are trimmed with scissors along the dotted lines as shown.

C.   Two double-needled mattress sutures are placed at each end and tied, unless one limb is a synthetic prosthesis, in which case the suture (a) is first tied before putting in the suture (b) and one-half of the anastomosis is completed. When dealing with two blood vessels, both sutures (a) and (b) are tied. A short segment of a plastic catheter the same size as the lumen of the blood vessels that are to be anastomosed is inserted at the site of the anastomosis. This is used as a stent so that the lumen at the site of this long type of anastomosis will be of the same caliber as that of the blood vessel. It will also prevent puckering and wrinkling at the suture line and give a much better streamlined effect.

D.   The major part of the anastomosis has been completed and the stent is being removed, which means there will be a short segment that will have to be sutured without the stent, but this should be no greater in length than the diameter of the stent.

E.   This shows an excellent streamlined end-to-end type of anastomosis constructed in this manner. If done carefully there will be no evidence of stenosis or aneurysmal dilatation at the site of the anastomosis. The suturing is all done by a simple over-and-over type of stitch, which is very hemostatic, and there are few if any troublesome leaks in the anastomotic suture line. It will be found to be an extremely useful method of restoring continuity in blood vessels and implanting synthetic prostheses as grafts, such as the restoration of continuity after excision of peripheral arterial aneurysms.

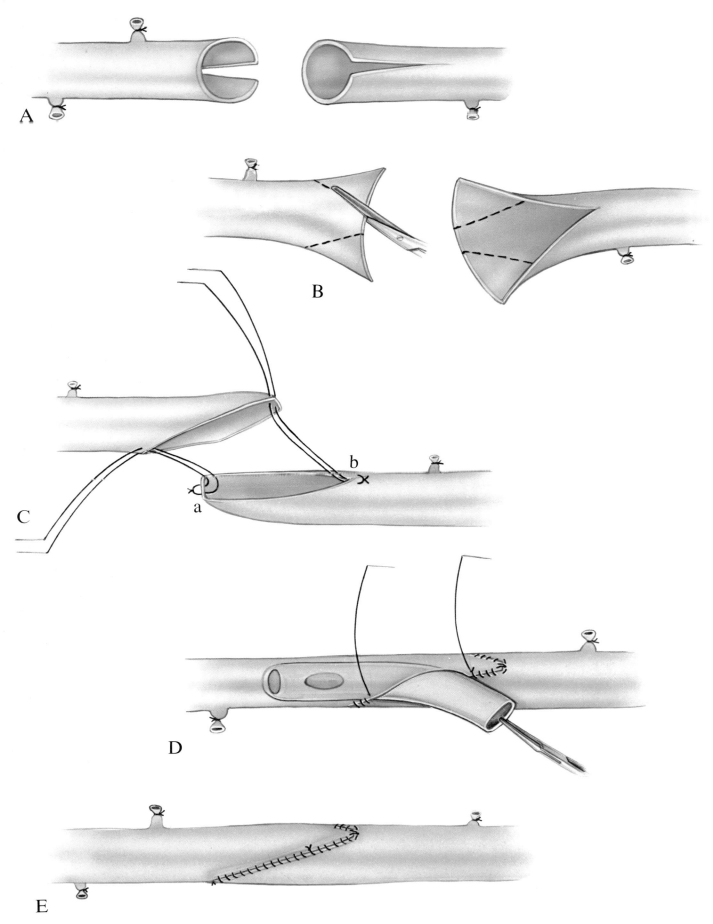

A

B

C

a

b

D

E

471

Plate 209

EXCISION OF A POPLITEAL ANEURYSM WITH IMPLANTATION OF A SAPHENOUS VEIN AUTOGRAFT THROUGH A MEDIAL APPROACH

A.   The leg is placed with slight hip flexion and external rotation and the knee is bent at a 15 degree angle. It is held in this position with a sterile towel placed around the foot and held to the sterile sheet beneath it with a clamp. The line in the left groin indicates the site of the incision made to excise the long saphenous vein for the autograft to replace the popliteal aneurysm. The superficial femoral vein is also interrupted at its junction with the profunda femoris vein through this incision. This is because the popliteal vein is excised with the aneurysm, which leaves a long blind venous segment of the superficial femoral vein without major branches. The blood in it becomes stagnant and clots, and since pulmonary emboli may arise from it, proximal interruption of the vein at its junction with the profunda femoris vein is the best safeguard against them. It should be interrupted before removing the aneurysm, as it may increase the venous pressure in the limb with a resulting increase of venous bleeding at the site of the aneurysmectomy; this is easier to control during the dissection of the aneurysm than if the superficial femoral vein is interrupted after removing it. The excision of the saphenous vein is performed later, after determination of the length that will be necessary. The more distal line indicates the location of the incision to remove the aneurysm. This approach gives the best exposure of the arteries distal and proximal to the aneurysm in order to obtain adequate control of the arterial inflow and outflow.

B.   Adequate exposure is essential for excision and grafting of popliteal aneurysms. This requires division of the tendons of the sartorius (a), the gracilis (b), the semitendinosus (c) and the semimembranosus (d) muscles, and the medial head of the gastrocnemius (e). The proximal ends of the gracilis and the semitendinosus tendons retract during the operation so 0 black silk ligatures are tied to them as markers to facilitate finding them. Excellent exposure of the aneurysm and especially of the popliteal artery distal and proximal to it is obtained with little danger of injuring the posterior tibial nerve (f). A bulldog clamp should be placed on the popliteal artery distal to the aneurysm after injection of 3000 units of heparin intravenously prior to dissecting the proximal end of the aneurysm. The clamp prevents embolization of the distal arteries by dislodged pieces of the intrasaccular clot. After proximal control is obtained, the aneurysm is readily excised. The popliteal vein is usually ribbon-like, so it is best to resect it with the aneurysm. Complete excision of the aneurysmal sac is accomplished by keeping the plane of dissection close to it. This method for large aneurysms gives more rapid healing and return of function than if the aneurysm is not excised.

C.   The aneurysm has been completely removed. The popliteal vein has been resected and each end ligated. A saphenous vein autograft has been implanted end-to-end by the end-to-side technique to the distal popliteal artery (a), and the proximal anastomosis (b) is under construction. The severed tendons of the muscles are sutured back together with interrupted mattress sutures of linen or cotton. This method of repair results in a normal stable knee. The skin is closed with interrupted mattress sutures of silk or synthetic thread. Drainage for 24 hours with a Penrose tubing may be advisable for large aneurysms.

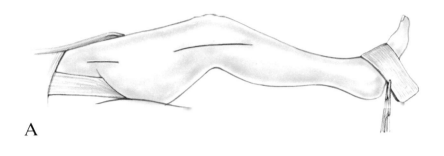

A

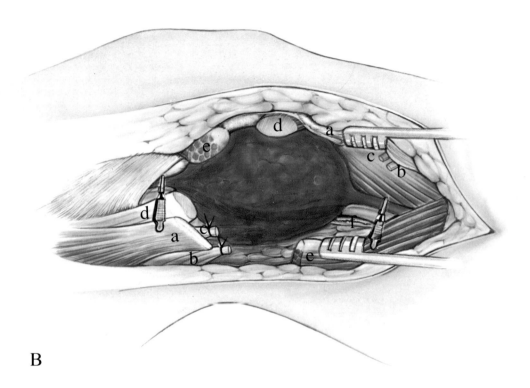

B

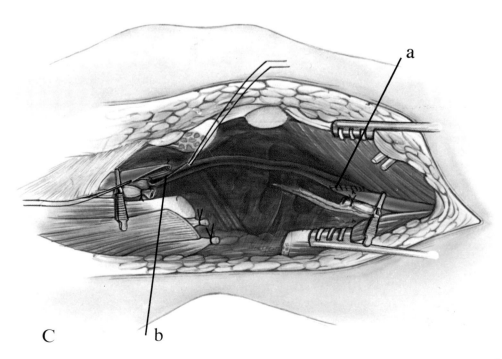

C

473

Plate 210

EXCISION OF A POPLITEAL ANEURYSM WITH IMPLANTATION OF SAPHENOUS VEIN AUTOGRAFT THROUGH THE POSTERIOR APPROACH

A. This demonstrates the posterior approach to popliteal aneurysms with the patient lying prone. It is routine with this exposure of the aneurysm to first explore the groin with the patient supine in order to obtain a section of the long saphenous vein for use as the graft to reconstitute the popliteal artery. At the same time the superficial femoral vein is interrupted just distal to the profunda femoris vein to avoid thromboembolic disease. The patient is then turned in the prone position. This method is most useful when the aneurysm is relatively small, as the exposure can be done without division of muscles so that recuperation is more rapid than by the medial approach. The incision is made in the midline posteriorly as a straight incision across the popliteal crease because it gives better exposure. It will heal without contracture if the outlined technique is followed. The incision should be a generous one to permit exposure of the popliteal artery distal and proximal to the aneurysm.

B. This demonstrates the structures encountered after dividing the popliteal fascia. The first important structure that should be searched for is the sciatic nerve, which branches into the posterior tibial (a) and the peroneal (b) nerves. A 1-inch Penrose tubing is placed around the sciatic nerve to mark it and to help to avoid injury to it.

C. The dissection is carried further so that more of the posterior tibial nerve is exposed. Coursing over the aneurysm and parallel with it is the popliteal vein, which is usually flattened out to a thin ribbon-like structure. Heparin, 3000 units, is given intravenously at this stage of the procedure. The next step is to isolate the popliteal artery distal to the aneurysm; then the dissection is performed proximal to the aneurysm to isolate the popliteal artery. By this time the heparin will have taken effect so that the two arteries can be occluded with bulldog clamps. It is important to do this before freeing up the aneurysm because of the danger of dislodging an intrasaccular blood clot that would embolize the distal arterial tree.

D. The aneurysm has been resected with the popliteal vein. An autogenous saphenous vein graft has been implanted end-to-end to the proximal popliteal artery or the distal superficial femoral artery, and distally to the distal end of the popliteal artery by the end-to-side technique. (See Plate 208.) The sciatic nerve and the posterior tibial and peroneal nerves have been carefully preserved.

E. The closure of the incision is with interrupted sutures of fine linen or cotton in the popliteal fascia, as shown, and with interrupted mattress sutures of silk or a synthetic thread in the skin. Drainage is seldom necessary. A large gauze dressing and a well padded posterior plaster splint are applied to keep the knee in full extension. This is removed in five days. The splinting of the knee prevents the development of a flexion contracture of the knee and subsequent keloid formation in the longitudinal incision.

F. This shows the neat scar, without contracture or keloid formation five years postoperative that is obtained when the incision is closed and splinted as described.

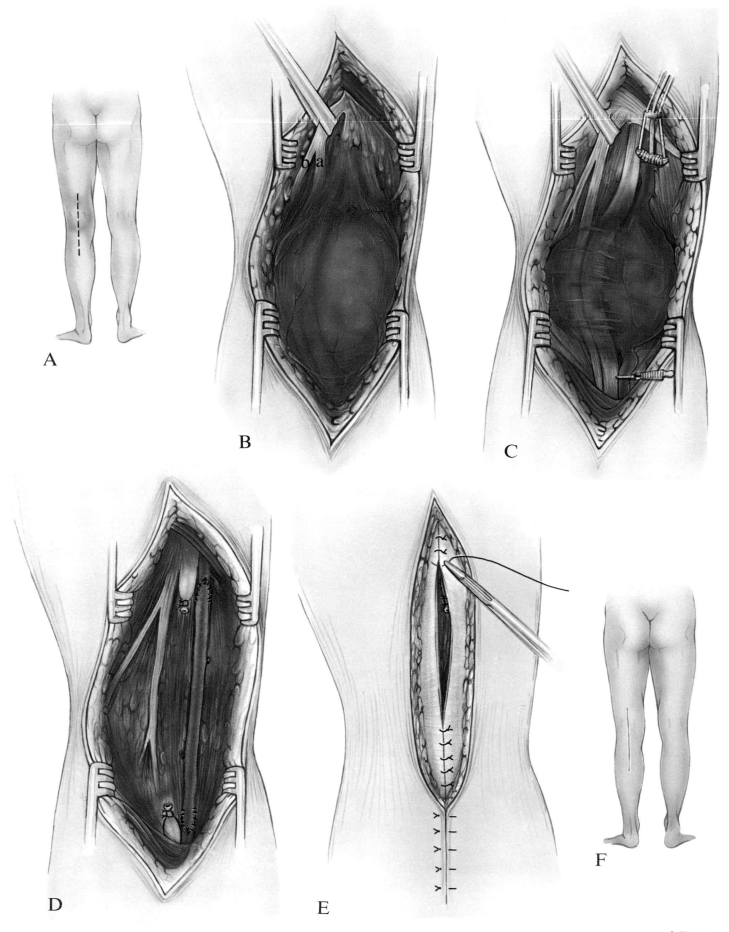

A

B

C

D

E

F

475

Plate 211

ABDOMINAL AORTIC EMBOLECTOMY

A and B.   This demonstrates a large embolus lodged at the bifurcation of the abdominal aorta. Arterial emboli invariably lodge at bifurcations of major arteries. This makes the diagnosis and localization of them easy even without the use of angiograms if the patient is seen early. The direct exposure of the site of embolization permits the best method of embolectomy in most peripheral arteries if the patient is seen within a few hours. The Fogarty catheter has simplified the removal of aortic bifurcation emboli and emboli lodged in arteries difficult to expose, as the procedure can be performed under local anesthesia through arteriotomies in arteries readily exposable. Both common femoral, superficial and profunda femoris arteries must be isolated and controlled to perform an aortic embolectomy by this technique. The common femoral arteries may be opened by longitudinal arteriotomies if they are of large size or, as shown in *B,* by using a transverse one. A Fogarty catheter is first passed up on the left into the common iliac artery and inflated to prevent fragments of embolus from being swept down this side as the Fogarty catheter on the right is withdrawn. The second Fogarty catheter is then passed up the right side into the abdominal aorta, inflated and withdrawn. Several passages of the balloon catheter may be needed to clear the bifurcation. The one on the left should also be passed into the aorta and withdrawn to be sure that this side is cleared. After obtaining a good arterial flow on both sides, the femoral arteries are occluded as dilute heparin solution is injected proximally. The distal arteries are checked for flow and, if necessary, small Fogarty catheters are passed to remove clots in them. The arteriotomies are closed with 5-0 synthetic sutures and the groin incisions in layers without drainage.

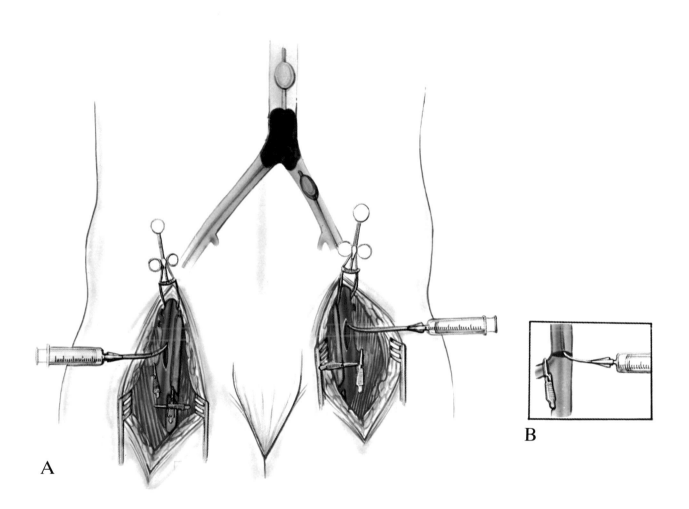

A

B

477

Plate 211 (Continued)

COMMON FEMORAL EMBOLECTOMY AND THROMBECTOMY WITH RETROGRADE FLUSH TECHNIQUE

C.   This demonstrates a thrombus that has occluded the bifurcation of the right common femoral artery. Because of a delay of 12 hours in removing the embolus a distal secondary thrombus has formed that occludes the entire arterial tree. Note the marked degree of vasoconstriction in these arteries. If the thrombi, in addition to the embolus, are not removed, gangrene of the leg will develop, requiring amputation. The removal of the embolus and the proximal thrombus is readily accomplished, and the fresh thrombi in the superficial femoral and the popliteal arteries may be readily removed with Fogarty catheters. However, it may be difficult to clear the arteries in the lower leg. For this reason a retrograde flush may be necessary to clear these vessels.

D.   This is accomplished by exposing the posterior tibial artery at the ankle or, in some patients, the dorsalis pedis artery. A 20-gauge needle with an olive tip is ligated in place in the artery with distal control. A 50-cc. syringe filled with dilute heparin and normal saline solution (200 units per cc.) is connected to it with plastic tubing.

E.   A transverse arteriotomy is made in the popliteal artery distal to the knee joint between the bulldog clamps. One hundred cubic centimeters of dilute heparin-saline solution is injected forcefully through the needle to distend the arteries of the lower leg and to loosen the clots in them. The solution is allowed to remain in the arteries for several minutes and then the distal bulldog clamp on the popliteal artery is removed. More dilute heparin saline solution is injected, which forces the clots out through the arteriotomy aided by gentle traction on it. After clearance the popliteal, femoral and posterior tibial arteriotomies are closed with fine synthetic sutures. The results of this method can be very gratifying, but it is a more difficult way to obtain success when the problem can be solved so easily by the embolectomy alone if performed within a few hours after the embolus has lodged.

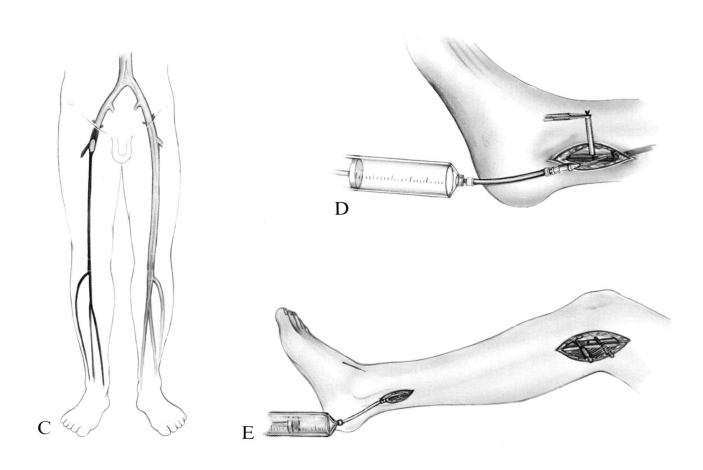

C

D

E

479

Plate 212

COARCTATION OF
THE THORACIC AORTA

A. The patient is placed in the right lateral decubitus position and rotated slightly posteriorly. An oblique left thoracic incision is made. The pleural space is entered by a subperiosteal excision of the fifth rib, or through the fourth intercostal space.

B. The lung is displaced forward. The posterior pleura is divided over the aorta and the left subclavian artery to expose a portion of the transverse arch of the aorta (a), the subclavian artery (b), the descending aorta distal to the coarctation (c), and the hypertrophied first and second intercostal arteries (d). The dissection is carried medialward to expose the vagus nerve crossing over the arch of the aorta. The ligamentum arteriosum is isolated leading off from the point of the coarctation. The left recurrent laryngeal nerve arising from the left vagus nerve is seen circling around behind the aorta.

C. All the arterial structures are isolated; a tourniquet clamp is placed on the arch of the aorta proximal to the subclavian artery, another on the distal thoracic aorta beyond the coarctation and the hypertrophied intercostal arteries. The latter are very thin-walled and fragile so they must be handled with extreme care. The proximal ligature on the largest one should not be placed too close to the aorta or it will tear and cause serious hemorrhage. The ligamentum arteriosum is ligated and divided, carefully preserving the recurrent laryngeal nerve. The narrowed portion of the aorta with the coarctation is excised.

D. This demonstrates the type of coarctation that can be resected, with an end-to-end anastomosis performed between the proximal and distal descending aorta.

E. This demonstrates the completed aortic anastomosis made with interrupted mattress stitches of Teflon-coated Dacron sutures. These are double-needled sutures that are tied together, which explains why there are knots on both sides of the suture line.

F. In some patients the coarctation will involve a longer section of the aorta. The occluding clamps are placed in a similar manner as they are in *B*, but farther apart. The proximal occluding clamp on the transverse arch is placed between the left common carotid (a) and the left subclavian artery (b). A patent ductus arteriosus (c) with the recurrent laryngeal nerve passing around it posteriorly is seen; the descending aorta is considerably dilated, demonstrating poststenotic dilatation (d), and there are some very large proximal intercostal arteries (e). The left subclavian artery is controlled with a bulldog clamp.

G. The narrowed coarctation area is excised after ligating the ductus arteriosus with a transfixion ligature of linen or cotton and also ligating the two hypertrophied proximal left and right intercostal arteries. A knitted Dacron prosthesis that has been preclotted is then inserted end-to-end to the proximal and distal ends of the aorta, using interrupted mattress sutures of 4-0 Teflon-coated Dacron. It is advisable to try to cover the graft with the adjacent pleura to obviate the lung's becoming adherent to it. The chest incision is closed with interrupted nonabsorbable sutures of linen or cotton, and the skin with interrupted silk sutures. A No. 24 Foley catheter is brought out through the seventh or eighth interspace for drainage of the pleural space for 24 to 48 hours.

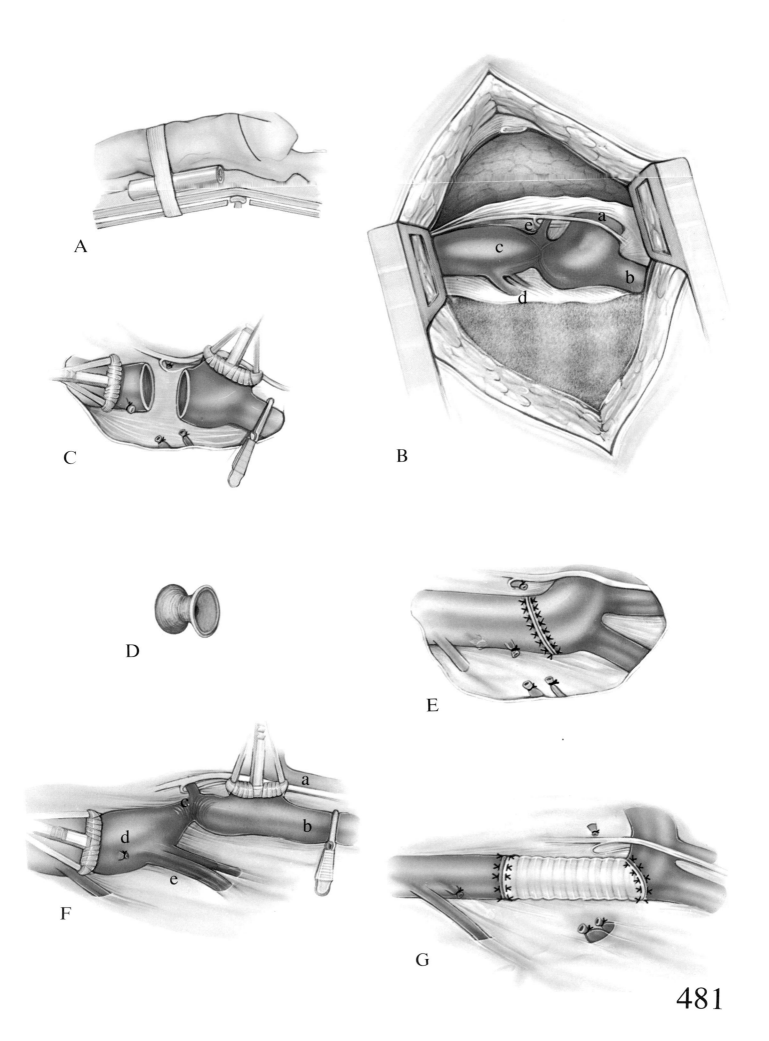

A

B

C

D

E

F

G

481

Plate 213

COARCTATION OF THE ABDOMINAL AORTA WITH BILATERAL RENAL AORTIC ANEURYSM

A.   Coarctation of the abdominal aorta is a rare congenital anomaly. In the case presented here an additional complication was bilateral renal artery aneurysm. The patient was a 31 year old married female with a blood pressure of 240/130 mm. of Hg. The location of the thoraco-abdominal incision that was used is shown. It was a long, left paramedian type, which cut across the rectus muscle opposite the eighth rib, which was removed, so that both the abdominal and pleural cavities were entered. Hypotensive spinal anesthesia was used. The left colon, spleen and pancreas were freed up and retracted to the right.

B.   This diagrammatic drawing demonstrates the location of the coarctation, the origin of the celiac axis (a), the superior mesenteric artery (b), the renal artery aneurysms 2 by 3 cm. in size and a small aortic aneurysm (c) at the level of the two renal arteries. The coarctation was most marked at the origin of the renal arteries. The aorta distal to them was small, measuring about 8 to 9 mm. in diameter.

C.   This is an operative view demonstrating the two renal artery aneurysms (a) and (b) and the small aortic aneurysm (c). The distal aorta (d) is small in comparison to the large distal thoracic aorta (e). The origins of the superior mesenteric artery (f) and the celiac axis (g) are seen. The left renal vein (h) is retracted cephalad to demonstrate the origins of the left and right renal arteries and the small diameter of the aorta.

D.   An aortic homograft with its renal limbs is shown implanted by an end-to-side anastomosis (a) to the supradiaphragmatic aorta and distally to the infrarenal aorta (b), with resection of the left renal artery and small aortic aneurysms and the anastomosis of the left renal artery of the graft to the one of the left kidney.

E.   This is a diagrammatic illustration of the completed grafting procedure. The order in which the anastomoses were performed was as follows: First, the proximal aortic end-to-side anastomosis (a) was performed using a Statinsky type of clamp. Then the distal aortic end-to-side anastomosis (b) was constructed to the infrarenal aorta between bulldog clamps. The aortic graft was opened with the renal artery limbs occluded. Then the right renal artery aneurysm was resected and the renal artery continuity re-established, using a section of the external iliac artery (c) of the graft sutured to the right iliac limb of the graft to extend it to reach the distal section of the right renal artery. This artery was then opened. Then the left renal artery aneurysm was resected and the final anastomosis was made between the renal artery limb of the graft and the distal portion of the left renal artery of the patient. The patient made a very satisfactory recovery, with both kidneys functioning well.

F.   This is an aortogram performed by the Seldinger technique 15 years postoperatively by Dr. Christos A. Athanasoulis. This shows the location of the proximal aortic anastomosis (a) and the distal one (b), the right renal artery (c), the superior mesenteric artery (d), the left gastric artery (e) and the splenic artery (f). It will be noted that the left renal artery is not visualized, as it has become occluded. The patient continues in satisfactory health with a normal blood pressure 15 years postoperative. If the procedure were performed today a knitted Dacron prosthesis would be used instead of the aortic homograft.

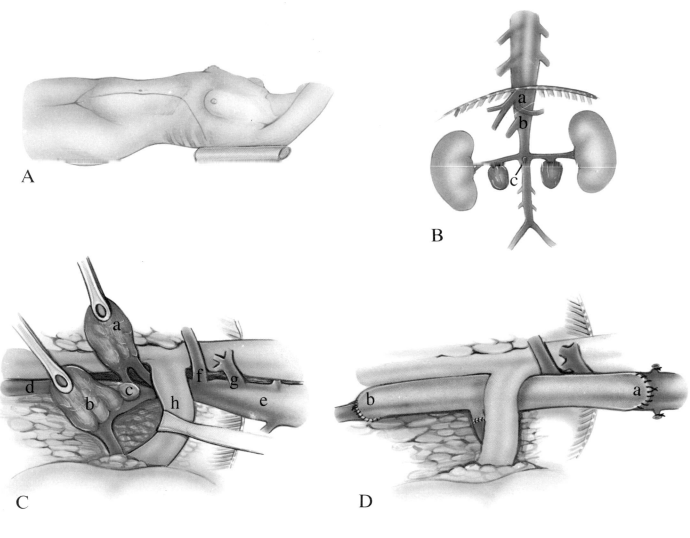

A

B

C

D

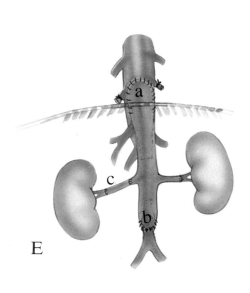

E

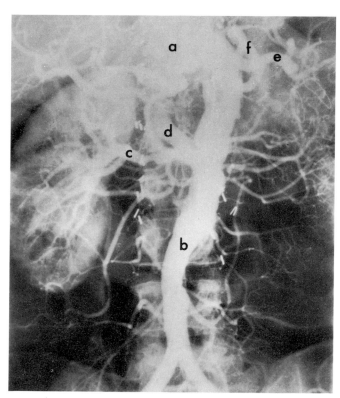

F

483

Plate 214

INTRASACCULAR WIRING
OF AORTIC ANEURYSMS

The first recorded intrasaccular wiring of an aneurysm was performed by Moore, an English surgeon, in 1864. Since then numerous reports have appeared in the surgical literature, but this method of treatment has been practically abandoned since 1950, when resection of aortic aneurysms with the implantation of a graft was first reported, which since then has been performed in thousands of patients.

A. The necessary equipment for intrasaccular wiring of aortic aneurysms consists of the Blakemore type of wiring trocar. It consists of a double needle so constructed that the inner one (c) fits snugly but not too tightly within the outer one (b), which is 14-gauge in caliber and 16 cm. in length. The sharp pointed stylet (a) fits the outer sheath (b) by means of which the trocar can be inserted into the aneurysmal sac. The wire that is used is a stainless steel alloy of 30-gauge which comes on wooden spools (e) in 200 ft. lengths. A metal rod is threaded through the spool so that it can be unwound easily. In order to increase the clotting factor of the wire it is roughened with fine emery cloth (f) before being sterilized. Several feet of the wire are passed first through the inner sheath (c) before this is inserted into the outer one. This length of the wire is pulled over a firm edge to make it coil. The wire is then withdrawn until its end is at the tip of the inner sheath. It is then inserted into the outer sheath after withdrawing the stylet (a).

B. This demonstrates the method of inserting the wire. The trocar is directed at right angles to the aneurysmal lumen, and about 10 cm. of wire are first pushed through the inner sheath into the aneurysmal sac. The inner sheath is grasped with the thumb and forefinger and pulled up on the wire, then the inner sheath and the wire are grasped together and pushed forward, advancing approximately 15 cm. of wire. This step is repeated many times so that in a short time several hundred feet of wire can be inserted into the aneurysmal sac. When no more wire will pass it is cut off flush, with the inner sheath fully advanced. The inner sheath is then pulled back and the blunt pointed stylet (d) (in *A*) is inserted into it and both advanced to push in the last few centimeters of wire. The trocar is then withdrawn from the aneurysm, and bleeding from the trocar puncture site stops shortly with finger pressure on it. The spool of wire should be held directly over the trocar to facilitate the wiring procedure. The direction and depth of the outer trocar sheath within the aneurysm is changed frequently in order to obtain a wide and even distribution of the wire. Care should be taken not to direct it into the main axis of the aorta, since this may result in the wire passing up or down the aorta.

C. This is a copy of a roentgenogram of a man aged 72 years and shows 200 feet of 30-gauge stainless steel wire that was inserted into an aneurysm of the transverse arch of the aorta 21 years ago in 1952, because of dyspnea, dysphagia and hoarseness. The procedure was performed by direct exposure of the aneurysm through a transthoracic exposure. Following the wiring his symptoms soon disappeared, and since then he has led a healthy normal existence. It is recommended that wiring be done under direct vision of the aneurysm to obtain a more complete wiring of it. This procedure may be carried out for aneurysms in the ascending and transverse portions of the aortic arch at the site of the take-off of the major branches of the arch, as has been demonstrated in this patient. It would seem, therefore, that this method is justifiable in some poor risk patients with aneurysms that are considered inoperable, especially those of the thoracic aorta.

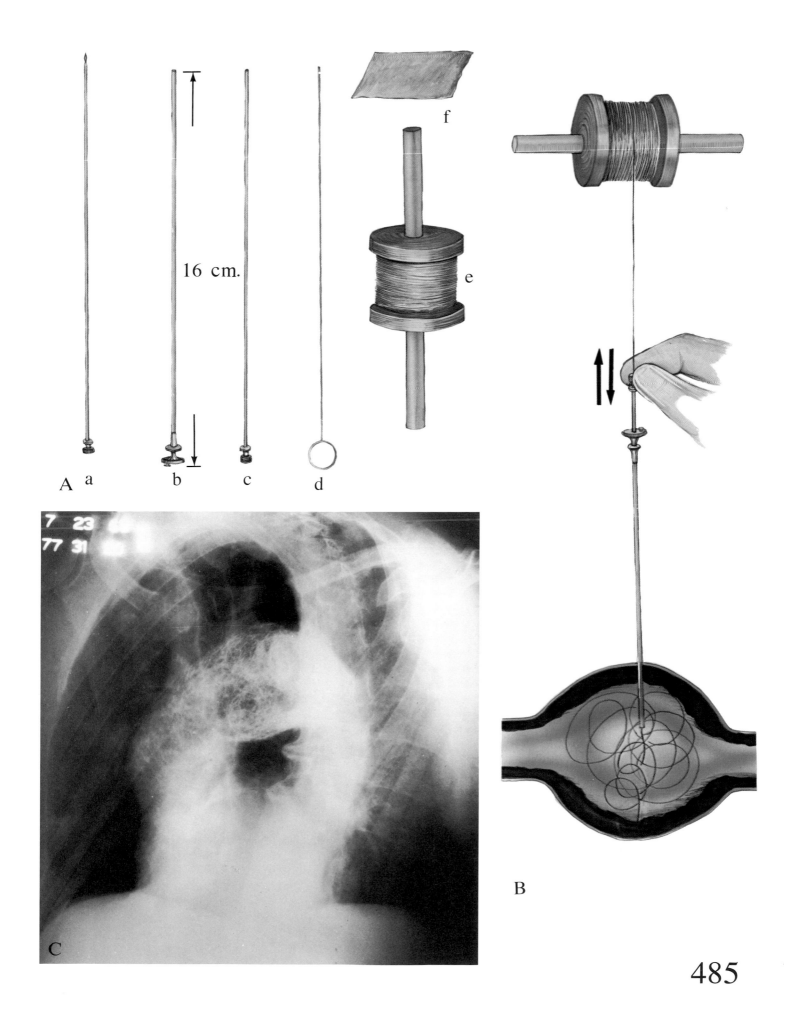

A

a   b   c   d

16 cm.

f

e

B

C

485

Plate 215

DORSAL SYMPATHETIC GANGLIONECTOMY FOR THE UPPER EXTREMITY

I. TRANSTHORACIC METHOD

A. This demonstrates a patient in the right decubitus position with the right arm elevated for a left dorsal sympathectomy. An oblique thoracic incision is made below the scapula, then carried through the muscles so that the scapula can be elevated to expose the fourth rib.

B. This demonstrates the exposure after resection of the fourth rib subperiosteally. The pleural space is entered. The left upper lobe is retracted to expose the thoracic sympathetic chain beneath the pleura along the bodies of the upper thoracic vertebrae. The "sine qua non" of the most effective sympathetic ganglionectomy for severe Raynaud's disease is that it must include the stellate ganglion consisting of C-8 and T-1 ganglia, which will produce a Horner's syndrome, and in addition the removal of the sympathetic ganglia through T-4 or T-5. The vertebral artery (a) is closely associated with the eighth cervical ganglia, so that adequate exposure of this area is necessary to avoid injury to this artery. In addition to the ganglionectomy, spinal nerves D2 (c) and D3 (d) are removed along with their intraspinal roots. This of necessity means the removal of the nerve of Kuntz (b), which if left intact may facilitate a return of symptoms. The chest incision is closed in the routine manner, with drainage of the pleural space with a No. 24 Foley catheter for 48 hours.

C. This drawing shows the upper five thoracic ganglia, the eighth cervical ganglia and the second and third spinal nerves with their intraspinal roots that are removed in this radical sympathetic denervation, which has given better long-term results for severe Raynaud's disease than any less extensive procedure.

II. TRANSAXILLARY METHOD

D. For a right dorsal sympathetic ganglionectomy through a transaxillary approach the patient is placed in a left lateral decubitus position with the arm extended. An oblique incision is made in the axilla over the third or fourth intercostal space between the pectoralis major muscle anteriorly and the latissimus dorsi muscle posteriorly. These muscles are retracted and sometimes the edges of them incised to give a larger field. The long thoracic nerve lying on the serratus anterior muscle and the thoracodorsal nerve on the axillary margin of the subscapularis muscle should be carefully protected from injury.

E. The pleural space is opened through the third or fourth interspace and the right upper lobe of the lung is retracted to the left. The sympathetic chain is seen lying against the bodies of the thoracic vertebrae and in close association with some branches of the azygos venous system. A ganglionectomy is performed, removing ganglia T-1, T-2 and T-3. As a rule, the eighth cervical ganglia is not removed as it is more difficult than through a larger transthoracic approach. The chest wall is closed in the routine manner after completion of the ganglionectomy, with drainage of the pleural space using a No. 24 Foley catheter for 48 hours.

F. This demonstrates the extent of the ganglionectomy. It is less radical than through the transthoracic approach and spinal nerves two and three are not removed. Its main disadvantage is that the exposure is more limited and, although it ablates effectively the sudomotor innervation of the upper extremity, it does not the vasomotor innervation, so for severe Raynaud's disease the more extensive procedure is recommended; for hyperhidrosis, however, it gives excellent results.

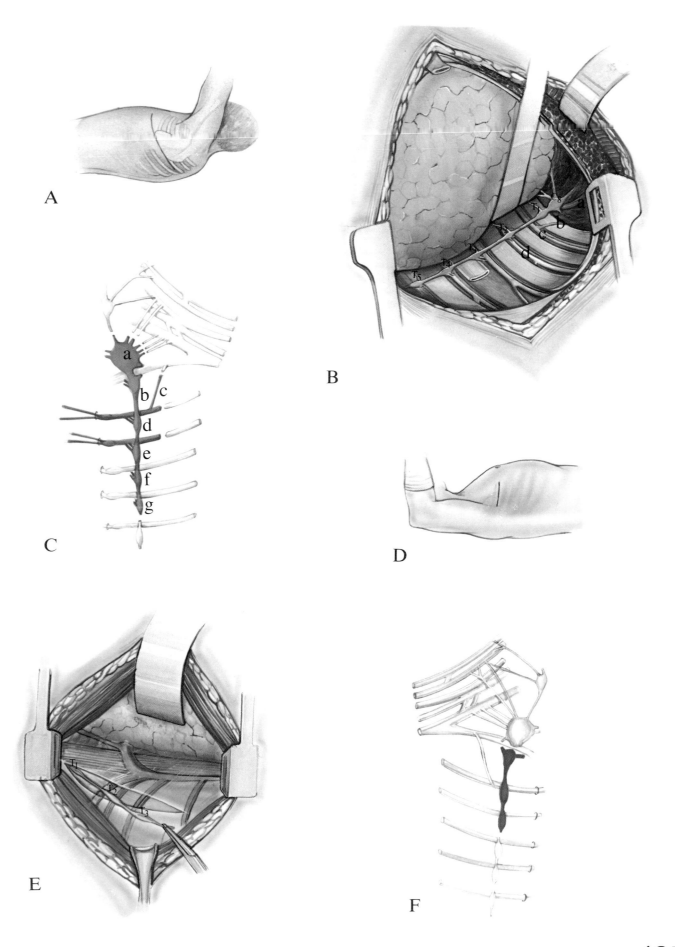

A

B

C

D

E

F

487

Plate 216

RIGHT LUMBAR
SYMPATHETIC GANGLIONECTOMY

A. This demonstrates the position of the patient on the operating table in the left lateral decubitus position with the table flexed and the kidney bar elevated opposite the left twelfth rib. The patient is maintained in this position with two back rests, one against the thorax and the other against the gluteal region. The right thigh is flexed to 45 degrees and is held in that position with a blanket roll behind the thigh held in place with a strip of adhesive tape. The left lower extremity is in full extension. This position places the muscles of the right flank on tension and separates the twelfth rib from the iliac crest. The flexion of the right thigh relieves tension on the iliopsoas muscle, thus making it easier to dissect out the lumbar sympathetic ganglia. The anesthesia is by intravenous pentothal and a muscle relaxant, with nitrous oxide and oxygen inhalation anesthesia administered through an endotracheal catheter.

B. The incision is an oblique one over the course of the distal portion of the twelfth rib, cutting partially across the latissimus dorsi (a), and the external oblique (b) muscles. This exposes the distal end of the twelfth rib (c).

C. The distal portion of the twelfth rib is removed subperiosteally. The internal oblique muscle (d) is then cut partially transversely.

D. The posterior rib bed, some of the diaphragm (e) and the transversalis muscle (f) are separated in the line of their fibers. This opens the retroperitoneal area. As the portion of the twelfth rib is removed, care should be taken to avoid opening the pleura, but if it is opened, no attempt should be made to suture it. It is not serious, as the anesthetist can easily institute positive pressure with the endotracheal tube to keep the lung inflated. As the incision is being closed, a catheter is placed in the pleural space, aspirated after closure and then removed.

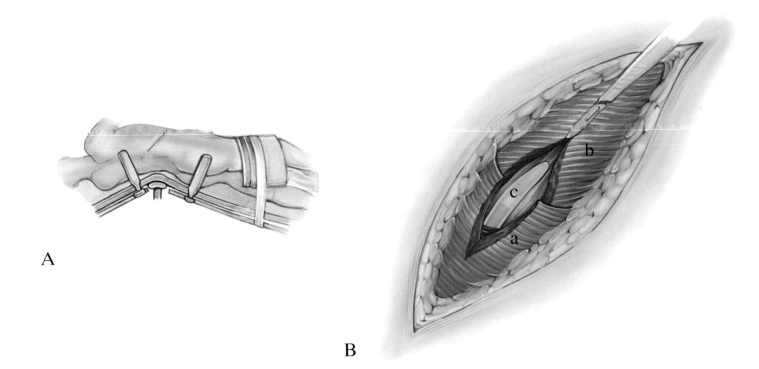

A

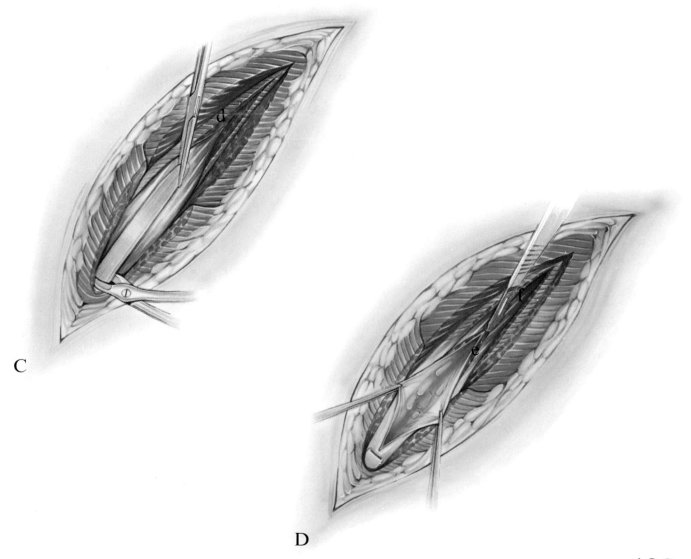

B

C

D

489

Plate 217

RIGHT LUMBAR SYMPATHETIC GANGLIONECTOMY (*Continued*)

A. The right kidney and retroperitoneal fat are separated from the quadratus lumborum and the iliopsoas muscles with finger dissection. Several gauze sponges are inserted over this fatty tissue, then a large Deaver retractor is used to retract it medially and anteriorward. The fingers of the right or left hand are then inserted along the posterior musculature, being careful not to dissect between the iliopsoas muscle and the quadratus lumborum, but carrying them over the former to the bodies of the vertebrae. The inferior vena cava is seen. The lumbar sympathetic ganglia (a) are palpated under the ends of the fingers against the bodies of the lumbar vertebrae, which is the easiest way to locate them. The angled Hartmann forceps (b) is a great help in working in the depths of this wound.

B. With the forefinger of the left hand resting on the lumbar sympathetic chain, it is very simple in many instances to pick up the chain without seeing it, by means of a nerve hook, as shown. The chain lies very close to the bodies of the vertebrae so the nerve hook should be inserted in the manner shown.

C. After the sympathetic chain has been elevated with the first nerve hook another one is placed in the reverse direction to avoid possible injury to the large lumbar veins because, if torn, they may be difficult to secure. It is fortunate that in most instances the lumbar ganglia lie over the veins, although occasionally they may pass behind them, which makes it a little more difficult to remove them. An additional Deaver retractor has been placed in the upper end of the incision and this exposes the right crus of the diaphragm (a) through which the sympathetic chain can be seen entering. It is readily possible to remove the twelfth dorsal ganglion by separating the fibers of this muscle for a more complete ganglionectomy. A dural clip is placed on the chain at the upper end of the dissection usually proximal to D-12 ganglion and the trunk divided between the clip and the ganglion.

D. The chain is then picked up with a Kelly clamp and the dissection is carried caudad, removing lumbar ganglia one, two and three. The distal ganglia are readily exposed by an assistant holding a narrow Deaver retractor against the iliopsoas muscle and pushing the vena cava in the opposite direction with a gauze pledget on the end of a long curved clamp. The gray and white rami and some visceral branches are readily isolated and divided. It is usually unnecessary to clip these since the rami seldom carry blood vessels with them. One clip is placed on the trunk distal to the point it is divided. The advantage of this twelfth rib approach for a lumbar sympathetic ganglionectomy is that it is possible to remove the lumbar sympathetic ganglia from D-12 through L-3 inclusive. It is recommended that this extensive resection be carried out in those patients in whom a reconstructive arterial procedure cannot be performed because of poor distal outflow tract in the lower extremity. It is, therefore, a very important operative procedure with which the vascular surgeon should be well acquainted. The extensive resection gives a more complete and longer lasting vasomotor denervation than removing a shorter section, as is done when using a transverse muscular incision with the patient lying supine. The incision is closed in layers, suturing each divided muscle back together with interrupted sutures of linen or cotton. The skin is closed with interrupted mattress sutures of silk or synthetic material, without drainage.

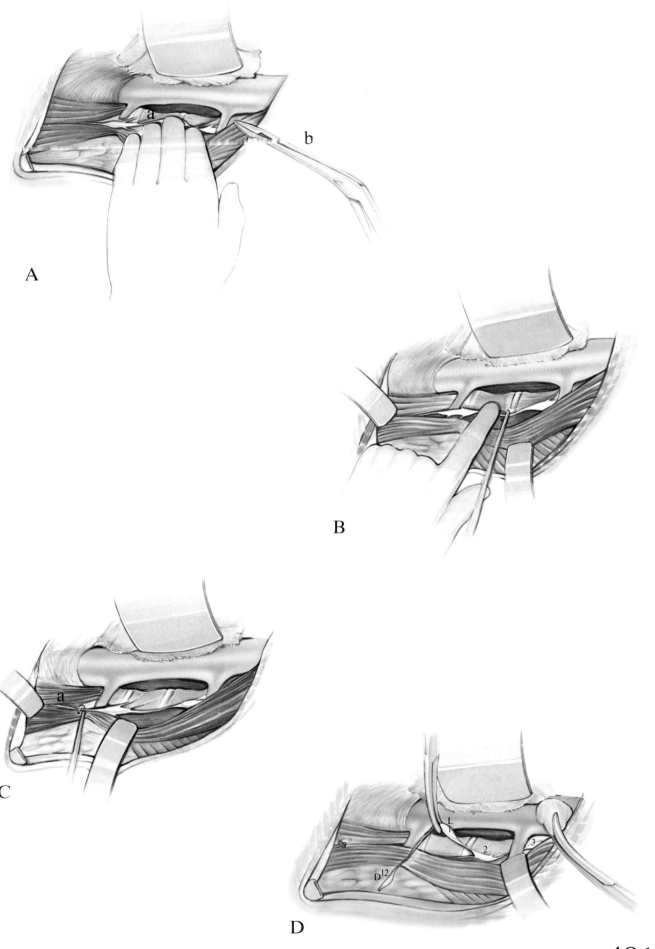

491

Plate 218

TRANSMETATARSAL AMPUTATION

During the past 20 years reconstructive arterial surgery has reduced greatly the incidence of major amputations in patients with obliterative atherosclerotic arterial disease of the lower extremity with gangrene and ischemic lesions of the foot and lower leg. It is important, however, that surgeons doing vascular surgery should also know how to perform satisfactory amputations of ischemic limbs. In addition to the encouraging results from reconstructive arterial surgery, it has been possible to perform more transmetatarsal and below the knee amputations, thereby saving a patient's foot in the former cases, and the knee joint in the latter. Both these amputations, of course, can be performed in patients who have sufficient collateral circulation but who cannot have reconstructive arterial surgery.

A. This shows the foot of an elderly patient with gangrene of the second and third toes of the right foot and ischemic color changes in the first, fourth and fifth toes. In the dependent position, marked rubor does not develop more proximally than shown, indicating a satisfactory collateral circulation in the body of the foot.

The distal portion of the foot which is to be amputated should be covered with Steridrape before making the incision. (For the sake of clarity this was omitted in the illustrations.) The slightly curved line proximal to the base of the toes shows the location of the dorsal portion of the amputation incision.

This type of amputation is best performed with the patient in slight reversed Trendelenburg position, with the feet six inches lower than the heart. This fills the veins so that they will bleed, thereby obtaining better isolation and ligation of them for better hemostasis.

B. This shows the location of the plantar portion of the incision, which is more distal than the dorsal one, in order to form a long plantar flap.

C. The plantar portion of the incision is continued through the plantar tissues of the foot, near the heads of the metatarsal bones, interrupting the tendons with a sharp knife as shown and allowing the proximal ends of them to retract. The dissection is then carried down to the metatarsal bones. The soft tissues of the plantar flap are dissected proximally away from these bones to make the long plantar flap. This should be carried a short distance more proximal than the incision on the dorsum of the foot. Bleeding is controlled with 4-0 chromic catgut ligatures and the diathermy.

D. The metatarsal bones are divided with a Gigli saw or a bone forceps. The proximal ends are then shortened with a rongeur so that they will be slightly shorter than the proximal skin flap.

E. The closure of the amputation stump is by stitches of 36-gauge stainless steel wire. These should be made with small bites of skin and subcutaneous tissue and tied loosely without tension but with approximation of the edges. Drainage should not be necessary, but if bleeding is difficult to control a small Penrose tube can be brought out through the medial end of the incision to be removed in 24 hours.

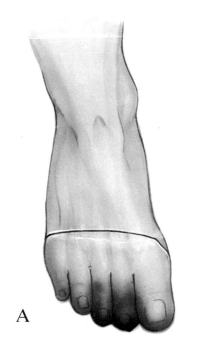

A

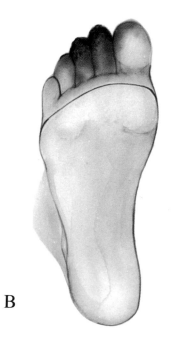

B

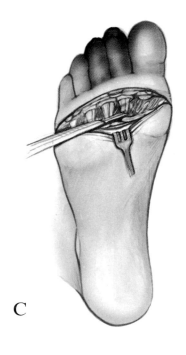

C

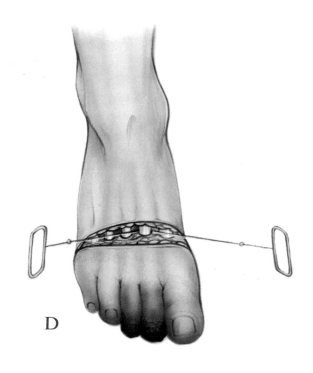

D

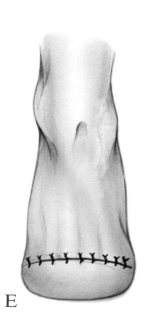

E

493

Plate 219

BELOW-KNEE AMPUTATION

A. When gangrene involves the dorsum of the foot or if there is marked rubor up to the mid part of the foot or ankle level, it is not possible to perform a transmetatarsal amputation. Under these conditions the next best site of amputation is below the knee at the site of election in order to preserve the knee joint. This is performed in a manner similar to a transmetatarsal amputation, namely, it has a very short anterior skin flap and a long dermal and musculofascial posterior flap.

B. The anterior portion of the incision is made just slightly distal to the point where the tibia is divided, 10 to 14 cm. below the knee joint. The periosteum on the tibia is incised carefully with a knife and the distal part pushed distally with a periosteal elevator. The bone is divided with a Gigli saw just distal to the proximal cut edge of the periosteum. The bone is irrigated with normal saline solution to counteract the heat of the sawing process. It is important to have the proximal edge of the periosteum clean cut, as osteophytes may develop if there are ragged torn edges.

C. The anterior edge of the tibia is smoothed off carefully with a bastard file. The fibula must be divided 1.0 to 1.5 cm. shorter than the tibia. This is done with a Gigli saw or a rongeur. The muscles medial and lateral to the fibula are divided and a long musculofascial dermal flap is developed posteriorly, as shown. The anterior tibial and posterior tibial arteries and veins are ligated and the posterior tibial nerve is crushed with a Kocher clamp and ligated with a 3-0 plain catgut ligature. It is then necessary to excise a large amount of the gastrocnemius and soleus muscles to fashion a thin musculofascial flap of some of the posterior part of these muscles and their distal tendinous portions. Careful hemostasis is obtained with fine ligatures of catgut. The tendinous portion of the musculofascial flap is then brought anteriorly over the ends of the bones and sutured with interrupted stitches of fine chromic catgut to the deep anterolateral fascia and a few sutures in the anterior tibial periosteum a little proximal to its cut edge.

D. The long posterior skin flap is then fashioned to fit the short anterior skin flap. The edges are approximated neatly but without tension with interrupted 36-gauge stainless steel wire sutures; subcutaneous sutures should not be used. A large pressure dressing is applied. The knee is held in full extension with a posterior molded plaster splint that is removed in five days. Some surgeons prefer to apply an immediate temporary prosthesis, which permits earlier ambulation but may, in some patients, interfere with primary wound healing. I prefer to wait for healing, usually two weeks, then measure the amputation stump for a temporary prosthesis and have the patient walking with it three weeks postoperatively.

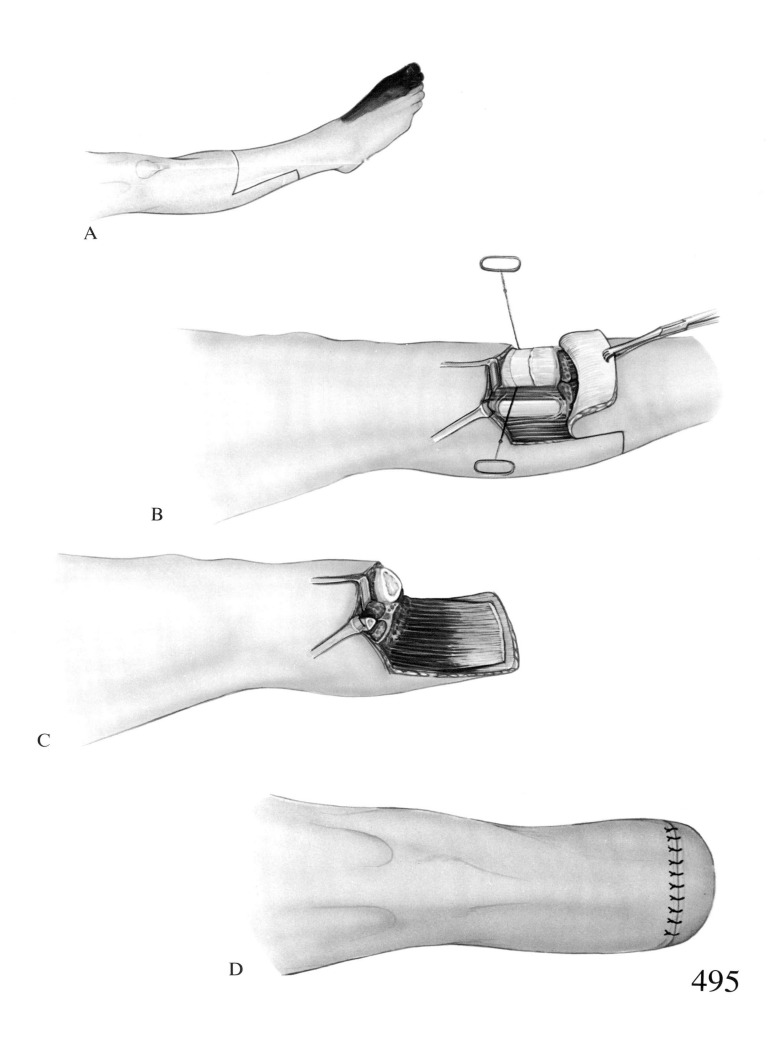

A

B

C

D

495

Plate 220

LOW THIGH AMPUTATION

A. The location, the type of incision and the level that the femur is divided are shown for a low thigh amputation with a short posterior flap and a medium long anterior flap. It is performed when it is impossible to amputate below the knee because of insufficient arterial blood supply at that level. It is a very serviceable type of amputation and seldom gives trouble postoperatively.

B. This demonstrates the location of the anterior portion of the incision. A groin incision is also made to interrupt the superficial femoral vein just distal to the profunda femoris vein, to prevent pulmonary emboli that may arise from the superficial femoral vein. This should be performed before doing the amputation to prevent a pulmonary embolism at the time of amputation and also to obtain better hemostasis in the amputation site.

C. The incision is carried through the deep fascia. The quadriceps tendon is divided just proximal to the patella.

D. The quadriceps tendon is retracted up and proximally with a double hook. The periosteum of the femur is incised cleanly with a knife. The distal portion is pushed distalward. The femur is divided with a Gigli saw, keeping the bone moistened and cool with normal saline solution.

E. The amputation has been completed. The popliteal artery and vein are ligated separately. The muscles medial, lateral and posterior to the femur are divided approximately at the same level as the bone. The sciatic nerve is grasped with a Kocher clamp to retract it distally. It is crushed with a similar clamp that is shown open at the level of the divided femur. The nerve is ligated with a 3-0 plain catgut ligature at the point it is crushed, to control the blood vessels that are usually found in the sciatic nerve. It is then cut with a sharp knife just distal to the ligature, allowing it to retract proximally away from the site of the amputation, which avoids a painful amputation stump. The crushing of the nerve also tends to prevent formation of a neuroma.

F. The end of the femur always lodges at the lateral edge of the amputation stump unless some step is taken to fix it in the mid portion of the stump. This is readily accomplished by placing three large stitches of 0 chromic catgut between the vastus lateralis and the biceps muscles just lateral to the femur. The proximal one should be placed 4 or 5 cm. proximal to the end of the femur. A similar fixation is not necessary on the medial side.

G. In the closure of the stump the quadriceps tendon is first sutured with 0 chromic catgut to the hamstring muscles and their fascia posteriorly to cover the end of the femur. This also helps to reduce the tension on the skin flaps. The deep fascia is sutured transversely with interrupted sutures of 4-0 chromic catgut. The skin is closed with interrupted fine sutures of 36-gauge wire or fine plastic sutures without drainage. The first postoperative dressing is performed in a week. Healing is invariably per primam, so measurements for a temporary ischial bearing prosthesis are taken then. The patient starts walking with the artificial limb two weeks postoperatively and usually is discharged home three weeks postoperatively. Gait training for this type of prosthesis is more necessary than for a below the knee amputation. No patient who is able to be out of bed should go home after an above-knee amputation without a prosthesis and sufficient instruction for walking on it properly. The surgeon who performs the amputation should help in the gait training.

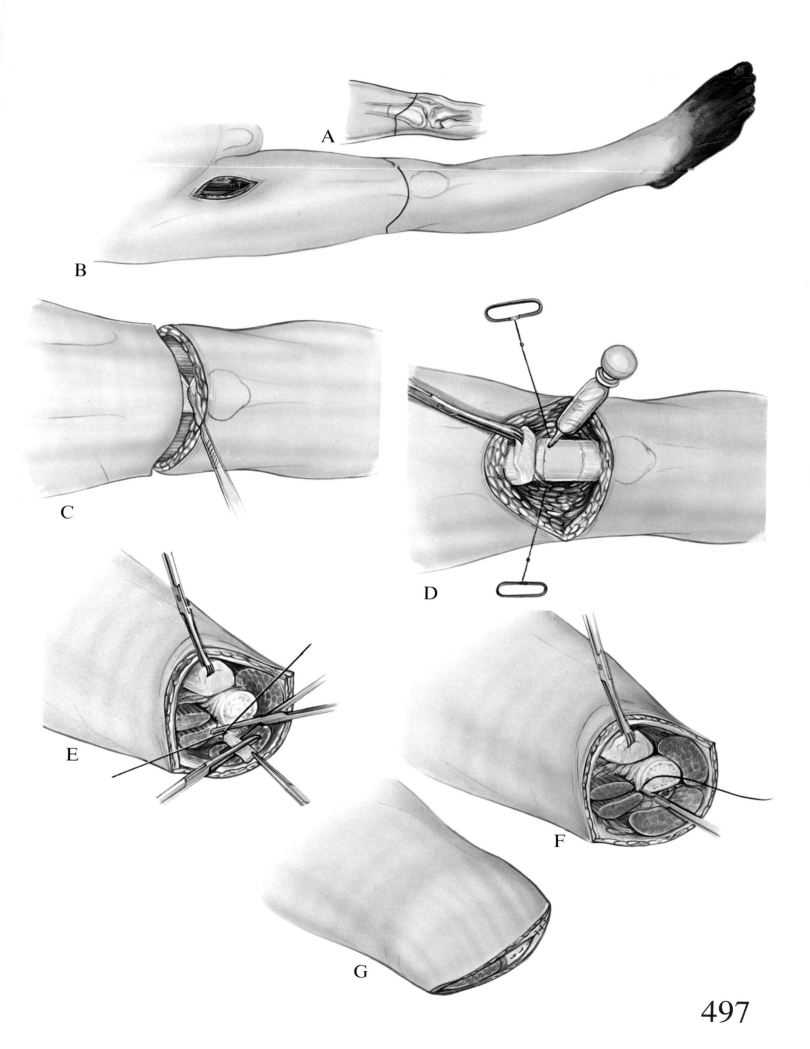

A

B

C

D

E

F

G

497

INDEX